The Science and
Clinical Application of Manual Therapy

Commissioning Editor: Sarena Wolfaard/Alison Taylor
Development Editor: Fiona Conn
Project Manager: Nayagi Athmanathan
Designer: Stewart Larking
Illustration Manager: Gillian Richards
Illustrator: Martin Woodward

The Science and Clinical Application of Manual Therapy

Edited by

Hollis H. King DO PhD

Professor of Osteopathic Principles and Practice
AT Still University School of Osteopathic Medicine in Arizona
USA

Wilfrid Jänig MD

Professor of Physiology
Physiologisches Institut
Christian-Albrechts-Universität zu Kiel
Kiel, Germany

Michael M. Patterson PhD

Professor of Osteopathic Principles and Practice, Retired
College of Osteopathic Medicine
Nova Southeastern University
Florida, USA

Illustrations by Martin Woodward

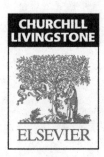

Edinburgh London New York Oxford Philadelphia St Louis Sydney Toronto 2011

CHURCHILL
LIVINGSTONE
ELSEVIER

ISBN 978-0-7020-3387-2

British Library Cataloguing in Publication Data
A catalogue record for this book is available from the British Library

Library of Congress Cataloging in Publication Data
A catalog record for this book is available from the Library of Congress

Notices
Knowledge and best practice in this field are constantly changing. As new research and experience broaden our understanding, changes in research methods, professional practices, or medical treatment may become necessary.

Practitioners and researchers must always rely on their own experience and knowledge in evaluating and using any information, methods, compounds, or experiments described herein. In using such information or methods they should be mindful of their own safety and the safety of others, including parties for whom they have a professional responsibility.

With respect to any drug or pharmaceutical products identified, readers are advised to check the most current information provided (i) on procedures featured or (ii) by the manufacturer of each product to be administered, to verify the recommended dose or formula, the method and duration of administration, and contraindications. It is the responsibility of practitioners, relying on their own experience and knowledge of their patients, to make diagnoses, to determine dosages and the best treatment for each individual patient, and to take all appropriate safety precautions.

To the fullest extent of the law, neither the Publisher nor the authors, contributors, or editors, assume any liability for any injury and/or damage to persons or property as a matter of products liability, negligence or otherwise, or from any use or operation of any methods, products, instructions, or ideas contained in the material herein.

ELSEVIER your source for books, journals and multimedia in the health sciences

www.elsevierhealth.com

Working together to grow libraries in developing countries

www.elsevier.com | www.bookaid.org | www.sabre.org

 ELSEVIER   BOOK AID International   Sabre Foundation

The Publisher's policy is to use paper manufactured from sustainable forests

Printed in China

Contents

Contributors

Brian S Budgell, DC PhD
Professor, Graduate Education and Research
Programmes, Canadian Memorial Chiropractic College,
Toronto, Ontario, Canada

Kari Guinn Clark, DO PhD
Research Associate, Department of Integrative
Physiology University of North Texas Health Science
Center Fort Worth, Texas, USA

Robert D Foreman, PhD
Professor and Chair, George Lynn Cross Research
Professor, Department of Physiology, University of
Oklahoma Health Sciences Center, Oklahoma City, USA

Steven Z George, PT PhD
Assistant Professor and Chair, Department of Physical
Therapy, University of Florida, Gainesville, Florida, USA

Lisa E Goehler, PhD
Research Associate Professor,
Department of Neuroimmunology & Behavior,
Center for the Study of Complementary & Alternative
Therapies School of Nursing, University of Virginia
Charlottesville, VA

M Ram Gudavalli, PhD
Associate Professor, Palmer Center for Chiropractic
Research, Palmer College of Chiropractic,
Davenport, Iowa, USA

Cheryl Hawk, DC PhD
Vice President of Research and Scholarship, Cleveland
Chiropractic College, Kansas City, USA

Charles N R Henderson, DC PhD
Associate Professor, Palmer Center for Chiropractic
Research, Palmer College of Chiropractic,
Davenport, Iowa, USA

Charles H Hubscher, PhD
Professor, Department Anatomical Sciences &
Neurobiology, University of Louisville School of Medicine,
Louisville, Kentucky, USA

Wilfrid Jänig, MD
Professor of Physiology, Physiologisches Institut,
Christian-Albrechts-Universität zu Kiel, Kiel, Germany

Chuan Chau Jerry Jou, DO PhD FAAP
Fellow in Pediatric Cardiology, University of Utah, Utah, USA

Janet R Kahn, PhD NCBMT
Research Assistant Professor, Department of Psychiatry,
University of Vermont College of Medicine; and Executive

Director, Integrated Healthcare Policy Consortium,
Burlington, Vermont, USA

Michael J Kenney, PhD
Professor, Department of Anatomy and Physiology,
Kansas State University, Manhattan, Kansas, USA

Hollis H King, DO PhD
Professor of Osteopathic Principles and Practice, AT Still
University School of Osteopathic Medicine in Arizona,
Arizona, USA

Michael M Patterson, PhD
Professor of Osteopathic Principles and Practice, Retired,
College of Osteopathic Medicine, Nova
Southeastern University,
Florida, USA

Maria Petersson, MD PhD
Department of Molecular Medicine and Surgery,
Endocrine and Diabetes Unit, Karolinska Institutet,
Stockholm, Sweden

Joel G Pickar, DC PhD
Professor, Palmer Center for Chiropractic Research,
Palmer College of Chiropractic, Davenport,
Iowa, USA

Chao Qin, MD
Associate Professor of Research, Department of
Physiology, University of Oklahoma Health Science
Center, Oklahoma, USA

Xiangrong Shi, PhD
Associate Professor, Department of Integrative
Physiology, University of North Texas Health Science
Center Fort Worth, Texas, USA

Michael L Smith, PhD
Professor, Department of Integrative Physiology,
University of North Texas Health Science Center Fort
Worth, Texas, USA

John J Triano, DC PhD
Professor, Department of Research, Canadian Memorial
Chiropractic College, Toronto, Ontario, Canada

Kerstin Uvnäs-Moberg, MD PhD
Department of Animal Environment and Health,
Swedish University of Agricultural Sciences,
Skara, Sweden

It is with pleasure that the editors present this book based on the International Research Symposium on 'Somato-Visceral Interactions and Autonomic Mechanisms of Manual Therapy' held March 31-April 1, 2008 in Fort Worth, Texas.

The symposium was a landmark event for the field of manual treatment and therapy. It brought together clinicians and scientists from the fields of osteopathic medicine, chiropractic, massage therapy and physical therapy, as well as scientists from laboratories around the world. Never before have all the major groups of practitioners who use manual procedures been together in such a meeting.

The program was originally conceived as a follow up to the 1989 International Symposium 'The Central Connection: Somatovisceral/Viscerosomatic Interaction' held in Cincinnati, Ohio and sponsored by the American Academy of Osteopathy. The goals of the symposium were to assess the state of knowledge of the effects of somatic stimulation and movement on visceral and autonomic function at all levels of the neuraxis. In this regard, the symposium was more inclusive than the 1989 meeting, which looked mainly at spinal level influences.

This book, like the 2008 symposium, aims to bring together the latest information on somato-visceral interactions at the spinal level and to expand the information to include the effects on these interactions of the brainstem and cortex. In addition, information from all major manual therapy professions is presented to give a much broader perspective to the effects of somatic stimulation on visceral and somatic functions. Information from each profession on its practice perspectives and views on effects of somatic therapy is presented, as is basic science data on neural processing at all levels of the nervous system. In addition, in the last two chapters, the editors have attempted to summarize current evidence on central processing of somato-visceral interactions, and to challenge current thinking on how neural processing of manual therapy may affect function. The book is a challenge to practitioners and scientists to rethink long held dogmatic beliefs about dysfunction and to expand and reformulate these beliefs in light of current knowledge.

The program committee for the symposium was composed of Michael M Patterson, PhD; Robert D Foreman, PhD; Hollis H King, DO PhD; John J Triano, DC PhD; and Cynthia D Myers, LMT PhD. Participation in the 2008 program by Robert D Foreman, PhD; Fernando Cervero, MD PhD DSc; Robert Schmidt, MD PhD; and Wilfrid Jänig, MD, all of whom also presented at the 1989 symposium, provided continuity and focus to the program.

The event was hosted and sponsored by the Osteopathic Research Center, located on the campus of the University of North Texas Health Science Center-Texas College of Osteopathic Medicine. Major funding for the symposium came from the National Center for Complementary and Alternative Medicine of the NIH in the form of a Research Conference Grant (R13-AT004669-01) 'Delineating the Evidence-base for Somato-Visceral Interactions'. There was also broad support from manual therapy professions in the form of financial sponsorship by Orthopaedic Section-American Physical Therapy Association, American Academy of Orthopaedic Physical Therapists, Canadian Memorial Chiropractic College, NCMIC Insurance, Massage Therapy Foundation, Osteopathic Heritage Foundation, American Osteopathic Association, American Academy of Osteopathy, American Association of Colleges of Osteopathic Medicine, and the University of North Texas Health Science Center. Representatives of the sponsors who provided invaluable assistance were Major John D Childs, PT PhD; Kathleen Sluka, PT PhD; Gini Ohlson; Diana Thompson, LMT; James Irrgang, PT PhD; Andy Crim and Cathleen Kearns.

The Symposium event was staffed by ORC and UNTHSC personnel under the coordination of Cathleen Kearns, ORC Administrative Director. The Program Committee and Editors express a special thanks to Cathy Kearns whose effort and oversight made the symposium a successful event and a contribution to the science and clinical application of manual therapy.

The editors thank the symposium participants who have authored chapters in this book for the hard work and dedication they have provided to bring the insights and knowledge to the practitioners of manual therapy. It is our hope that the information provided proves useful to all fields of manual treatment and therapy.

HHK, WJ, MMP

The concepts of osteopathic medicine: past and present

Hollis H King • Michael M Patterson

Introduction

Among the professions that emphasize the use of manual therapy in healthcare the osteopathic medical profession is unique because it bridges the traditions of allopathic and alternative medicine. The practice of osteopathic medicine has followed a set of concepts that is arguably the most complete of all the manual therapy and healthcare professions. Osteopathic concepts provide rationale for the efficacy of manual therapy and at the same time encourage a broader perspective to the practice of medicine through its 'whole-person' approach to patient care.

At a recent research symposium dealing with synergistic goals in manual therapy research, the first author presented the set of osteopathic concepts as they related to research priorities (Langevin et al. 2009). During the panel discussion, presenters from the chiropractic, physical therapy, massage therapy and body worker professions all said that their respective professions taught similar concepts within their scope of practice. Therefore, this chapter reflects inclusiveness for all manual therapy professions as far as concepts are concerned while acknowledging the longer history of osteopathy and the emphasis placed on underlying concepts by the osteopathic medical profession. The authors of Chapters 13 Chiropractic, 14

Physical Therapy and 15 Massage Therapy present some elaboration on the concepts presented in this chapter as well as the background of their respective professions.

Apart from licensure and certification issues, both in the United States and internationally, there are nomenclature differences between the manual therapy professions that are described below in order to minimize any confusion readers unfamiliar with this area of research may have. However, as the careful reader will see, there are far more similarities with regard to manual therapy research than differences between the professions represented in this book, a fact necessitated by common interests and adherence to the principles of good scientific research.

Indeed, the accumulated research accomplishments of manual therapy over the past 15 years have resulted in the inclusion of spinal manipulation into federal agency medical practice guidelines (Bigos et al. 1994). Osteopathic and manual therapy research has also contributed to the inclusion of diagnostic codes for somatic dysfunction (defined and discussed below) in the definitive reference source for medical diagnoses, the *International Classification of Diseases* (ICD-9-CM, 2008) and procedure codes for osteopathic manipulative treatment (OMT) in *Current Procedural Terminology* (American Medical Association, 2009) both essential for the process of physician reimbursement for manual therapy services. Inclusion of these diagnostic and procedure codes in definitive reference books places osteopathic and manual therapy in the mainstream of modern medical practice.

Osteopathic medicine – background and comparison with allopathic medicine

'Osteopathic medicine has from its beginnings been a profession based on ideas, tenets that have lasted through all sorts of adversity and have been credited with bringing the profession to its present level of success' (Peterson 2003, p. 19). This set of concepts and their associated applications to medical practice originate with a 19th century itinerant, apprentice-trained American physician, Andrew Taylor Still, who served as a military physician on the side of the North in the American Civil War. After the deaths of three of his children from spinal meningitis, Still eschewed the common medical practices of the day such as purging, blistering and bloodletting in search of a better form of healthcare. In 1874, a personal experience in which he received relief from a headache by resting his neck over a sling of rope hung between two trees started still on the path of discovery of what he called osteopathy. *From its very beginning the neuromusculoskeletal system evaluation and treatment has been central to the osteopathic profession.* After years of successful practice of osteopathy, in 1892 he established the American School of Osteopathy.

Following the Flexner Report of 1910, which sought to standardize medical education and was responsible for the closure or merging of many medical schools (Flexner 1910), eight osteopathic medical schools survived the reforms in American medical training, as they were deemed by Flexner to have curricula sufficiently consistent with the new standards of the time. This was a very important event, as it set the stage for the development of osteopathic medicine as a distinct school of medicine coexistent with allopathic medicine. In America, the DO – Doctor of Osteopathic Medicine degree – and the MD – Doctor of Medicine – permit licensure for the 'full scope of medical practice,' and as such both degrees are equivalent in practice privileges.

The adversity that Peterson (2003) speaks of was due primarily to lack of understanding of, and resistance to, osteopathic concepts, which emphasized the evaluation and treatment of the musculoskeletal system in healthcare, in contrast to the modern allopathic profession (defined below), or 'regular' internal medicine, which emphasized a pharmacological approach. Stated another way, osteopathic concepts emphasize the use of the biological mechanisms of the brain/body in its treatment strategies, whereas traditional modern medicine has the tendency to influence them through the use of chemical agents as the first line of treatment. As for the practice of surgery, which technically is not considered allopathic medicine, both medical and osteopathic professions have been virtually identical since the 1940s. Since the 1960s osteopathic physicians have had full medical practice rights in all the states and in the military medical services.

Although there remains a lively debate on the primacy of allopathic pharmacologically based practices with regard to osteopathic musculoskeletal/anatomically based practices, in recent times the two professions have worked toward a rapprochement. This increased cooperation stems partly from the fact that osteopathic physicians meet a critical need for healthcare in the United States. Also, in the last decade, the publication of research on osteopathic manipulative medicine (Chapter 12), as well as the research on other manual therapies (Chapters 13–15) has increased acceptance of these practices in medical practice, as mentioned above.

Another important factor meriting mention in this discussion is the trend towards public interest in and acceptance of the type of philosophy enunciated by the osteopathic profession. This trend is perhaps best defined by the terms 'holistic' and 'integrative' medicine. Whereas practices defined by these terms may be embraced by many allopathic physicians, these ideas are a part of the 'hard copy' of the osteopathic profession and are explicitly taught and reiterated from the first year and throughout osteopathic medical training. So what is this philosophy?

Osteopathic medical philosophy

The modern version of osteopathic philosophy was published in 1953 (Special Committee on Osteopathic Principles and Osteopathic Technic, 1953) and has become known as the Four Tenets (Box 1.1). Because it relates to the theoretical underpinning of much of the research presented in this book, the elaboration of the Four Tenets published in 2003 (Seffinger et al. 2003, p. 5) is presented in Box 1.2. Still's fundamental concepts of osteopathy can be organized in terms of health, disease, and patient care, which gives a statement of broader application of healthcare from the osteopathic perspective.

Osteopathic principles – heuristic implications and development

Somatovisceral and viscerosomatic interactions

The statement in Box 1.2, for emphasis, under #3 'Health,' #5 'Disease,' and #8 'Patient Care' that 'illness is often caused by mechanical impediments to normal flow of body fluids and nerve activity,' has led to the development of specific OMT and

---

Box 1.1 Basic tenets of osteopathic medicine

- The body is a unit; the person is a unit of body, mind, and spirit.
- The body is capable of self-regulation, self-healing, and health maintenance.
- Structure and function are reciprocally interrelated.
- Rational treatment is based upon an understanding of the basic principles of body unity, self-regulation, and the interrelationship of structure and function.

Box 1.2 Application of the basic tenets of osteopathic medicine categorized in terms of health, disease, and patient care

Health

- Health is a natural state of harmony.
- The human body is a perfect machine created for health and activity.
- A healthy state exists as long as there is normal flow of body fluids and nerve activity.

Disease

- Disease is an effect of underlying, often multifactorial causes.
- Illness is often caused by mechanical impediments to normal flow of body fluids and nerve activity.
- Environmental, social, mental, and behavioral factors contribute to the etiology of disease and illness.

Patient care

- The human body provides all the chemicals necessary for the needs of its tissues and organs.
- Removal of mechanical impediments allows optimal body fluid flow, nerve function and restoration of health.
- Environmental, cultural, social, mental, and behavioral factors need to be addressed as part of any management plan.
- Any management plan should realistically meet the needs of the individual patient.

manual therapy procedures to accomplish the reversal or elimination of mechanical impediments. As described briefly below and more extensively in Chapter 12, OMT has been shown effective in the treatment of musculoskeletal disorders. These finding stem from Still's development of the concept of the removal of mechanical impediments by OMT for musculoskeletal disorders, such as pain, and can be considered the mechanical peripheral component of his theory. From Still's writings it appears that simultaneously or very shortly

thereafter he postulated the concept of viscerosomatic and somatovisceral interactions as an integration of peripheral (afferent and efferent) nervous system activity and central nervous system activity. This aspect of Still's concepts has also led to research on nervous system functions such as viscerosomatic interactions and alterations of spinal reflex excitability.

The earliest osteopathic account of somatovisceral interaction is an anecdotal story reported by Still and later published in his autobiography. Still writes in detail of the treatment of a child with 'bloody flux,' as severe diarrhea was called in the 19th century. The OMT was to several sites on the child's vertebral column that Still described as 'warm to the touch,' compared to the child's 'cold' stomach. Still's treatment apparently corrected the problem, bringing relief to the child and expressions of gratitude from the child's mother (Still 1908, p. 104–106). Still later described the pathophysiology and treatment for this condition, and in so doing was among the first to connect musculoskeletal dysfunction with systemic disorders.

The 2008 symposium 'Somato-visceral Interactions and Autonomic Mechanisms of Manual Therapy' (see Foreword), upon which this volume is based, focused on somatovisceral and viscerosomatic reflexes at all levels of the neuraxis. Albeit neither unique to nor 'discovered' by the osteopathic profession, the development of somatovisceral interactions for use clinically and as a possible explanation of mechanism of action for manual therapy is one of the major contributions of osteopathic concepts to research and science.

Citing the work of Claude Bernard in 1850 as impetus, Louisa Burns, an early osteopathic physician and researcher, published research in 1907 that influenced osteopathic thinking and research over the last century. Burns described experiments on cats and dogs demonstrating a viscerosomatic interaction: '*For the experiments upon the abdominal viscera, the abdominal wall was cut, and the viscera exposed to view with as little manipulation as possible. The stimulation of the inner wall, the muscular coat and the peritoneal covering of the cardiac end of the stomach or of the fundus was followed by the contraction of the spinal muscles near the sixth to the ninth thoracic vertebrae'* (Burns 1907, p. 54). For a somatovisceral interaction, she stated: *'The stimulation of the tissues near the fifth to the eighth thoracic vertebrae was followed by muscular and secretory activity in the stomach, and stimulation near the eighth to the twelfth thoracic vertebrae was followed by activity of the intestines.'* (Burns 1907, p. 55). In the same article she describes stimulation of the spine in humans that appeared to change blood pressure readings in 37 'healthy individuals.'

As is documented in this book (Chapters 2–4, 7–8, 10), the concept of somatovisceral and viscerosomatic interactions is a well-studied and useful concept in the neurosciences, most notably found in the work of Akio Sato (e.g., Sato & Schmidt 1971, Sato 1972), some of which is described in Chapter 2. Figure 1.1 is a schematic representation of the viscerosomatic reflex wherein a visceral dysfunction, due, for example, to an infection or other disease process, causes a reflex

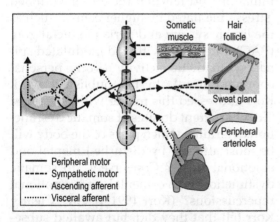

Figure 1.1 Schematic representation of the viscerosomatic reflex. (From Beal M C 1985 Viscerosomatic reflexes: a review. Journal of the American Osteopathic Association 85:786–801, reprinted with permission.)

activation of some kind in somatic or musculoskeletal structures. The early work of Denslow and Korr (Denslow 1944, Denslow et al. 1947, Korr et al. 1962) established the scientific credibility for osteopathic treatment based on the concept of somatovisceral interactions and a related concept of the facilitated segment(s)/area.

The concept of the facilitated segment(s)/area: Korr's theory

The integration of research on viscerosomatic interactions with the theory of facilitated areas provides a possible explanation of a neuromusculoskeletal mechanism of action for the impact of OMT and manual therapy. Denslow, Korr and their collaborators carried out and published research in which they concluded that chronic facilitation could develop in human motor neuron pools which resulted in measurable physiological manifestations such as electrical skin resistance changes in portions of the body related to specific spinal segments (Denslow et al. 1947, Korr et al. 1962, 1964, Wright & Korr 1965). These research findings formed a possible neurophysiological basis for the so-called 'osteopathic lesion' now termed 'somatic dysfunction' (described below), which served to advance and maintain the utilization of OMT by osteopathic physicians faced with increasing demands by medical insurance underwriters for statements of proof of the rationale and benefits of their treatment.

Korr's theory of the facilitated area(s) postulated that the chronic facilitation could start with either a visceral or musculoskeletal disorder of some kind. The presence of a systemic disorder such as hypertension or gallbladder infection could eventually cause musculoskeletal discomfort and palpable changes to spinal paravertebral tissues, along with patient perceptions of pain in the distribution of dermatomes and myotomes associated with specific vertebral segments.

Likewise, a vertebral or somatic dysfunction or problem – usually due to trauma or consistent poor posture – which was not corrected could bring about the maintenance of pools of neurons (e.g. premotor interneurons, motor neurons, or preganglionic sympathetic neurons in one or more segments of the spinal cord) in a state of constant partial or subthreshold excitation. In this state, less afferent stimulation is required to trigger impulse generation. The state of heightened nerve activity could cause and maintain abnormal muscle contraction (including even vascular muscle contraction, which could contribute to further worsening of the paravertebral muscle environment), leading to maintenance of vertebral biomechanical aberration and increased likelihood of perceived nociception (Johnston 1992, Ward 2003).

Thus, Korr's theory essentially describes 'spinal facilitation' as an increased spinal neural excitability. Facilitation may be due to a sustained increase in afferent input, aberrant patterns of afferent input, or changes within the affected neurons or their chemical environment. Once established, the heightened spinal neural excitation is analogous to a memory and has been shown to be a self-sustaining temporary or permanent change in neural function (Patterson 2003, 2010).

From the osteopathic perspective the application of OMT brought benefit by restoring normal structural configuration to the musculoskeletal system in the spinal and other somatic areas, which in turn diminished or eliminated the effects of the facilitated segments. Korr (1979) extended his formulation to include possible body-wide consequences, with the yet to be fully tested hypothesis that musculoskeletal trauma or stress produced contiguous areas of segmental sympathetic nervous system hyperexcitability. Korr suggested that a hyperactive sympathetic system also influenced the response of tissues to noxious external agents as well as inflammatory and immune processes. As a logical extension of his theory, Korr further suggested that chronic sympathetic hyperactivity is an often critical factor in such diverse clinical syndromes as neurogenic pulmonary edema, peptic ulcer, arteriosclerosis, cardiac lesions, and osteodystrophies. According to Korr, these abnormal reflexes become chronic and self-sustaining and often impair healing and recovery. OMT is proposed to be important in that such manual therapy, may restore normality to the dysfunctional reflexes and support normal healing and regulatory physiological function.

In Chapters 3 and 4, Pickar and Budgell describe centrally mediated aspects of viscerosomatic and somatovisceral interaction consistent with Korr's concept of facilitation. Korr's concept is consistent with and updated by current neuroscience findings which describe more widespread activity of both the sympathetic and parasympathetic nervous system functions related to somatovisceral and viscerosomatic interactions (Jänig 2006, Porges 2007, and Chapters 2 and 12). As noted above, Korr mentions 'stress' as a cause of sympathetic hyperactivity. Korr also embraced the holistic osteopathic 'body–mind–spirit' formulation and felt that the aforementioned 'stress,' mediated by higher centers such as the limbic system and periaqueductal gray (PAG), interacted with and modulated spinal sympathetic activity (Korr, personal communication). In his published work Korr addressed this matter with questions: 'To what extent do sites of somatic dysfunction determine which parts of the body will be most affected by disturbed mental and emotional states? Conversely, do somatic dysfunctions have mental and emotional repercussions?' (Korr 1991, p. 161). Clearly Korr felt that they did, but awaited subsequent research to test his hypotheses and formulations; and some research which appears to support Korr's theory is provided in Chapters 2 and 10 of this book in the description of higher center control over and interaction with segmentally mediated functions.

Current status of osteopathic medicine

Today the osteopathic medical profession embraces all that science and evidence-based medicine have to offer the public in the delivery of healthcare. Osteopathic physicians deliver state-of-the-art healthcare, adhering to the standard of practice applicable to all physicians in the United States. Even the distinctive osteopathic concepts have received empirical support. Chapter 12 details the research related to systemic disorders and physiologic functions.

In addition, a number of clinic trials have been conducted on the impact of OMT for musculoskeletal disorders and low back pain (Andersson et al. 1999, Burton et al. 2000, Cleary et al. 1994, Gibson et al. 1985, Hoehler et al. 1981, Licciardone et al. 2003). A systematic review and meta-analysis based on these clinical trials established the benefit of OMT in the treatment of musculoskeletal disorders, including low back pain (Licciardone et al. 2005).

The osteopathic medical profession has bolstered the research effort for OMT and manual therapy by establishing The Osteopathic Research Center (ORC) located on the campus of the University of North Texas Health Science Center. This book is based on a research symposium funded in part by an NIH-NCCAM grant to the ORC. The ORC continues a number of externally funded research projects related to OMT and is another example of how the osteopathic medical profession is in the mainstream of modern experimental medicine.

Nomenclature for manual therapy

Manipulation versus mobilization

As mentioned above, it is important for the reader to have some understanding of the nomenclature used in this book. Perhaps the most confusing nomenclature issue, and one that needs clarification from the outset, is the use of the terms 'manipulation' and 'mobilization.' From the osteopathic glossary, 'manipulation' includes all OMT techniques which involve manually guided forces applied to patients. This includes the high-velocity, low-amplitude (HVLA) 'thrust' techniques as well as much gentler soft tissue, myofascial release and cranial manipulations, defined below (ECOP, 2006).

From the chiropractic, physical therapy and massage perspective there are five grades or levels of 'mobilization' or application of manually guided forces, described in Table 1.1:

Table 1.1 Grades of mobilization

Grade	Definition
I	Small-amplitude movement performed at the beginning of the passive range of motion
II	Large-amplitude movement performed within the passive range of motion
III	Large-amplitude movement performed up to the point of limitation in the passive range of motion
IV	Small-amplitude movement performed at the limit of the passive range of motion
V	Small-amplitude, high-velocity thrust performed at the end of the passive range of motion (manipulation)

- The highest level, grade 5, is 'manipulation,' which is defined as 'controlled, judiciously applied dynamic thrust of high- or low-velocity and low-amplitude force directed toward one or more spinal joint segments within patient tolerance that puts the joint within the paraphysiologic space' (Hurwitz & Haldeman 2004, p. 66).
- 'Mobilization' levels comprise grades 4–1, depending on the amount of manually applied force, and are described as 'A controlled, judiciously applied force of low velocity and variable amplitude directed to one or more spinal segments. Mobilization procedures usually take place within the joint's physiologic space, that is, they do not take joints beyond the passive range of motion and do not typically result in joint cavitation [a 'popping sound, Ed]' (Hurwitz & Haldeman 2004, p. 66).

Throughout this book the contributors have attempted to define the particular techniques mentioned in the various research publications. However, when the word 'manipulation' is used in an osteopathic context, it may refer to a number of different types of manually applied techniques and forces. When used in the context of chiropractic, physical therapy and massage therapy research, 'manipulation' means a thrust of some kind (see Chapter 13).

For the reader unfamiliar with the research and terminology in manual therapy, Table 1.2 is presented for reference. Unless otherwise noted, all terms are defined according to the *Glossary of Osteopathic Terminology* (ECOP, 2006). Box 13.1 in Chapter 13 also gives definitions of chiropractic treatment techniques.

Table 1.2 Terminology used in this book

Allopathy – allopath – allopathic medicine	1. Allopathy is a therapeutic system in which a disease is treated by producing a second condition that is incompatible with or antagonistic to the first 2. Substitutive therapy 3. A traditional medical physician, as distinguished from eclectic or homeopathic practitioners 4. Conventional or orthodox medical practice (Stedman's Medical Dictionary 2006)
Somatic dysfunction	As stated above, another contribution to the understanding of the mechanism of action for OMT is the concept of somatic dysfunction. Originally termed 'osteopathic lesion' based on Denslow and Korr's research, the current definition is 'impaired or altered function of related components of the somatic (body framework) system: skeletal, arthrodial, and myofascial structures, and their related vascular, lymphatic, and neural elements. Somatic dysfunction is treatable using osteopathic manipulations. The positional and motion aspects of somatic dysfunction are best described using at least one of three parameters: 1. The position of a body part as determined by palpation and referenced to its adjacent defined structure 2. The direction in which motion is freer, and 3. The direction in which motion is restricted. See also TART

Table 1.2 Terminology used in this book—Cont'd

TART	TART is a mnemonic for four diagnostic criteria for somatic dysfunction: **T**issue texture abnormality, **A**symmetry, **R**estriction of motion, and **T**enderness, any one of which must be present for the diagnosis to be made. Virtually all of the manual therapy professions use the terms somatic dysfunction and TART in their research publications

Specific OMT or Manual Therapy Technique Abbreviations

ART	Articulatory treatment system – a low-velocity/moderate-to-high-amplitude technique where a joint is carried through its full motion, the activating force is either a repetitive springing motion or repetitive concentric movement of the joint through the restrictive barrier
BMT	Balanced membrane tension – similar to balanced ligamentous tension (BLT) in which the palpated tension of the ligaments or membranes guide the positioning provided by the practitioner until a release (improvement) occurs
CV-4	Compression of the fourth ventricle – a cranial manipulation technique directed to affect the flow of cerebral spinal fluid through the fourth ventricle in the brainstem
FT	Functional technique – an indirect treatment approach that involves finding the dynamic balance point and holding the position or adding compression to allow for spontaneous readjustment
ME	Muscle energy technique – a system in which the patient voluntarily moves the body as specifically directed by the osteopathic practitioner; this directed action is from a precisely controlled position against a defined resistance by the practitioner
MFR	Myofascial release – any technique directed at the muscles and fascia, and requires continual palpatory feedback to achieve release of myofascial tissues
OCF	Osteopathy in the cranial field – system of diagnosis and treatment by an osteopathic practitioner. [Gentle cranial manipulation, Ed.]
OMT	Osteopathic manipulative treatment – the therapeutic application of manually guided forces to improve physiologic functions and/or support homeostasis that has been altered by somatic dysfunction
Rib raising	An ART applied to the area of the rib angles and paravertebral muscle area
SCS	Strain-Counterstrain – system of diagnosis and indirect treatment in which the patient's somatic dysfunction is treated by using a passive position, resulting in spontaneous tissue release and reduction in tenderness at a specific point
SP	Splenic pump technique – rhythmic compression applied over the spleen for the purpose of enhancing the patient's immune response
ST	Soft tissue technique – a direct technique directed toward tissues other than skeletal or arthrodial elements and involves stretching, deep pressure, traction while monitoring tissue response and motion changes by palpation
TLP	Thoracic lymphatic pump – term used to describe the impact of OMT on intrathoracic pressure changes on lymphatic flow
VST	Venous sinus technique – a cranial manipulation in which gentle forces are applied with the purpose of improving blood flow in the intracranial venous dural sinuses

References

American Medical Association, 2009. Current Procedural Terminology (CPT) 2009. American Medical Association, Chicago, IL.

Andersson, G.B.J., Lucente, T., Davis, A.M., et al., 1999. A comparison of osteopathic spinal manipulation with standard care for patients with low back pain. N. Engl. J. Med. 341, 1426–1431.

Beal, M.C. J. Am. Osteopath. Assoc. December 1985.

Bigos, S.J., Bowyer, O.R., Braen, G.R., et al., 1994. Acute low back problems in adults: assessment and treatment. Clinical practice guideline number 14. Publication no. 95-0643. US Department of Health and Human Services, Public Health Services, Agency for Health Care Policy and Research, Rockville, MD, December, 1994.

Burns, L., 1907. Viscero-somatic and somato-visceral spinal reflexes. J. Am. Osteopath. Assoc. 7, 51–57.

Burton, A.K., Tillotson, K.M., Cleary, J., 2000. Single-blind randomized controlled trial of chemonucleolysis and manipulation in the treatment of symptomatic lumbar disc herniation. Eur. Spine J. 9, 202–207.

Cleary, C., Fox, J.P., 1994. Menopausal symptoms: an osteopathic investigation. Complement Ther. Med. 2, 181–186.

Denslow, J.S., 1944. An analysis of the variability of spinal reflex thresholds. J. Neurophysiol. 7, 207–216.

Denslow, J.S., Korr, I.M., Krems, A.D., 1947. Quantitative studies of chronic facilitation in human motoneuron pools. Am. J. Physiol. 105, 229–238.

Flexner, A., 1910. Medical education in the United States and Canada; a report to the Carnegie Foundation for the Advancement of Teaching. Merrymount Press, Boston, MA.

Gibson, T., Grahame, R., Harkness, J., et al., 1985. Controlled comparison of short-wave diathermy treatment with osteopathic treatment in non-specific low back pain. Lancet 1, 1258–1261.

ECOP, 2006. Glossary of Osteopathic Terminology Educational Council on Osteopathic Principles (ECOP) of the American Association of Colleges of Osteopathic Medicine. Bethesda, MD.

Hoehler, F.K., Tobis, J.S., Buerger, A.A., 1981. Spinal manipulation for low back pain. J. Am. Med. Assoc. 245, 1835–1838.

Hurwitz, E.L., Haldeman, S., 2004. Manual therapy including manipulation for acute and chronic neck pain. In: Fischgrund, J.S. (Ed.), Neck pain. Monograph Series #27. American Academy of Orthopaedic Surgeons, Rosemont, IL.

International Classification of Diseases, 9th Revision, Clinical Modification (ICD-9-CM), 2008. National Center for Health Statistics and the Centers for Medicare & Medicaid Services.

Jänig, W., 2006. The Integrative Action of the Autonomic Nervous System. Neurobiology of Homeostasis. Cambridge University Press, Cambridge, New York.

Johnston, W.L., 1992. Osteopathic clinical aspects of somatovisceral interaction. In: Patterson, M.M., Howell, J.N. (Eds.), The Central Connection: Somatovisceral/viscerosomatic Interactions. American Academy of Osteopathy, Indianapolis, IN, pp.30–46.

Korr, I.M., 1979. The spinal cord as organizer of disease process: the peripheral autonomic nervous system. J. Am. Osteopath. Assoc. 79, 82–90.

Korr, I.M., 1991. Osteopathic research: the needed paradigm shift. J. Am. Osteopath. Assoc. 91, 156–171.

Korr, I.M., Wright, H.M., Thomas, P.E., 1962. Effects of experimental myofascial insults on cutaneous patterns of sympathetic activity in man. Journal of Neurotransmission 23, 329–355.

Korr, I.M., Wright, H.M., Chase, J.A., 1964. Cutaneous patterns of sympathetic activity in clinical abnormalities of the musculoskeletal system. J. Am. Osteopath. Assoc. 24, 589–606.

Langevin, H., Goertz, C., King, H.H., et al., 2009. Synergistic research goals for manual treatments of musculoskeletal and soft tissue disorders. Symposium presented at North American Research Conference on Complementary and Integrative Medicine, Minneapolis, MN, May 12–15, 2009.

Licciardone, J.C., Stoll, S.T., Fulda, K.G., et al., 2003. Osteopathic manipulative treatment for chronic low back pain: a randomized controlled trial. Spine 28, 1355–1362.

Licciardone, J.C., Brimhall, A., King, L.N., 2005. Osteopathic manipulative treatment for low back pain: a systematic review and meta-analysis of randomized controlled trials. BMC Musculoskelet. Disord. 6, 43–54.

Patterson, M.M., 2003. Foundations of Osteopathic Medical Research. In: Ward, R.C. (Ed.), Foundations for Osteopathic Medicine, second ed. Lippincott Williams & Wilkins, Philadelphia.

Patterson, M.M., 2010. Foundations for Osteopathic Medical Research. In: Chila, A.G. (Ed.), Foundations for Osteopathic Medicine, third ed. Lippincott Williams & Wilkins, Philadelphia.

Peterson, B.E., 2003. Major events in osteopathic history. In: Ward, R.C. (Ed.), Foundations for Osteopathic Medicine, second ed. Lippincott Williams & Wilkins, Philadelphia, pp. 19–29.

Porges, S.W., 2007. The polyvagal perspective. Biol. Psychol. 74, 116–143.

Sato, A., 1972. Somato-sympathetic reflex discharges evoked through supramedullary pathways. Pflugers Archiv. 332, 117–126.

Sato, A., Schmidt, R.F., 1971. Spinal and supraspinal components of reflex discharges into lumbar and thoracic white rami. J. Physiol. 212, 839–850.

Seffinger, M.A., King, H.H., Ward, R.C., Jones, J.M., Rogers, F.J., Patterson, M., 2003. Osteopathic philosophy. In: Ward, R.C. (Ed.), Foundations for Osteopathic Medicine, second ed. Lippincott, Williams & Wilkins, Philadelphia.

Stedman's Medical Dictionary 28th ed 2006. Philadelphia: Lippincott Williams & Wilkins.

Still, A.T., 1908. Autobiography of Andrew T. Still. revised ed. A.T. Still, Kirksville, MO.

Ward, R.C. (Ed.), 2003. Foundations for Osteopathic Medicine, second ed. Lippincott Williams & Wilkins, Philadelphia.

Wright, H.M., Korr, I.M., 1965. Neural and spinal components of disease: progress in the application of 'thermography.' J. Am. Osteopath. Assoc. 64, 918–921.

Section One
Peripheral and spinal viscerosomatic mechanisms

Functions of the autonomic nervous system: current concepts

Wilfrid Jänig

Introduction

The body's motor activity is only possible when its internal milieu is controlled to keep the component cells, tissues, and organs (including brain and skeletal muscles) maintained in an optimal state for their functioning. This enables the organism to adjust its performance to the varying internal and external demands placed on it. The control of the internal milieu is exerted by the brain acting on many different types of peripheral target tissue (smooth muscle cells of various organs, cardiac muscle cells, exocrine glands, endocrine cells, metabolic tissues, immune cells, etc.). The *efferent signals* from the brain to the periphery of the body by which this control is achieved are *neural* (by the autonomic nervous systems) and *hormonal* (by the neuroendocrine systems). The *afferent signals* from the periphery of the body to the brain are neural, hormonal (e.g., hormones from endocrine organs including those in the gastrointestinal tract, cytokines from the immune system, leptin from adipocytes), and physicochemical (e.g., blood glucose level, body core temperature, etc.).

The maintenance of physiological parameters such as concentrations of ions, blood glucose, arterial blood gases, body core temperature, etc. in a narrow range is called *homeostasis* (Cannon 1929, 1939). This process of maintaining the stability of the internal milieu during changes in the body and in the environment requires systems that have a large range of activity, such as the cardiovascular system, the thermoregulatory system, the metabolic system (involving the gastrointestinal tract and endocrine systems releasing insulin, glucagon, leptin and thyroxin) or the immune system. The autonomic and endocrine homeostatic regulations are represented in the brain (i.e., in the hypothalamus, brain stem, and spinal cord) and under the control of the telencephalon. They are integrated at all central neural levels with the somatomotor and sensory representations of the body, leading to tight coordination of autonomic and somatomotor regulation. Thus the brain contains autonomic 'sensorimotor programs' for the regulation of the internal environment of the body and sends efferent commands to the peripheral target tissues through the autonomic and endocrine routes.

Autonomic regulation of body functions requires specific neuronal pathways in the periphery and a specific organization of neural circuits connected to these pathways in the central nervous system (CNS); otherwise it would be impossible to understand the precise rapid and slow adjustments of the body during various behaviors. The effector cells of the autonomic nervous system are diverse, whereas those of the somatic efferent system are not. Thus the autonomic nervous system is the major efferent component of the peripheral nervous system and outweighs the somatic efferent pathways in diversity of function and size.

The model in Fig. 2.1 outlines the role of the autonomic nervous system in the generation of behavior. Behavior is defined as purposeful motor action of the body in the environment. It is generated by coordinated activation of the three divisions of the motor system: the somatic, the autonomic, and the neuroendocrine motor systems (Swanson 2000, 2008). The somatomotor system moves

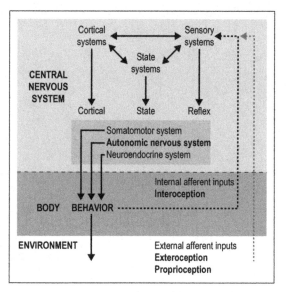

Figure 2.1 Functional organization of the nervous system to generate behavior. The brain controls behavior by way of the motor system, consisting of the somatomotor, the autonomic (visceromotor) and the neuroendocrine systems. The motor system is hierarchically organized in spinal cord, brain stem, and hypothalamus. It receives three general types of synaptic input: (a) from the sensory systems monitoring processes in the body (interoception) or the environment (exteroception) to all levels of the motor system generating reflex behavior (reflex); (b) from the cerebral hemispheres responsible for voluntary control of the behavior based on neural processes related to cognitive and affective–emotional processes (cortical); (c) from the behavioral system controlling attention, arousal, sleep/wakefulness, circadian timing (state). These three input systems communicate bidirectionally with each other (upper part of the figure). (Modified from Swanson (2000, 2008).)

the body in the environment. The autonomic and neuroendocrine motor systems prepare and adjust the internal milieu and body, enabling the body to move. Both are also important to protect the body against real and potential short- and long-term injuries occurring continuously from outside as well as from within the body.

- The motor neuron pools of the somatomotor and autonomic nervous systems extend from the midbrain to the caudal end of the spinal cord, with gaps in the cervical and lower lumbar spinal cord for the autonomic nervous system.

The neuroendocrine motor neurons are located in the periventricular zone of the hypothalamus.

- The three divisions of the motor system are hierarchically organized in spinal cord, brain stem, and hypothalamus, the neuroendocrine motor system being represented at the top of this hierarchy. They are integrated at each level of the hierarchy.
- The activity of the motor system generating behavior is dependent on three major classes of input: (1) the sensory systems, (2) the cortical system, and (3) the behavioral state system.
- The sensory systems innervating the body tissues are closely welded to the motor hierarchies and generate on all levels of these hierarchies reflex behavior (*reflex* in Fig. 2.1).
- Afferent neurons with C or Aδ fibers monitor the mechanical, thermal, and metabolic states of the body tissues and are involved in interoception (*internal* in Fig. 2.1).
- Afferent neurons with large-diameter (Aβ) fibers monitor events in the environment of the body or in the body related to movements. They are involved in extero- or proprioception (*external* in Fig. 2.1).
- The cerebral hemispheres initiate and maintain behavior based on cognition and affective–emotional processes (*cortical* in Fig. 2.1).
- The behavioral state system consists of intrinsic neural systems that determine the state of the brain in which it generates motor behavior. The behavioral state system controls sleep and wakefulness, arousal, attention, vigilance, and circadian timing (*state* in Fig. 2.1).
- The three global input systems to the motor system interact with each other.

This way of looking at the autonomic nervous system shows that the activity in the autonomic neurons is dependent on the intrinsic functional structure of the sensorimotor

programs of the motor hierarchies and on the three global input systems (sensory–reflex, cortical, state). Any change in these peripheral and central input systems is reflected in the activity of the autonomic pathways and therefore in the autonomic regulations. Brain and body are reciprocally 'glued' together by the autonomic nervous systems and by the small-diameter afferent systems innervating all tissues and being involved in interoception.

Based on this concept I will discuss (1) the principles of the organization and functioning of the autonomic nervous system in the periphery and in the CNS (Jänig 2006, Jänig & McLachlan 2002) and (2) the role of the sympathetic nervous system in body protection (including pain, hyperalgesia, and inflammation)(Jänig & Levine 2006, Jänig 2009a).

Organization of peripheral autonomic pathways

Definition of the autonomic nervous system and visceral afferent neurons

Langley (1921) originally proposed the generic term 'autonomic nervous system' to describe the innervation of virtually all tissues and organs except striated muscle fibers and the brain. Langley's division of the autonomic nervous system into the sympathetic, parasympathetic, and enteric nervous systems is now universally applied. The definition of the sympathetic and parasympathetic nervous systems is primarily anatomical (the thoracolumbar system or sympathetic system; the craniosacral or parasympathetic system). The enteric nervous system is intrinsic to the wall of the gastrointestinal tract and consists of interconnecting plexuses along its length (Furness 2006, Jänig 2006).

The peripheral sympathetic and parasympathetic pathways consist of two populations of neurons. The cell bodies of the postganglionic neurons are grouped in *autonomic ganglia*. Their axons are unmyelinated and project from these ganglia to the target organs. The cell bodies of the preganglionic neurons lie in the spinal cord and brain stem. They send axons from the CNS into the ganglia and form synapses on the dendrites and cell bodies of the postganglionic neurons. Their axons are myelinated as well as unmyelinated. The peripheral sympathetic and parasympathetic pathways are synaptically linked to distinct central circuits in the spinal cord, brain stem, and hypothalamus; the principle of organization of these circuits will be discussed below (Fig. 2.2).

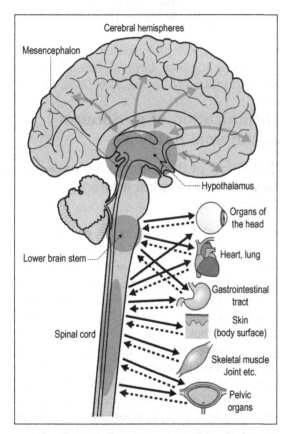

Figure 2.2 Reciprocal communication between brain and body tissues by efferent autonomic pathways and afferent pathways. The global autonomic centers in the spinal cord, lower and upper brain stem, and hypothalamus are shaded. The brain sends efferent commands to the peripheral target tissues through the peripheral autonomic pathways. The afferent pathways consist of groups of afferent neurons with unmyelinated or small-diameter myelinated fibers. These afferent neurons monitor the mechanical, thermal, chemical, and metabolic states of the body tissues.

In the definition of the terms sympathetic and parasympathetic, afferent neurons are not included. About 85% of the axons in the vagus nerves and up to 50% of those in the (spinal) splanchnic nerves are afferent and are called vagal or spinal visceral afferents, respectively. They come from sensory receptors in the internal organs and have their cell bodies in the ganglia of the ninth and tenth nerves, and in the dorsal root ganglia of the spinal segments corresponding to the autonomic outflow. To label thoracolumbar and sacral afferents 'sympathetic' or 'parasympathetic,' respectively, is misleading. This does not conflict with the idea that visceral afferents are integral components of most autonomic reflexes and regulations (Jänig & Koltzenburg 1993, Cervero 1994, Undem & Weinreich 2005, Jänig 2005, 2006). In fact, visceral afferent neurons, together with small-diameter (Aδ, C) afferent neurons innervating almost all somatic tissues, monitor the mechanical, thermal, chemical, and metabolic states of the body tissues. These afferent neurons are also involved in homeostatic regulations and regulation of body protection (see pp. 39–43 [Sympathetic nervous system and body protection]). Their activation leads to interoceptive body sensations that include pain, heat, sensual touch, itch, various visceral sensations, respiratory sensations, and sensations of deep somatic tissues (e.g., during exercise). Thus, these body sensations belong to interoception 'as the sense of the physiological conditions of the entire body' and have a distinct primary cortical representation in the insular cortex (Craig 2002, 2003a,b,c). This concept of interoception extends the concept of Sherrington (1900), who limited it to the viscera (Jänig 2009a).

Functional characteristics and anatomy of peripheral autonomic pathways

Preganglionic neurons are the final integrative pathways of activity in neural circuits of the CNS that are involved in regulation of

autonomic functions. The diversity of autonomic body functions implies that these
central circuits are as diverse. Only a few of
these central circuits have been worked out
as far as the excitatory and inhibitory neurons and their synaptic interactions are concerned. The functional variety is reflected
in the reflex activity patterns of the autonomic pre- and postganglionic neurons, and
it is expected that these patterns are correlated with the functions (i.e., the target cells)
of the peripheral autonomic neurons. It is
important to emphasize that the differentiated reflex patterns are only visible when
the afferent neurons are stimulated physiologically (e.g., arterial baro- or chemoreceptors, cutaneous receptors, receptors of
internal organs, etc.). In this section I will
show that this is indeed the case, and that
the autonomic nervous system consists of
many subsystems that are both anatomically and physiologically different.

Many peripheral autonomic neurons
exhibit spontaneous activity and/or can
be activated or inhibited reflexly by appropriate physiological stimuli. This has been
shown (1) in anesthetized animals (mainly
cats and rats) for neurons of the lumbar
sympathetic outflow to skeletal muscle,
skin, and pelvic viscera (Jänig 1996, Jänig
& McLachlan 1987), and for neurons of the
thoracic sympathetic outflow to the head
and neck; (2) in awake humans for the
sympathetic outflow to skeletal muscles
and skin (Jänig 2006, Jänig & Häbler 2003,
Wallin 2002); and (3) in animals for some
parasympathetic systems innervating inner
eye muscles, heart, trachea and bronchi,
upper gastrointestinal tract, urinary bladder, and colon. The reflexes observed correspond to the effector responses which
are induced by changes in activity of these
autonomic neurons. The reflex patterns
elicited by physiological stimulation of various afferent input systems represent physiological 'fingerprints' (markers) for each
autonomic pathway.

Reflex Patterns in Sympathetic Neurons: Animal Experiments

Figures 2.3 and 2.4 illustrate examples of
reflex responses in sympathetic neurons
regulating blood vessels in skeletal muscle
(muscle vasoconstrictor neurons, MVC),
skin (cutaneous vasoconstrictor neurons,
CVC), possibly the nasopharyngeal mucosa
('inspiratory' neurons, INS) and sweat glands
(sudomotor neurons, SM) in the anesthetized cat. The overall results obtained on
sympathetic neurons are:

- Reflex patterns in muscle and visceral
  vasoconstrictor neurons consist of
  inhibition by arterial baroreceptors, but
  excitation by arterial chemoreceptors,
  cutaneous nociceptors, and spinal
  visceral nociceptors (Figs 2.3A, B, 2.4).
- Most cutaneous vasoconstrictor neurons
  are inhibited by stimulation of cutaneous
  nociceptors of the distal extremities,
  spinal visceral afferents, arterial
  chemoreceptors, and central warm-
  sensitive neurons in the spinal cord and
  hypothalamus (Figs 2.3A–D, 2.4).
- Sudomotor neurons are activated by
  stimulation of Pacinian corpuscles in
  skin and by certain other afferent stimuli
  (Fig. 2.3C).
- Motility-regulating neurons innervating
  pelvic organs are excited or inhibited
  by stimulation of sacral afferents from
  the urinary bladder, hindgut, or anal
  canal, but are not affected by arterial
  baroreceptor activation. Functionally
  different types of motility-regulating
  neurons can be distinguished by their
  reflex patterns.
- Neurons firing only during inspiration
  (i.e., during phrenic nerve discharge)
  which innervate effectors of the head
  (probably the vasculature of the
  nasopharyngeal and tracheal mucosa)
  are excited by noxious stimulation or
  stimulation of chemoreceptors, most
  of them not being under baroreceptor
  control (Fig. 2.4).

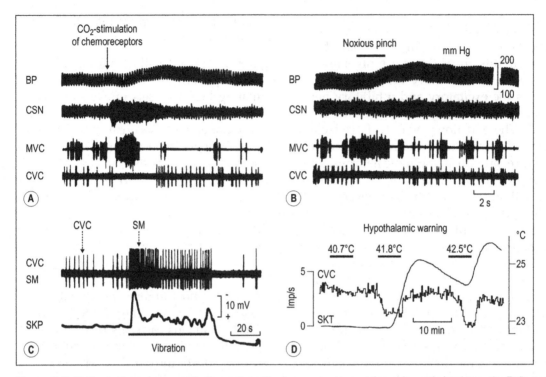

Figure 2.3 Reflex patterns in sympathetic postganglionic neurons innervating skin or skeletal muscle. Reflexes in muscle (MVC) and cutaneous (CVC) vasoconstrictor and sudomotor (SM) neurons recorded from postganglionic axons in bundles isolated from a skin nerve (medial plantar nerve) or muscle nerve (gastrocnemius–soleus nerve) of the hindlimb in anesthetized cats. **A.** Stimulation of the carotid chemoreceptors by a bolus injection of CO_2-enriched saline (arrow) activated the MVC neurons and inhibited the CVC neuron (recorded simultaneously). Increased activity in chemoreceptor afferents in the carotid sinus nerve (CSN) was monitored. **B.** Stimulation of cutaneous nociceptors by pinching the ipsilateral hindpaw (indicated by bar) also excited the MVC neurons and inhibited the CVC neuron. **C.** Simultaneous recordings of the activity in a single CVC neuron (small signal) and in a single SM neuron (large signal) and the skin potential (SKP) from the central paw pad. The SKP is an effector response generated by activation of sweat glands. Stimulation of Pacinian corpuscles in the hindpaws by vibration excited the SM neuron and inhibited the CVC neuron. SM activation was correlated with the changes in SKP. **D.** Inhibition of CVC neurons to warming of the anterior hypothalamus. Note the increase in skin temperature (SKT) on the central paw pad following depression of CVC activity. (Data for A–C from Jänig and Kümmel, unpublished; D modified from Grewe et al. 1995.)

- Some types of sympathetic neuron are only activated in special functional conditions: pilomotor neurons, vasodilator neurons to skeletal muscle or skin (Joyner & Halliwill 2000), neurons innervating the pineal gland, lipomotor neurons innervating brown adipose tissue in the rat (Morrison 1999, 2001), pupillomotor neurons, neurons innervating cells of the adrenal medulla releasing adrenaline (Morrison & Cao 2000), and neurons innervating pelvic erectile tissue and generating dilation of this tissue (de Groat 2002, Jänig 1996, 2006).

- Regulation of respiration and of peripheral sympathetic pathways is closely integrated in the medulla oblongata. This integration is reflected in respiratory rhythmicity of the activity in sympathetic neurons. The rhythmicity is not uniform, but varies in its pattern (respiratory activity profile) according to the function of the sympathetic neurons (Häbler et al. 1994, Jänig & Häbler 2003). Figure 2.4 illustrates an example. The muscle vasoconstrictor (MVC) neurons discharge in inspiration and expiration. The cutaneous vasoconstrictor (CVC) neurons discharge either only in

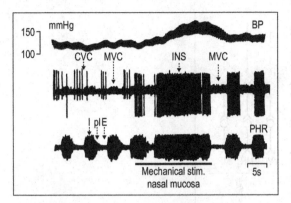

Figure 2.4 Reflexes in sympathetic preganglionic neurons generated by mechanical stimulation of the nasal mucosa. Simultaneous recording from three preganglionic axons in a strand isolated from the cervical sympathetic trunk and from a phrenic nerve in an anesthetized cat. Activity recorded from a cutaneous vasoconstrictor (CVC) neuron, an inspiratory (INS) sympathetic neuron and a muscle vasoconstrictor (MVC) neuron. Phrenic nerve activity indicates central inspiration (I), post inspiration (pI) and expiration (E). The mechanical stimulus was a shearing stimulus applied to the nasal mucosa; it probably was noxious. Note that this stimulus (1) activated the INS neuron, but only during phrenic nerve discharge (PHR; i.e., during inspiration), (2) inhibited the CVC neuron, which was otherwise only active during expiration, and (3) excited the MVC neuron, which was active in inspiration and expiration before the stimulus. The reflexes in these neurons outlasted the stimulus. The increase in blood pressure (BP) was correlated with the continuous MVC discharge during and after the stimulus. (Modified from Boczek-Funcke et al. 1992.)

expiration or in inspiration, or do not exhibit respiratory modulation of their activity. The inspiratory sympathetic neurons discharge only in inspiration. Sudomotor neurons discharge in postinspiration. Most motility-regulating neurons exhibit no respiratory modulation in their activity; a few discharge preferentially in postinspiration.

More than 10 different functional groups of post- and preganglionic sympathetic neurons have been identified in the lumbar sympathetic outflow to skin, skeletal muscle, and viscera, and in the thoracic sympathetic outflow to the head or neck of the cat (see Fig. 2.5 for the lumbar sympathetic outflow to skin, skeletal muscle, and pelvic organs). The same

types of reflex patterns have been observed in both pre- and postganglionic neurons. Most neurons in several of these pathways (e.g., the vasoconstrictor, sudomotor, and motility-regulating pathways) have ongoing activity, whereas in four investigated pathways (e.g., the pilomotor and vasodilator pathways) the neurons are normally silent. Other functionally distinct groups of sympathetic neurons which have not been studied so far are likely to innervate other autonomic target cells (e.g., the kidney [blood vessels, juxtaglomerular cells], the urogenital tract [urinary bladder, vas deferens, erectile tissue, glandular tissue], the hindgut [nonvascular smooth musculature or glandular tissue via the enteric nervous system], the spleen [immune tissue], the heart, the brown adipose tissue [Morrison 1999, 2001], etc.).

Reflex patterns in sympathetic neurons: studies in humans

Activity in bundles with few or single discriminated sympathetic postganglionic axons in human skin or muscle nerves can be recorded in the awake subject with tungsten electrodes inserted manually into the nerve. Using this microneurographic recording technique, it has clearly been shown that muscle vasoconstrictor, cutaneous vasoconstrictor, and sudomotor neurons have the same distinct activity patterns as in the cat or rat, and that there is also evidence for the existence of sympathetic vasodilator neurons supplying skin or skeletal muscle in humans (Jänig & Häbler 2003, Wallin 2002). However, in humans we have no recordings from sympathetic neurons innervating viscera or head, and no recordings from preganglionic neurons (Jänig 2006).

Reflex patterns in parasympathetic neurons

Several systematic studies have been carried out on the functional properties of the parasympathetic pre- and postganglionic neurons involved in the regulation of pelvic organs, gastrointestinal tract, heart, airways,

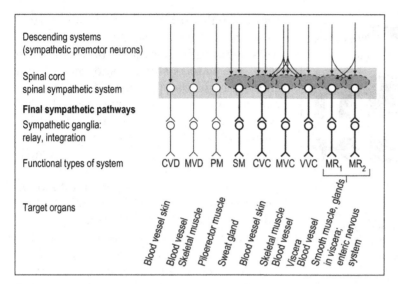

Figure 2.5 Lumbar sympathetic systems supplying skeletal muscle and skin of the hindlimb and pelvic organs (including distal colon) in the cat. The preganglionic neurons of these systems are largely located in the lumbar segments L1 to rostral half L5 (the cat has seven lumbar segments) and project in the lumbar sympathetic trunk distal to paravertebral ganglion L5 or in the lumbar splanchnic nerves and the hypogastric nerves. The first group projects (with a few exceptions related to pelvic organs) to postganglionic neurons innervating somatic tissues, and the second group to postganglionic neurons innervating pelvic organs or colon. The second group includes other sympathetic pathways associated with the internal sexual organs, and probably other target cells in the pelvic organs which are not shown in the figure. Preganglionic neurons are associated with spinal circuits (shaded areas) and are under multiple supraspinal control via sympathetic premotor neurons (see Fig. 2.12). Sympathetic neurons with spontaneous activity in bold. CVC, cutaneous vasoconstrictor; CVD, cutaneous vasodilator; MR, motility-regulating; MVC, muscle vasoconstrictor; MVD, muscle vasodilator; PM, pilomotor; SM, sudomotor; VVC, visceral vasoconstrictor. (Modified from Jänig (2006).)

salivary glands, and inner eye muscles. There are good reasons to assume that the principle of organization into functionally discrete pathways is the same as in the sympathetic nervous system, the main difference being that some targets of the sympathetic system are widely distributed throughout the body (e.g., blood vessels, sweat glands, erector pili muscles, fat tissue), whereas the targets of parasympathetic pathways are more restricted (for details and references see Jänig 2006).

Functional implications of the neurophysiological studies of autonomic neurons in vivo

These neurophysiologic studies in animals and humans argue that the peripheral autonomic nervous system consists of many separate pathways. This separation is supported by a substantial amount of histochemical evidence demonstrating that, depending on

their function, peripheral autonomic neurons may contain neuropeptides or combinations of neuropeptides in addition to the classic transmitters noradrenaline and acetylcholine. The co-localized peptides in autonomic neurons are to a certain degree correlated with the function of the autonomic neurons, although this correlation is not straightforward and absolute; although there are species differences; and although the function of almost all peptides in these neurons is unknown (Gibbins 1995, 2004).

The separation of the peripheral autonomic nervous system into many functionally discrete channels is fundamental to an understanding of how the autonomic nervous system works and why autonomic regulation of all effector systems by the brain is always precisely adapted to the behavior of the organism, depending on the environmental conditions and on the conditions within the body. The concept that the sympathetic nervous system operates in an 'all-or-none' fashion, without distinction between different effector organs, is misleading. The same applies to the idea of a simple functional antagonism between the sympathetic and parasympathetic nervous systems. This is corroborated by the finding that circulating noradrenaline has no detectable function under physiological conditions. Circulating adrenaline, the release of which from the adrenal medulla is regulated by a distinct sympathetic pathway, is a metabolic hormone and may have some other functions, but does not otherwise elicit autonomic effector responses under physiological conditions. Thus, these findings refute the idea that the sympathetic nervous system functions in a generalized fashion.

Signal transmission in peripheral autonomic pathways

The transmission of signals from spinal cord or brain stem to autonomic targets is function specific. Thus, the messages generated in the brain in the context of different autonomic regulations are transmitted by specific mechanisms from preganglionic to postganglionic neurons in the autonomic ganglia, and from the postganglionic axons to the effector cells.

Autonomic ganglia

In peripheral autonomic ganglia preganglionic axons diverge to and converge on postganglionic neurons. Both divergence and convergence occur within, but not between, functionally distinct autonomic pathways. A major function of peripheral autonomic ganglia is to distribute the centrally generated signals by connecting each preganglionic neuron with several postganglionic neurons. In this way a small number of preganglionic neurons connect with a large number of postganglionic neurons. The extent of divergence varies significantly, the ratio of pre- to postganglionic axons being, in pathways such as in the ciliary ganglion

to the iris and ciliary body, as low as 1:4, and in others, such as in the superior cervical ganglion with many vasoconstrictor neurons, as high as 1:150. A limited divergence and much divergence are not characteristics of the parasympathetic or sympathetic systems, respectively. Probably, by analogy with somatic motor units, limited divergence is common in pathways to small targets with discrete functions (e.g., in autonomic pathways to the inner muscles of the eye, or the parasympathetic cardiomotor pathway to cardiac pacemaker cells), whereas widespread divergence is a feature of pathways to anatomically extensive effectors that act more or less simultaneously (e.g., of cutaneous, muscle, or visceral vasoconstrictor pathways) (McLachlan 1995, Jänig 2006).

Sympathetic paravertebral ganglia

Most postganglionic neurons in sympathetic paravertebral ganglia (in the sympathetic chains) innervate autonomic targets in somatic tissues; some innervate viscera (e.g., the heart) or targets of the head (e.g., the intracranial blood vessels, salivary and nasopharyngeal glands, intraocular smooth muscles). Within these ganglia, ganglionic neurons have uniform properties. Each convergent cholinergic preganglionic axon produces excitatory postsynaptic potentials by activating cholinergic nicotinic receptor channels. The amplitude of the potentials ranges from a few millivolts (subthreshold weak synaptic inputs) to 10–40 mV (suprathreshold strong synaptic inputs). In most cases, one or a few strong preganglionic synaptic inputs are always suprathreshold, such as the endplate potential at the skeletal neuromuscular junction. They have a high safety factor and always initiate an action potential. Thus, these ganglion cells relay the incoming CNS-derived signals in only a few of their converging preganglionic inputs (McLachlan et al. 1997, 1998). The function of weak preganglionic synaptic inputs generating small subthreshold potentials in paravertebral ganglia is not clear (Fig. 2.6A).

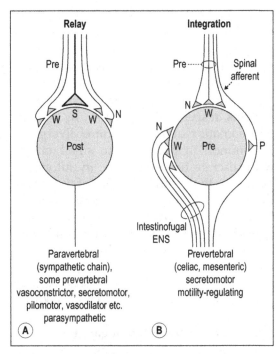

Figure 2.6 Signal transmission in peripheral autonomic pathways: Transmission through autonomic ganglia. **A.** Relay functions of autonomic ganglion cells. Postganglionic neuron with one or a few strong (S; suprathreshold) preganglionic synaptic inputs (generating postsynaptic potentials of 10–30 mV) and several weak (W; subthreshold) synaptic inputs (generating synaptic potentials of a few mV). This connectivity occurs in almost all neurons in paravertebral sympathetic ganglia, in some neurons of prevertebral ganglia, and in parasympathetic ganglia. These connections function mainly to transmit the activity from pre- to postganglionic neurons (McLachlan et al. 1997, 1998). **B.** Relay and integrative functions of autonomic ganglion cells in prevertebral ganglia. Postganglionic neuron with weak synaptic inputs from both preganglionic neurons and interneurons of the enteric nervous system (ENS; intestinofugal neurons), and also from collaterals of spinal visceral afferents. The first two are nicotinic cholinergic (N). The afferent collaterals are peptidergic and use substance P (SP) as transmitter. These postganglionic neurons innervate neurons of the enteric nervous system and possibly other target organs in the viscera (but not blood vessels). They fire only after integration of several subthreshold cholinergic synaptic inputs and/or a slow afferent-induced depolarization. (Modified from Jänig & McLachlan (2002).)

Sympathetic prevertebral ganglia

Neurons in prevertebral (sympathetic) ganglia innervate viscera (gastrointestinal tract, pelvic organs, kidney, and spleen). These postganglionic neurons do not have uniform properties. Three broad groups differ electrophysiologically (by the K^+ channels that control excitability), morphologically (by their size and dendritic branching), and neurochemically (by their neuropeptide content). Two groups, e.g., paravertebral neurons, have suprathreshold synaptic connections with one or a few preganglionic axons which determine the firing pattern of these neurons, one of them having vasoconstrictor function and the other being involved in regulation of motility or secretion. The mode of synaptic transmission in the third group is different. These neurons receive weak preganglionic synaptic inputs and many weak cholinergic nicotinic inputs from intestinofugal neurons of the enteric nervous system, which can be activated by mechanical stimulation of the gastrointestinal tract. Summation of synaptic potentials from peripheral and preganglionic inputs is necessary to initiate their discharge. These postganglionic neurons do not have vasoconstrictor function, but are involved in regulation of motility or secretion. Some of them, possibly the secretomotor neurons, also receive synaptic input from collaterals of visceral primary afferent neurons (which have their cell bodies in the dorsal root ganglia) and depolarize slowly when these inputs are activated at relatively high frequency. The slow responses are generated by the neuropeptide substance P released from the afferent collaterals. This third group of prevertebral neurons therefore depends on temporal and spatial integration of incoming synaptic signals and may establish peripheral (extraspinal) reflexes (Jänig & McLachlan 1992, 2002, Jänig 2006) (Fig. 2.6B).

Parasympathetic ganglia

The structure of many parasympathetic ganglion cells, with few dendrites, is simpler than that of sympathetic neurons. The preganglionic input is correspondingly simple, often consisting of a single suprathreshold input. However, in addition to postganglionic neurons, some parasympathetic ganglia in the body trunk (e.g., cardiac ganglia) contain neurons that behave as primary afferent neurons or interneurons. These ganglia may have the potential for reflex activity independent of the CNS, like the enteric nervous system (McLachlan 1995, Jänig 2006).

The pelvic or hypogastric plexuses contain the neurons that innervate the pelvic organs. Some of these ganglion cells are noradrenergic and are innervated by lumbar sympathetic preganglionic axons; others are cholinergic and receive sacral parasympathetic inputs. A small proportion of pelvic neurons receive synaptic connections from both sympathetic preganglionic neurons projecting through the hypogastric nerves and parasympathetic preganglionic neurons projecting through the pelvic nerves (Keast 1995).

Transmission of signals at the autonomic neuroeffector junctions

In peripheral tissues the transmission of activity in autonomic nerve terminals onto autonomic effector cells is complex and depends on the release of several different compounds and on the presence and distribution of the receptors in the effector membranes for these compounds. Anatomical investigations of neuroeffector junctions at arterioles, veins, pacemaker cells of the heart, cells of the vas deferens, the iris dilator myoepithelium, and the longitudinal muscle of the gastrointestinal tract have demonstrated that varicosities of autonomic nerve fibers which are not surrounded by Schwann cells form close synaptic contacts with the effector cells (Hirst et al. 1992, 1996). These structures are the morphological substrate for the transmission of the centrally generated signals by the postganglionic neurons to the effector cells (Fig. 2.7). The close synaptic contacts occur on <1% of the surface of effector cells. Neuroeffector transmission on arterioles, small arteries, the heart, the vas deferens, the iris dilator myoepithelium, and the longitudinal musculature of the

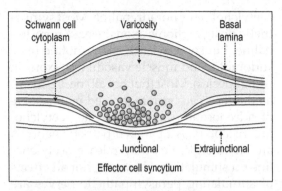

Figure 2.7 Simplified scheme of neuroeffector transmission to autonomic target cells (arterioles, heart, non-vascular smooth muscle cells, secretory cells). Subjunctional (subsynaptic) receptors mediate the effect of transmitter released by the nerve terminals during excitation under physiological conditions. The cell surface at which this nerve–effector communication occurs is ≤1% of the total cell surface. The subsynaptic receptors are ligand-coupled or second messenger-coupled to cellular effectors (e.g., ionic channels). Extrasynaptic receptors for the transmitter are either different from the subsynaptic ones and/or are coupled by different intracellular second-messenger pathways to the cellular effectors. The function of the extrajunctionally located receptors is unclear for most innervated effector cells. Small vesicles containing the transmitter are located close to the synaptic cleft. Large vesicles are also present in many varicosities (not shown). In these vesicles neuropeptides are co-localized with 'classic' transmitter. Large vesicles are not located close to the synaptic cleft. The physiological role of the neuropeptides is in most cases unclear. (Modified from Jänig (2006).)

gastrointestinal tract has been studied in in-vitro preparations using neurophysiological and other methods. These investigations show that signal transmission from postganglionic axons to autonomic effector cells occurs via close neuroeffector junctions and postjunctional receptors, but not – or only to a limited degree (as far as vascular target cells are concerned) – via extrajunctional receptors. This specific method of neuroeffector transmission is the basis upon which signals generated in specific central circuits (see below) are channeled to the appropriate autonomic target cells.

Chemical transmission at these neuroeffector junctions is based on the release of one of the 'conventional' transmitters, acetylcholine or noradrenaline. Most sympathetic postganglionic axons release noradrenaline, but some release acetylcholine (e.g., sudomotor and muscle vasodilator axons in some species). Most (but not all) nerve-mediated effects can be antagonized by blockade of adrenoceptors or muscarinic acetylcholine receptors. All parasympathetic neurons are cholinergic, i.e., they release acetylcholine on stimulation. However, not all effects of stimulating parasympathetic nerves are blocked by muscarinic antagonists. This clearly implies that other transmitters and/or other receptors may be involved. It is now clear that several chemical substances, often contained within individual autonomic neurons, can be released during excitation and can have multiple actions on effector tissues (Furness et al. 1989, Morris & Gibbins 1992). The compounds which may be involved are nitric oxide (NO), adenosine triphosphate (ATP), or a neuropeptide (e.g. vasoactive intestinal peptide [VIP], neuropeptide Y [NPY], galanin [GAL] and other peptides). Immunohistochemistry has revealed the presence of many peptides, although only a few of these have been demonstrated to modify the function after release from nerve terminals in vivo (e.g., NPY or VIP) (Gibbins 1995, 2004, Gibbins et al. 2003).

The response of autonomic target tissues to nerve-released noradrenaline or acetylcholine or other compounds usually only follows repetitive activation of many axons. High-frequency stimuli, particularly in bursts, may produce effector responses owing to the concomitant release of a neuropeptide. Alternatively, when the effects of nerve activity are not completely blocked by an adrenoceptor or muscarinic antagonist at a concentration that entirely abolishes the response to exogenous transmitter, it may not necessarily be the case that a transmitter other than acetylcholine or noradrenaline is involved (as the subjunctional receptors may be different from the extrajunctional ones; and as the concentration of transmitter released into the junctional cleft may reach millimolar concentrations). Although the effects of exogenously applied substances, which have putative transmitter function, on cellular functions are known for many tissues, the consequences of activation of postjunctional receptors by neurally released transmitters have rarely been investigated. When they have, the mechanisms of neuroeffector transmission have been found to be diverse, involving a range of cellular events (Jänig & McLachlan 2002). One important concept that has emerged is that the cellular mechanisms utilized by an endogenously released transmitter are often not the same as when this transmitter substance or its analogue is applied exogenously. The endogenously released transmitter acts primarily or exclusively on the subjunctional receptors, whereas the exogenously applied transmitter acts on the extrasynaptically located receptors (Fig. 2.7, Hirst et al. 1996).

Conclusions

The experimental studies of the peripheral autonomic systems show that (Fig. 2.8):

- The peripheral autonomic nervous system is composed of many distinct pathways that are characterized functionally by their reflex patterns and immunohistochemically by their peptides and other compounds. These reflex patterns are the result of integrative processes in spinal cord, brain stem, and hypothalamus.
- Preganglionic and postganglionic neurons of the same functional type are synaptically connected in autonomic ganglia, with no 'cross-talk' between functionally different types of peripheral pathway. Thus, the centrally generated reflex patterns are transmitted through the autonomic ganglia without distortion. In prevertebral sympathetic ganglia the central messages may be modulated by extraspinal synaptic inputs from the enteric nervous system in pathways involved in the

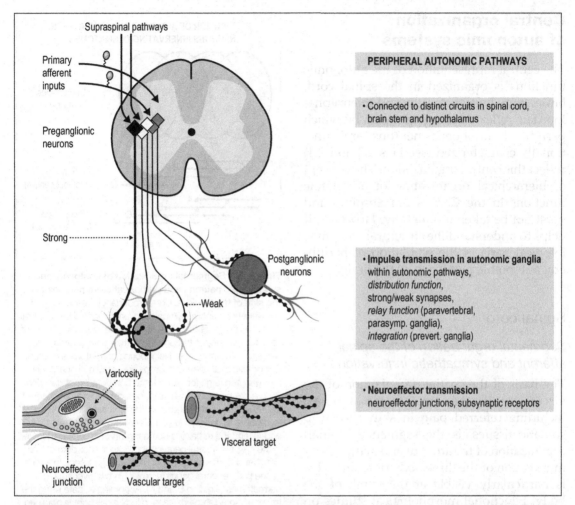

PERIPHERAL AUTONOMIC PATHWAYS

- Connected to distinct circuits in spinal cord, brain stem and hypothalamus

- **Impulse transmission in autonomic ganglia** within autonomic pathways, *distribution function,* strong/weak synapses, *relay function* (paravertebral, parasymp. ganglia), *integration* (prevert. ganglia)

- **Neuroeffector transmission** neuroeffector junctions, subsynaptic receptors

Figure 2.8 Organization of spinal autonomic systems into functional pathways. Separate functional pathways extend from the spinal cord to the effector organs. Preganglionic neurons located in the intermediate zone of the thoracolumbar spinal and sacral cord integrate signals descending from the brain stem and hypothalamus and segmentally from primary afferent fibers. This integration involves several classes of autonomic interneurons in the spinal cord. A similar organization exists for parasympathetic pathways originating from the brain stem. The preganglionic neurons project to peripheral ganglia and converge onto postganglionic neurons. Some preganglionic inputs to postganglionic neurons are always suprathreshold (or strong; see Fig. 2.6A). Others are subthreshold (weak). Subthreshold (weak) postganglionic potentials must either summate to generate an action potential (in some postganglionic neurons of prevertebral ganglia) or their functions are unknown (see Figs 2.6A, B). The postganglionic axons form multiple neuroeffector junctions with their target cells. Many varicosities of the terminal axons which contain the synaptic vesicles with the transmitter(s) form close contacts with the target cells (neuroeffector junctions; see Fig. 2.7). For details of this concept see Jänig (2006) and Jänig & McLachlan (2002). (Modified from Jänig & McLachlan (1992).)

regulation of motility or secretion of the gastrointestinal tract.
- The messages in these functional pathways are transmitted to the autonomic effector cells by distinct neuroeffector mechanisms. This has been shown for the transmission of impulses from parasympathetic and

sympathetic postganglionic axons to various effector cells.
- The composition of the peripheral autonomic nervous system into anatomically and functionally distinct pathways is one important basis for the precise regulation of autonomic body functions.

Central organization of autonomic systems

The central representation of the autonomic functions is organized in the spinal cord, brain stem, hypothalamus, and telencephalon. The reflex discharge patterns by which peripheral autonomic neurons are functionally characterized (see Figs 2.3 and 2.4) reflect this central organization. The concept of hierarchical organization of autonomic functions in the CNS is not absolute and must not be taken too literally. However, it helps to understand the structural and physiological basis of the regulation of peripheral autonomic pathways by the brain.

Spinal cord

Segmental organization of the spinal afferent and sympathetic innervation

The basis of the spatial organization of the viscerosomatic and somatovisceral reflexes, including referred pain in skin and deep somatic tissues, is the segmental (spinal) organization of the afferent and sympathetic innervation of the three body domains. This is particularly visible at the trunk of the body. Functional morphological studies on rats using tracers such as horseradish peroxidase applied either to a dorsal cutaneous nerve or an internal intercostal nerve have shown that about 90% of all sympathetic postganglionic neurons that project to the skin of the trunk through the dorsal or ventral ramus of a spinal nerve have their cell bodies in the paravertebral ganglia of the corresponding segment and of the adjacent caudal segment, the remaining postganglionic cell bodies being located in the two rostral paravertebral ganglia. For example, the cell bodies of the postganglionic neurons innervating dermatome C and projecting through segmental nerve C in Figure 2.9 are located in paravertebral ganglia 3 and 4 (90%) and 1 and 2 (10%). The cell bodies of the primary afferent neurons that innervate dermatome C and project through

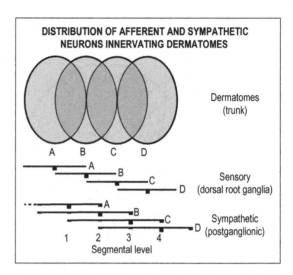

Figure 2.9 Segmental organization of postganglionic sympathetic neurons and primary afferent neurons to the skin of the trunk. A. Dorsal root ganglia (sensory) and paravertebral ganglia (sympathetic) are indicated by vertebral bars. The height of the bars indicates the relative numbers of neurons that project through the corresponding segmental nerve to the dermatome. Neighboring dermatomes overlap. Cell bodies of all afferent neurons are located in one dorsal root ganglion (e.g., for dermatome C in dorsal root ganglion 3). The cell bodies of the postganglionic neurons are located to 90% in the corresponding or the next caudal paravertebral (sympathetic) ganglion (e.g., for dermatome C in ganglions 3 and 4), and the remaining postganglionic neurons are located in the next two rostral paravertebral ganglia (for dermatome C in 1 and 2). This means that most postganglionic neurons in one paravertebral ganglion project in two overlapping dermatomes (e.g. 2 in B and A). According to data using the tracer horseradish peroxidase to locate cell bodies obtained in the rat from Baron et al. (1995).

the segmental spinal nerve C are located in spinal ganglion 3 (Baron et al. 1995). All preganglionic neurons of a spinal segment project through the ventral root and the corresponding white ramus of this segment. In the spinal cord the preganglionic neurons are arranged in rostrocaudal columns and in clusters in the intermediate zone. There is some topical organization with respect to the type of target (Baron et al. 1985, Jänig 2006). Preganglionic axons preferentially form synapses with postganglionic neurons that innervate effector cells in the corresponding dermatome, myotomes, or sclerotome. The degree of branching of individual preganglionic axons is unknown. However, individual preganglionic neurons do not seem to project up and down into the sympathetic chain, and do not project into functionally different nerves (e.g., both into a splanchnic nerve innervating viscera and into the sympathetic chain to ganglia projecting to somatic tissues).

Primary afferent neurons innervating individual visceral organs project through several spinal nerves to the spinal cord. Single visceral afferent neurons with C fibers project to the dorsal horn rostrocaudally over several segments and mediolaterally over the whole width of the dorsal horn (in particular in laminae I and V; Fig. 2.10). These projections extend into the contralateral dorsal horn. The densest projection occurs into lamina I and other projections into lamina V. Laminae II, III, and IV are almost spared by the projections of spinal visceral afferents. The wide spinal rostrocaudal and mediolateral projections of spinal visceral afferent neurons are in contrast to the central projections of myelinated or unmyelinated cutaneous afferent neurons (Fig. 2.9). Myelinated afferents exhibit functionally characteristic spatial spinal projections (Brown 1981; Willis & Coggeshall 2004). Projections of single unmyelinated cutaneous afferents are rostrocaudally and mediolaterally restricted and occur largely to laminae I and II (Willis & Coggeshall 2004).

Spinal autonomic reflex pathways

The spinal cord is an integrative organ in its own right and determines various components of the discharge pattern in the spinal autonomic pathways when the spinal cord is intact. Important constituents in this integration are groups of spinal interneurons that are function specific and which have been postulated on the basis of the study of the reflex patterns in sympathetic neurons (see above and Figs 2.3 and 2.4), and on the basis of reflex patterns in sacral parasympathetic preganglionic neurons being involved in the regulation of pelvic organs (de Groat 2002, Fowler et al. 2008, Shefchyk 2001). However, at present only a few spinal autonomic interneurons (in the sacral spinal cord) have been functionally

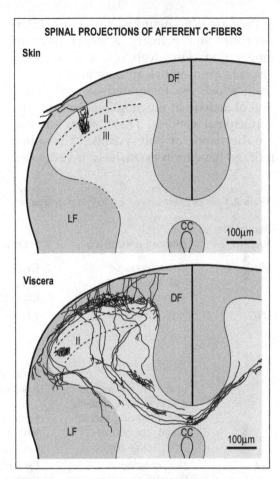

Figure 2.10 **Projections of primary afferent C-fibers to the dorsal horn.** Camera lucida drawing of the central projections of single primary afferent neurons with unmyelinated axons that innervate either visceral organs or the skin. Horseradish peroxidase was injected through a micropipette into single dorsal root ganglionic cells that were identified to project to skin or viscera in the guinea pig. I, II, and III show the superficial laminae of the dorsal horn. Transverse sections. CC, central canal; DF, dorsal funiculus; LF, lateral funiculus. (Modified after Sugiura et al. (1989).)

identified by direct recording – that is, they have been characterized by their functional types of synaptic input and by the functional type(s) of preganglionic neurons with which they form synapses (Jänig 2006, Chapter 9). The interneurons are excitatory or inhibitory. Excitatory interneurons use glutamate as transmitter and inhibitory interneurons use γ-amino-butyric acid (GABA) as transmitter, which may be co-localized with the inhibitory transmitter glycine.

Preganglionic neurons, autonomic interneurons, and primary afferent neurons innervating skin, deep somatic tissues or viscera, form spinal autonomic reflex circuits which are integrated in the regulation of activity in preganglionic neurons by supraspinal centers. These reflex circuits are disynaptic or polysynaptic. The spinal reflexes have been extensively investigated in the lumbar sympathetic outflow of the cat using animals with an intact spinal cord, animals in which the spinal cord was transected between segmental level T7 and T13 30–135 days before the experiments (chronic spinal cats), and animals in which the spinal cord was transected acutely at T10 (for references see Table 2.1). The functional types of spinal reflex were inferred on

Table 2.1 Reflex pathways in the spinal cord associated with lumbar sympathetic systems

Sympathetic system	Afferent neuron	Reaction[a]	References
MVC	Nox. cutaneous	Excitation	Horeyseck & Jänig (1974b) Kümmel (1983)
	Hair follicle	Inhibition	Horeyseck & Jänig (1974b)
	Viscera, sacral	Excitation	Jänig (1985); Kümmel (1983)
CVC	Nox. cutaneous	Inhibition il[b]	Grosse & Jänig (1976); Horeyseck & Jänig (1974b); Jänig (1975); Jänig (1985); Jänig & Kümmel (1981); Jänig & Spilok (1978); Kümmel (1983)
		Excitation cl.	Grosse & Jänig (1976); Jänig (1975)
	Low threshold mech., (Pacinian c., hair follicle)	Inhibition[c]	Horeyseck* Jänig (1974b); Kümmel (1983)
	Viscera mech., sacral	Excitation[d]	Jänig (1985); Kümmel (1983)
	Warm, spinal cord	Inhibition	Jänig and Kümmel (1981)
	Cold, spinal cord	Excitation	Jänig and Kümmel (1981)
SM	Nox. cutaneous	Excitation[b]	Jänig & Spilok (1978); Kümmel (1983)
	Pacinian corp. paw	Excitation	Jänig & Spilok (1978); Kümmel (1983)
	Viscera mech., sacral	Excitation	Jänig (1985); Kümmel (1983)
MR1	Urinary blad. mech., sacral	Excitation	Bartel et al. (1986)
	Colon mech., sacral	Inhibition[e]	Bartel et al. (1986)
	Anus mech., sacral	Excitation[f]	Bartel et al. (1986)
MR2[g]	Urinary blad. mech., sacral	Inhibition	Bartel et al. (1986)
	Colon mech., sacral	Excitation	Bartel et al. (1986)
	Anus mech., sacral	Excitation[f]	Bartel et al. (1986)

All data obtained on chronic spinal (MVC, CVC, SM) or acute spinal (MR) cats. Spinal cord transected between segmental level T7 and T13 30–135 days before the experiments; cl, contralateral; il, ipsilateral.
MVC, muscle vasoconstrictor neurons; CVC, cutaneous vasoconstrictor neurons; SM, sudomotor neurons; MR, motility-regulating neurons.
[a]*All reflexes which are present in the sympathetic neurons after transection of the spinal cord are also present, with two exceptions (see[c,d]), in animals with intact spinal cord under standardized experimental conditions.*
[b]*Inhibition and excitation outlast stimulus.*
[c]*In cats with intact spinal cord, stimulation of hair follicle receptors elicits excitation mostly followed by depression of activity in many CVC neurons (Horeyseck & Jänig, 1974a; Grosse & Jänig, 1976).*
[d]*In cats with intact spinal cord, inhibition in most CVC neurons (see Häbler et al. 1992).*
[e]*Probably more pronounced in spinal preparation (acute) than in the intact preparation.*
[f]*After discharge sometimes present, but shorter in duration than in intact preparation (Bahr et al. 1986); sometimes also inhibition present in acute spinal preparation to mechanical stimulation of the anal canal.*
[g]*This pattern seems to be rare.*

the basis of neurophysiological recordings from functionally identified postganglionic or preganglionic sympathetic neurons (cutaneous vasoconstrictor neurons, muscle vasoconstrictor neurons, sudomotor neurons, motility-regulating neurons). The populations of spinal primary afferent neurons were stimulated physiologically (cutaneous nociceptors, hair follicle receptors, Pacinian corpuscles, sacral mechanosensitive afferents from the anal canal, hindgut or urinary bladder, warm receptors from the spinal canal). The functional types of reflex mediated by the upper lumbar spinal cord are listed in Table 2.1. These reflexes are not only present (and functioning) in anesthetized chronically spinalized animals, but also in anesthetized cats with an intact spinal cord. They show (1) that the thoracolumbar spinal cord isolated from supraspinal regulation centers contains many differentiated autonomic reflex circuits; and (2) that these reflex circuits are functioning during the regulation of activity in the sympathetic pathways.[1]

The same principle applies to the parasympathetic systems of the sacral spinal cord in the regulation of pelvic organs. Here, various groups of excitatory or inhibitory functionally distinct segmental or (sacrolumbar) propriospinal interneurons are postulated to explain the fine-tuned regulation of these organs. Only a few types of these interneurons are known (Jänig 2006, Chapter 9.3).

A similar arrangement exists for parasympathetic autonomic pathways in the brain stem. The preganglionic neurons are located in dorsal vagal motor nuclei (gastrointestinal tract[2]), in the salivary nuclei (salivary glands, nasopharyngeal glands), in the external formation of the nucleus ambiguus (heart; smooth muscles and glands of airways) or in the Edinger–Westphal nucleus (eye). The afferent inputs occur to second-order neurons (interneurons) located in the nucleus tractus solitarii or close to the Edinger–Westphal nucleus.

Supraspinal control of spinal autonomic reflex pathways

The sympathetic or parasympathetic premotor neurons in brain stem or hypothalamus that project to the spinal autonomic circuits connect to the preganglionic neurons either monosynaptically, disynaptically, or polysynaptically. This arrangement of preganglionic neurons, interneurons, primary afferent neurons, and autonomic premotor neurons in supraspinal centers constitutes the basic building blocks of spinal autonomic systems and is probably present in all central autonomic pathways (Fig. 2.11).

Neurons projecting from brain stem or hypothalamus (autonomic premotor neurons) to the spinal autonomic circuits are located in the rostral ventrolateral medulla or the caudal raphe nuclei of the medulla oblongata and lateral to these nuclei, in the A5 area of the caudal ventrolateral pons, in the lateral hypothalamus, or in the paraventricular nucleus (parvocellular parts) of the hypothalamus (Fig. 2.12). The same is true for parasympathetic premotor neurons for autonomic circuits in the brain stem. The primary excitatory transmitter of

[1]Electrical stimulation of spinal afferents (e.g., in the dorsal roots or white rami) elicits short- and long-latency reflexes in sympathetic preganglionic neurons that are mediated by spinal and supraspinal pathways. The spinal reflexes are most powerful when the afferents of the same or a neighboring segment in which the preganglionic neurons are located are stimulated. Although there seem to be some general organizing principles for reflexes in the sympathetic system at the spinal segmental and supraspinal level, it is unclear from these investigations (1) which *functional* types of afferent neurons are involved in these reflexes, and (2) which functional types of sympathetic neuron exhibit segmental (spinal) and/or suprasegmental reflexes (Sato & Schmidt 1971, 1973; Sato et al 1997).

[2]Some parasympathetic preganglionic neurons with unmyelinated fibers projecting to the heart are located in the dorsal vagal motor nucleus. Their function is unknown (see Jänig 2006). These neurons may be involved in coronary vasodilation or control of ventricular contractility (Geis & Wurster 1980).

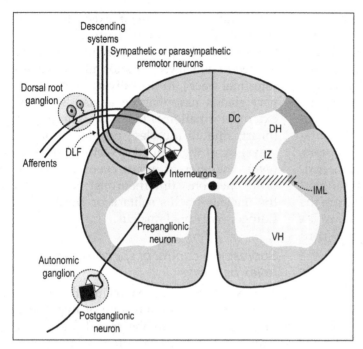

Figure 2.11 The spinal autonomic reflex pathway as the building block between supraspinal centers and peripheral autonomic pathways. There is usually at least one (excitatory or inhibitory) interneuron between (visceral or somatic) primary afferent neurons and preganglionic neurons. Supraspinal centers in brain stem and hypothalamus project through the dorsolateral funiculus (DLF) of the spinal cord and connect synaptically to autonomic interneurons and preganglionic neurons. DC, dorsal column; DH, dorsal horn; IML, nucleus intermediolateralis; IZ, intermediate zone; VH, ventral horn. (Modified from Jänig (2006).)

the sympathetic premotor neurons probably is glutamate. GABA is the primary inhibitory transmitter in some groups of sympathetic premotor neurons. The functions of the monoamines in the sympathetic premotor neurons (adrenaline in the sympathetic C1 premotor neurons of the rostral ventrolateral medulla (RVLM); noradrenaline in the A5 premotor neurons; serotonin in the sympathetic raphe premotor neurons) and of the neuropeptides (e.g., corticotropin-releasing hormone, enkephalin, substance P, thyrotropin-releasing hormone, oxytocin, vasopressin) regulating sympathetic final pathways remain unclear.

The discharge patterns in the autonomic neurons obtained under standardized experimental conditions show (Jänig 2006) that (1) the spinal cord contains distinct autonomic reflex pathways that are integrated with supraspinal reflex pathways during regulation of the autonomic target

organs; (2) the discharge pattern in the different types of sympathetic or (sacral) parasympathetic neuron consists of components that are associated with integration in the spinal cord as well as in the lower brain stem, upper brain stem, and hypothalamus; (3) reflex integration in the spinal cord is related to distinct afferent inputs from skin, viscera, and deep somatic structures; (4) signals arising in supraspinal systems (Fig. 2.12) are integrated with those from spinal circuits at the preganglionic neuron; and (5) spinal circuits are important in the coordination of different spinal autonomic systems as well as somatomotor and autonomic functions.

Thus spinal circuits, spinal afferent inflows, and descending influences from brain stem and hypothalamus always work together to produce the integrative activity of the preganglionic neurons. By analogy with the somatomotor systems (for

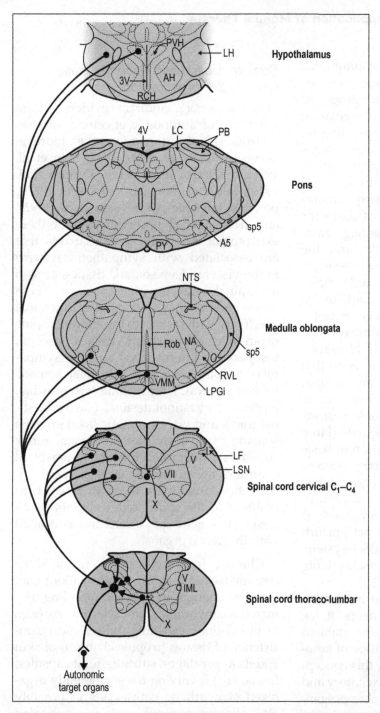

Figure 2.12 Sympathetic premotoneurons in brain stem and hypothalamus, spinal segmental interneurons and propriospinal neurons projecting to sympathetic preganglionic neurons. Sympathetic premotor neurons project to preganglionic neurons and to spinal autonomic interneurons. They are located in the rostral ventrolateral medulla (RVLM), in the caudal raphe nuclei of the medulla oblongata (raphe magnus, pallidus and obscurus [Rob]) and lateral to these nuclei, in the area A5 of the caudal ventrolateral pons, in the lateral hypothalamus (LH), and in the paraventricular nucleus of the hypothalamus (PVH). Autonomic interneurons are located in laminae I, II, V, VI, IX and X of the spinal cord. Propriospinal neurons are located in laminae I, V, VII and X of the cervical spinal segments C1–C6, in the lateral funiculus (LF) and in the lateral spinal nucleus (LSN) of the cervical segments C1–C4. Transverse sections according to Paxinos and Watson (2007). AH, anterior hypothalamus; LC, locus ceruleus; LPGi, lateral paragigantocellular nucleus; NA, nucleus ambiguus; NTS, nucleus tractus solitarii; PB, parabrachial nuclei; PY, pyramidal tract; RCH, retrochiasmatic area; sp5, spinal trigeminal tract; VMM, ventromedial medulla (includes the gigantocellular reticular nucleus alpha und ventral and the parapyramidal nucleus); 3V, third ventricle; 4V, fourth ventricle. (Modified from Jansen et al. 1995, 1997; Strack et al. 1989a, b.)

references see Jänig 2006), spinal autonomic interneurons and preganglionic neurons constitute spinal autonomic motor programs that are integrated in the normal regulation of autonomic target organs. Depending on function, the peripheral autonomic pathways are either under predominant control of the lower brain stem (e.g., muscle and visceral vasoconstrictor pathways innervating resistance vessels, the cardiomotor pathway), of the hypothalamus (e.g., cutaneous vasoconstrictor pathways and the pathway to the brown adipose tissue [in rodents], both probably via the caudal raphe nuclei [see below]), or of the circuits in the spinal cord (e.g., the sympathetic motility-regulating and secretomotor pathways supplying the gastrointestinal tract). However, in *all* spinal autonomic systems it seems that the spinal autonomic circuits are essential for this integration, because they determine the excitability of the preganglionic neurons and/or gate the supraspinal signals (Jänig 1996, 2006). A similar organization of basic reflex circuits, involving primary afferent neurons, interneurons, and preganglionic neurons, and their multiple control circuits, exists in the brain stem for the autonomic control of the gastrointestinal tract (including salivary glands), the respiratory system, the heart, and the inner eye muscles (Jänig 2006, 2009b, Travagli et al. 2006).

It is frequently assumed that autonomic reflexes are hardwired components of the nervous system that are enhanced or inhibited by 'higher' centers in the regulation of autonomic target organs. However, this concept is too narrow and misleading. Excitatory and inhibitory interneurons outnumber preganglionic neurons by an order of magnitude. The synaptic connections between autonomic premotor neurons, interneurons, and preganglionic neurons (including the synaptic connections between different groups of interneurons) are probably responsible for the adaptability and flexibility of autonomic regulation during behavioral changes in the organism.

Somatovisceral and viscerosomatic spinal reflex organization

There is strong indirect evidence from recording of autonomic effector responses or from spinal autonomic nerves (adrenal nerve [Araki et al. 1980, 1984, Sato et al. 1996], cardiac or renal nerve [Kimura et al. 1995], nerve to stomach [Sato et al. 1993], pelvic splanchnic nerve [Sato et al. 1992]) and from clinical observations that there exist spinal autonomic reflex circuits that are associated with sympathetic systems to the viscera, deep somatic tissues, or skin and spinal parasympathetic systems. These reflex circuits may also exhibit functional specificity with respect to the afferent inputs (from skin, deep somatic tissues, viscera), the putative interneurons and the sympathetic output systems (to skin, deep somatic tissues, viscera). They include cardiocardial, renorenal, intestinointestinal (gastrointestinal tract), and viscerosomatic (to skin, deep somatic tissues) and somatovisceral reflex circuits, all integrated into the supraspinal control of the autonomic targets. These spinal reflex circuits are listed in Box 2.1, in addition to the spinal reflex circuits mediated by the sacral spinal cord and associated with the pelvic organs.

Chronic irritation of viscera or deep somatic tissues (e.g., by inflammation) may generate changes in the corresponding dermatomes, myotomes, and sclerotomes (e.g., of blood flow, sweating, piloerection, consistency of tissues [trophic changes] of skin and its appendages, subcutis, joint capsules, fascia, etc.) involving the segmentally organized sympathetic pathways and possibly also afferent neurons with unmyelinated fibers. Interventions in the dermatomes or myotomes may influence, most likely via spinal reflex pathways linked to sympathetic outflows, motility, secretion, blood flow, or other processes in the viscera, as well as blood flow and other processes in deep somatic tissues (for details, see Chapters 3, 4, and 5). Furthermore, as reported in the

Box 2.1 Organ-specific spinal autonomic reflexes and their functions

- **Urinary bladder:** Regulation of micturition and continence: *sacrosacral reflexes, sacrolumbar reflexes*
- **Hindgut:** Regulation of defecation and continence: *sacrosacral reflexes, sacrolumbar reflexes*
- **Sexual organs:** Regulation of erection and ejaculation: *sacrosacral reflexes, sacrolumbar reflexes*
- **Gastrointestinal tract:** Regulation of motility and secretion: *intestinointestinal reflexes*
- **Kidney:** Regulation of kidney functions: *renorenal reflexes*
- **Heart:** Regulation of cardiac functions: *cardiocardial reflexes*
- **Reciprocal neural connections between viscera and somatic tissues*:** *cutivisceral, viscerocutaneous, viscerosomatomotor, deep somatovisceral reflexes*

Data based on indirect measurements of effector responses and some on neurophysiological experiments.
Visceral organs: afferents from and spinal autonomic pathway(s) to the respective organ (organ system).
*Afferents from the respective tissue (deep somatic tissues, skin or viscera) and sympathetic outflow to the respective tissue.

literature, the clinical diagnosis of a visceral disease (e.g., of the gastrointestinal tract, the evacuative [pelvic] organs, the heart, the lung, etc.) can be predicted from changes in the skin and subcutaneous tissues with a probability of about 70% (Beal 1983, 1985, Cox et al. 1983, Nicholas et al. 1985).

The changes in the autonomic effector organs in somatic tissues or viscera (e.g., blood vessels, sweat glands, intestinal smooth musculature, etc.) can be explained relatively easily by changes in the activity of neurons of the sympathetic pathways. The mechanisms underlying the trophic changes following injury to viscera or deep somatic tissues are still unknown. These trophic changes occur in regions (skin, subcutaneous tissue, deep somatic tissues) which are outside the site of this injury or trauma and can only be mediated by peripheral

(sympathetic and/or afferent) neurons. The first sign of theses trophic changes is probably the edema, and the severe signs develop relatively slowly and late. It is believed that these changes are also associated with the segmental sympathetic outflow to the visceral or deep somatic reference zones in the trunk. However, it may be questioned whether this can be the only explanation, as, for example, the sacral reference zones of pelvic organs do not have a segmentally organized sympathetic outflow from the sacral spinal cord. In theory, visceral or deep somatic trauma could induce the trophic changes in remote tissues via afferents with unmyelinated fibers. This idea is supported by experiments on rats showing that inflammatory injury to a hindlimb (paw, knee joint) or lesion of a hindlimb skin nerve leads to mechanical hyperalgesic behavior, edema, or a reduction in cutaneous plasma extravasation in corresponding territories of the contralateral hindlimb, i.e., remotely from the trauma site (for discussion and references see Jänig 1993, Jänig & Häbler 1995, Shenker et al. 2003). Experimental studies on humans have shown that intradermal injection of capsaicin into the volar skin of the forearm is followed by mechanical hyperalgesia and allodynia of the corresponding skin area of the contralateral forearm (Shenker et al. 2008). The local mechanisms underlying edema and trophic change and their dependence on the sympathetic and/or afferent innervation remain to be explored.

Lower brain stem

Homeostatic regulations of arterial blood pressure, respiration, and gastrointestinal function are represented in the lower brain stem. These regulations require a temporally precise coordination and adaptation to somatic body functions and are therefore closely integrated. This integration is reflected in the anatomy and physiology of the neural substrates of these homeostatic regulations in the lower brain stem. Included in this integration are the spinal autonomic circuits, the peripheral autonomic pathways, and the enteric nervous system (Jänig 2006):

- Neurons involved in the regulation of arterial blood pressure (regulation of heart and peripheral resistance blood vessels) and respiration are situated in rostrocaudally organized columns in the ventrolateral medulla oblongata (VLM) which extend from the facial nucleus to about 10 mm caudal to the obex. The VLM includes (a) the ventral respiratory groups of neurons; (b) the rostral ventrolateral medulla (RVLM) containing sympathetic premotor neurons and associated interneurons; and (c) various parts of the caudal ventrolateral medulla (CVLM) which contain excitatory and inhibitory interneurons and mediate several types of cardiovascular reflexes. The VLM is closely associated with parasympathetic preganglionic cardiomotor and bronchomotor neurons in the external formation of the nucleus ambiguus (Dampney 1994, Rekling & Feldman 1998).

- The RVLM is a sympathetic cardiovascular premotor nucleus mediating homeostatic reflexes to cardiovascular sympathetic preganglionic neurons. The sympathetic premotor neurons are topically arranged in the RVLM according to their function (muscle, visceral, renal vasoconstrictor, and cardiomotor). Spontaneous activity in the neurons of these cardiovascular pathways is also mediated by the RVLM. It originates in neuronal networks associated with the RVLM and possibly in the premotor neurons themselves (Guyenet 1990, 2006, Dampney 1994, Spyer 1994).

- Distinct arterial baroreceptor reflexes exist to sympathetic cardiovascular neurons and parasympathetic cardiomotor neurons. These baroreceptor reflex pathways consist of four synapses between the baroreceptor input to the nucleus tractus solitarii (NTS) and the preganglionic neurons in the spinal cord: excitatory interneurons in the NTS project to inhibitory interneurons in the CVLM; these project to the premotor neurons in the RVLM. The transmitter of the inhibitory interneuron is GABA; the transmitter at the other synapses is glutamate. The baroreceptor reflex pathway to the parasympathetic cardiomotor neurons in the external formation of the nucleus ambiguus is disynaptic, the transmitter at both synapses being glutamate (Guyenet 1990, 2006, Spyer 1994). All synapses of the baroreceptor reflexes are under modulatory influence from other nuclei in the lower and upper brain stem, hypothalamus, and telencephalon.

- Reflexes elicited in sympathetic cardiovascular preganglionic neurons by stimulation of arterial chemoreceptors are mediated via the NTS and the respiratory network, or independently of the respiratory network (Guyenet 2000).

- Reflexes in sympathetic cardiovascular neurons related to cardiac afferents, lung afferents, or afferents from the gastrointestinal tract are also mediated by the NTS and by sympathetic premotor neurons in the RVLM. However, their central pathways are unknown.

- Reflexes in sympathetic cardiovascular neurons generated by stimulation of somatic or spinal visceral afferent neurons may also be mediated by the RVLM. Again, their central pathways are unknown.

- The caudal raphe nuclei of the medulla oblongata (raphe magnus and pallidus) contain sympathetic premotor neurons to preganglionic cutaneous vasoconstrictor (CVC) neurons or to preganglionic lipomotor neurons (supplying brown adipose tissue in the rat). These premotor neurons are involved in thermoregulation and in regulation of energy balance (Morrison 2001, Rathner et al. 2001) and under powerful control of the hypothalamus. Other sympathetic premotor neurons functionally related to the heart or kidney may also be located in the caudal raphe nuclei.

- Sympathetic neurons exhibit respiratory rhythmicity in their activity. The respiratory pattern in cardiovascular autonomic neurons is probably mediated by the 'common cardiorespiratory network' in the VLM. This network represents a sensorimotor program that closely coordinates regulation of respiration and regulation of arterial blood pressure under all physiological conditions. The respiratory modulation in the other types of sympathetic neuron – e.g., being involved in thermoregulation, regulation of the gastrointestinal tract, or regulation of pelvic organs, etc. – is generated by other mechanisms, probably also in the medulla oblongata (Häbler et al. 1994, Jänig & Häbler 2003).

- Preganglionic parasympathetic neurons innervating the gastrointestinal tract (GIT) are viscerotopically arranged in the dorsal motor nucleus of the vagus (DMNX), which is the motor nucleus of the GIT. The DMNX, NTS and area postrema (a neurohemal organ that receives hormonal and humoral signals via the blood) constitute the dorsal vagus complex, which contains many vagovagal reflex pathways that are the basic building blocks in the neural regulation of the GIT by the upper brain stem, hypothalamus, and telencephalon (Jänig 2006, 2009c, Travagli et al. 2006).

- Preganglionic parasympathetic neurons to salivary and nasopharyngeal glands are situated in the salivary nuclei, and preganglionic parasympathetic neurons to the airways (smooth muscles, glands) in the external formation of the nucleus ambiguus. Also, these preganglionic neurons form basic – at least disynaptic – reflex circuits with afferent neurons projecting to the NTS (e.g., from taste receptors or afferents innervating the airways) that are under supramedullary control. However, these reflex pathways have been little explored (Canning & Mazzone 2005).

- Centers in the brain stem that are involved in neural regulation of pelvic organs (hindgut, sexual organs, urinary bladder) have been little investigated (or not at all) at the single neuron level (de Groat 2002, Fowler et al. 2008, Jänig 2006).

Upper brain stem and hypothalamus

The circuits in the medulla oblongata are under the control of the upper brain stem, hypothalamus, and telencephalon. They are neural building blocks of regulations represented in the supramedullary brain centers. Table 2.2 summarizes the data about functions of the hypothalamus (and upper brain stem) in which the autonomic systems are involved (Card et al. 2008). These complex integrative functions include somatomotor, neuroendocrine, and autonomic components. The important point to be made here is that these complex regulations require anatomically and functionally precisely organized peripheral autonomic pathways innervating various target organs (shaded column in Table 2.2); and precisely organized central autonomic circuits in the spinal cord and lower brain stem.

An important function in which hypothalamus and mesencephalon are involved, and which seems very much to depend on functioning sympathetic systems (in addition to the neuroendocrine systems), is the protection of body tissues during acute and chronic pain and stress; this includes the neuronal control of the immune system

Table 2.2 Integrative functions of the hypothalamus

Function	Behavior	Nuclei in hypothalamus	Afferent feedback: neural, hormonal, cytokines	Autonomic systems	Endocrine systems, hormones
Thermoregulation	Thermoregulatory behavior	Preopt. region, ant./posterior hypothalamus, OVLT (pyrogenic zone, fever)	Peripheral thermoreceptors, central thermosens. (preopt.), cytokines (fever)	SyNS (skin [CVC,SMI], [BAT [rodents]])	TRH/Thyr (anterior pituitary)
Reproduction, sexual behavior	Sexual behavior and sexual orientation	MPNl (male; human dimorphic) VMl (female), TU, PM	Afferents from sexual organs, afferents from other sensory systems	SyNS (thor.-lumb.), PaNS (sacral) (sexual organs)	GnRH, FSH/LH (anterior pituitary)
Volume-, osmoregulation (fluid omeostasis)	Drinking behavior, thirst	N. paraventr./supraopt., R. pre-opt. med., AVPV, OVLT, SFO	Osmorecept. in OVLT & liver, volume rec. ri. atrium (vagal) angiotensin II via SFO	NTS, SyNS (kidney)	Vasopressin (posterior pituitary)
Regul. of nutrition. Regul. of metabolism	Nutritive behavior, hunger/satiety	N. arcuatus, N. paraventr., N. ventromed. (regulation of insulin secretion)	Vagal afferents & hormones from GIT (CCK, ghrelin, GLP-1, insulin, glucagon), leptin from adipose tissue, nutritive signals	Enteric nervous system, PaNS (DMV), SyNS (BAT [rodents], WAT)	Insulin, glucagon, orexin, leptin
Temporal organization of body functions	Sleep–waking behavior, circadian/endogenous rhythm of body functions	N. suprachiasmaticus, SBPV	Afferents from retina (retinohypothalamic tract)	SyNS, PaNS, SyNS to gl. pinealis	Melatonin (gl. pinealis)
Body protection (acute, e.g. during pain and stress)	Defense behavior (fight, flight, quiescence)	AHN, VMH, PM; lateral and ventrolateral PAG	Nociceptive afferents (from body surface, deep somatic, viscera)	SyNS, PaNS, (cardio-vascular system [CMN, MVC, VVC, etc.])	CRH/ACTH (anterior pituitary gland), adrenaline (SA system)
Immune defense	Defense of toxic substances and situations (sickness behavior)	N. paraventr. hypothalami?	Cytokines	SyNS (to immune tissue)	CRH/ACTH (anterior pituitary gland), adrenaline (SA system)

The specific autonomic systems which are mainly involved in these functions are shown in the shaded column. Functions related to the protection of the body are shown in the horizontal shading. (Data after Jänig (2006).)

AH, anterior hypothalamus; AHN, anterior hypothalamic n.; AVPV, anteroventral periventricular n.; BAT, brown adipose tissue; CCK, cholecystokinin; CRH/ACTH, cortocotropin-RH/ adrenocorticotropic hormone; CVC, cutaneous vasoconstrictor neurons; CMN, cardiomotor neurons (symp., parasymp.); DMV, dorsal motor nucleus of the vagus; FSH/LH, follicle-stimulating hormone/luteinizing hormone; GIT, gastrointestinal tract; GLP-1, glucagon-like peptide 1; GnRH, gonadotropine RH; MPNl, lateral part of the medial preoptic nucleus; MVC, muscle vasoconstrictor neurons; N, nucleus; NTS, nucleus tractus solitarii; OVLT, organum vasculosum laminae terminalis (osmosensors); PAG, periaqueductal grey; PaNS, parasympathetic nervous system; PM, premammillary n.; R., regio; RH, releasing hormone; SA system, sympathoadrenal system (adrenal medulla); SBPV, subparaventricular zone; SFO, subfornical organ (angiotensin sensitivity); SM, sudomotor neurons; SyNS, sympathetic nervous system; thor.-lumb., thoraco-lumbar; TRH/Thyr, thyreotropin RH/thyroxin; TU, tuberal n.; VMH, ventromedial hypothalamus; VMvl, ventrolateral part of the ventromedial nucleus; VVC, visceral vasoconstrictor neurons; WAT, white adipose tissue.

(shaded horizontal column in Table 2.2). This will be further discussed in the section on Sympathetic nervous system and body protection (see below on this page).

Conclusions

Corresponding to the functionally distinct peripheral autonomic pathways, the central organization of autonomic systems shows that (Jänig 2006):

1. The spinal cord and brain stem contain many autonomic circuits characterized by their primary afferent inputs and their connections to the final autonomic pathways. Several distinct types of autonomic interneuron have to be postulated.

2. The brain stem and hypothalamus contain several types of autonomic premotor neurons that connect the supraspinal autonomic centers with the spinal autonomic circuits, and form synapses with the preganglionic neurons and/or the spinal autonomic interneurons. The same organizational principle applies to the control of parasympathetic reflex circuits in the brain stem.

3. The medulla oblongata and caudal pons contain complex circuits which are involved in homeostatic regulation of the cardiovascular system (blood pressure), respiratory system, and gastrointestinal tract, and in the integration of these three regulations. Some of the underlying circuits (e.g., those related to arterial baroreceptor and chemoreceptor afferents, and to respiration) have been worked out.

4. Hypothalamus and mesencephalon embody organized somatomotor systems, autonomic systems, neuroendocrine systems, and afferent systems to complex functions (stereotyped behaviors) that are important for the survival of the individual and the species. Integrated

in these functions are the homeostatic regulations organized in the lower brain stem and the simple autonomic reflex circuits in spinal cord and brain stem.

5. The cerebral hemispheres have multiple accesses to the autonomic regulations represented in the spinal cord, brain stem, and hypothalamus. In this way the homeostatic autonomic regulations are adapted to the behavior of the organism (see Fig. 2.2).

Sympathetic nervous system and body protection

A concept

The sympathetic nervous system is not only involved in the regulation of various target organs related to the cardiovascular system, cutaneous blood flow and sweating (control of body core temperature), gastrointestinal tract, pelvis organs, etc., but has functions that are conceptually best described in the context of regulating the protection of body tissues during ongoing challenges occurring within the body or from the environment. Responses of the organism during these challenges involve the autonomic, neuroendocrine, and somatomotor systems, including the corresponding afferent feedbacks from the body tissues. These systems serve to adapt organ functions to the changing behavior and the behavior to changing threatening environments. The coordinated responses shown by the organism are states of the organism that are represented in the brain (brain stem, hypothalamus, limbic system, and neocortex) and which prepare the organism to generate the appropriate responses against the threatening events. Autonomic responses, endocrine responses, somatomotor responses, and the interoceptive body sensations occur principally in parallel, and are therefore parallel readouts of these central representations (see Fig. 2.1). The central representations receive neuronal afferent, hormonal, and humoral signals that monitor continuously the mechanical, thermal, metabolic, and chemical states of the tissues. Control of inflammation and hyperalgesia by the CNS is an integral component in this scenario and requires sympathetic systems that function in a differentiated manner. During real or impending tissue damage this integrated protective system is activated by the brain, leading to illness responses that include pain, hyperalgesia, and other adverse sensations (Fig. 2.13).

The patterning of the neural afferent feedback in the small-diameter afferents from the body tissues may also particularly depend on the activity of the neurons of the autonomic pathway. In fact, in view of the functional differentiation of the autonomic pathways with respect to the target cells, and as reflected in the discharge pattern of the peripheral autonomic neurons (see Organization of peripheral autonomic pathways, pp. 17–23, and Signal transmission in peripheral autonomic pathways, pp. 23–26) it is hypothesized that autonomic outflows, target cells and afferent neurons

form feedback body loops that lead to spatially and temporally patterned activation of the central representations of the body tissues, and this autonomically dependent activation leads to the typical illness responses. If so, it would mean that also the (efferent) autonomic outflow determines the affective–emotional responses generated by the brain (Damasio 1999, 2003, Ellsworth 1994, James 1884, 1994, Lange 1922).

Regulation of pain and hyperalgesia is an integral component of the fast and the slow defense systems organized by the hypothalamomesencephalic system. During *fast defense*, two alternative strategies are taken by the organism:

1. Fight (confrontational defense) or flight (avoidance) is taken if the environmental threat is escapable. Both are characterized by mobilization of energy, activation of various sympathetic channels (including the sympathoadrenal system), activation of the hypothalamopituitary–adrenal

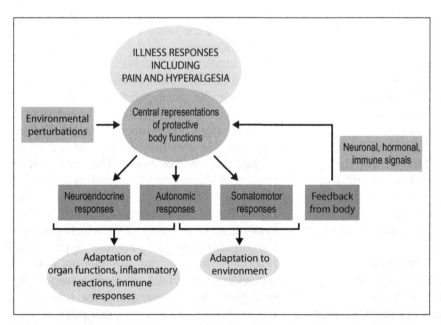

Figure 2.13 **Protective mechanisms of the body regulated by the brain: inputs, central representations, outputs.** Activation of the central circuits leads to neuroendocrine, autonomic, somatomotor, and illness responses (which include pain and hyperalgesia). The afferent feedback from the body tissues is neural and hormonal, and additionally mediated by cytokines from the immune system. The central circuits in the spinal cord, brain stem, and hypothalamus are adapted by the telencephalon to the environmental situations and to the situations in the body. (Modified after Jänig & Häbler 2000b.)

(HPA) axis and a fast non-opioid-mediated hypoalgesia (generated by active suppression of nociceptive impulse transmission from primary afferent nociceptive neurons to second-order neurons and by other supraspinal inhibitory processes). This fast defense is enhanced or can be triggered from the periphery of the body by stimulation of surface nociceptors. It is accompanied by increased vigilance, alertness, arterial blood pressure, and heart rate, and a vasodilation in skeletal muscle of the extremities (to fight or to run away).

2. A passive coping strategy is taken if the threat is inescapable. The organism is in a state of quiescence, rest, immobility, and decreased responsiveness to environmental stimuli. This state is characterized by low blood pressure, low heart rate, and an opioid-mediated hypoalgesia. It is enhanced by activation of deep (somatic or visceral) nociceptive afferents and during chronic activation of nociceptors.

During *slow defense* the organism is in a state of healing (recuperation). The physiological characteristics are similar to those of the passive coping strategy.

The neural representations of the integrative responses of the body during fast and slow defense are located in the periaqueductal gray (PAG) of the mesencephalon (Fig. 2.14) (Bandler & Shipley 1994, Keay & Bandler 2004, 2009):

- The neural mechanisms of confrontational defense and flight are represented in the dorsolateral and

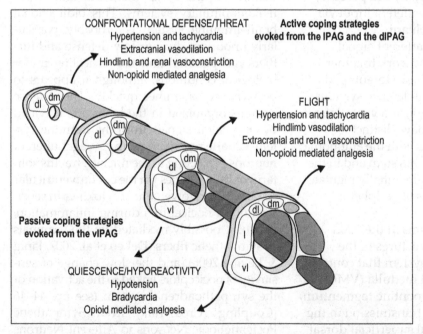

Figure 2.14 Representation of defense behaviors in the dorsolateral, lateral and ventrolateral periaqueductal gray. Schematic illustration of the dorsolateral (dl), lateral (l) and ventrolateral (vl) columns within the rostral, intermediate, and caudal periaqueductal gray (PAG). Stimulation of neuron populations in the dlPAG, lPAG, and vlPAG by microinjections of the excitatory amino acid glutamate, which excites only cell bodies of neurons but not axons, evokes distinct defense behaviors: confrontational defense is elicited from the rostral portion of the dlPAG and lPAG; flight is elicited from the caudal part of the dlPAG and lPAG; quiescence (cessation of spontaneous motor activity) is elicited from the vlPAG in the caudal portion of the PAG. These defense behaviors include typical autonomic cardiovascular reactions (changes in blood pressure, heart rate, blood flow) and sensory changes (non-opioid or opioid-mediated analgesia). The representations of confrontational defense and flight are the basis for active coping strategies produced by the cortex. The representation of quiescence is the basis for passive coping strategies produced by the cortex. dm, dorsomedial column. (Modified from Bandler and Shipley 1994 and Bandler et al. 2000a,b.)

lateral columns of the PAG. These behavioral patterns can be activated from the medial prefrontal cortex, either via direct projections to the PAG or via the dorsal or ventromedial hypothalamus, or reflexly from the body surface (skin) via the spinal or trigeminal superficial dorsal horn (mainly lamina I neurons) and the lateral column of the PAG.

- The neural mechanisms of passive coping strategies and slow defense are represented in the ventrolateral column of the PAG. These behavioral patterns can be generated from the orbital prefrontal cortex, either via direct projections to the ventrolateral PAG or via the lateral hypothalamus, and reflexly by afferent nociceptive inputs from the deep somatic or visceral body domains, and probably also by vagal visceral afferent input via the nucleus tractus solitarii.

- The cortical and the afferent signals from the body always work together in the activation of these stereotyped mesencephalic neural defense systems.

- The dorsolateral, lateral, and ventrolateral columns of the PAG have distinct reciprocal connections with the autonomic centers in the lower brain stem and in the hypothalamus that differentially regulate the activity in neurons of peripheral autonomic pathways.

- The neural mechanisms in the PAG are integral nodal structures of the endogenous neural system that controls, via the ventromedial medulla (VMM) and the dorsolateral pontine tegmentum, nociceptive impulse transmission in the spinal and trigeminal superficial dorsal horn, and possibly elsewhere. Thus, they are involved in mechanisms underlying centrally generated antinociception and pronociception, and therefore also in hypoalgesia and hyperalgesia (Fields et al. 2006, Heinricher & Ingram 2009). However, it must be emphasized that the PAG-VMM system is biologically primarily or mainly not involved in the control of nociception and pain. It has multiple and coordinated effector functions in the regulation of behavior which include sensory, somatomotor, and autonomic systems. The modulation of nociception and pain is only part of these functions and must be seen in a wider behavioral context (Mason 2001, 2005a,b).

- The neural circuits in the PAG represent active and passive coping strategies that are activated by the cortex during ('psychological' or 'physical') stress.

An important component of this protective system, promoting tissue repair and recuperation, is the bidirectionally functioning brain–immune system. The brain is continuously influenced by signals from the immune system (cytokines) and modulates its reactivity, mainly via the sympathoneural and hypothalamopituitary systems. This bidirectional brain–immune system is probably particularly important during slow defense and furthers recuperation and tissue healing under biological conditions, although it appears to be switched on rather quickly. The defense systems organized in the brain are activated by peripheral signals from the immune system via afferent neurons (e.g., vagal afferent neurons projecting to the nucleus tractus solitarii) or by cytokines via the circumventricular organs. The involvement of cytokines in sensitization of nociceptors during inflammation, part of it possibly mediated by the terminals of sympathetic fibers (DeLeo et al. 2007, Jänig & Levine 2006), and the slow change of sensitivity of nociceptors linked to the activation of the sympathoadrenal system (see pp. 44–46 [Coupling (Cross-Talk) from Sympathetic Postganglionic Neurons to Afferent Neurons in the Generation of Pain]), may also be components of the slow defense system (Maier & Watkins 1998, Watkins & Maier 2000).

It is unclear whether signaling from the brain to the immune system via the sympathetic nervous system occurs by a specific sympathetic channel which is anatomically and functionally different from sympathetic channels to other target cells (see pp. 17

Organization of peripheral autonomic pathways), or whether it is a general functional characteristic of the peripheral sympathetic nervous system (Besedovsky & del Rey 1995, Elenkov 2008, Hori et al. 1995, Madden & Felten 1995, Madden et al. 1995). Based on various experimental observations, I favor the more likely hypothesis that the brain modulates the immune system by way of a functionally and anatomically distinct sympathetic pathway. However, this has yet to be proven (Jänig & Häbler 2000a; Jänig 2006).

The contexts in which the sympathoneural and the sympathoadrenal systems may be involved in the generation of protective body reactions that includes nociception, pain, hyperalgesia, and inflammation are listed in Box 2.2 and graphically expressed in Fig. 2.15. This complex subject has been extensively discussed by Jänig (2009d) and Jänig and Levine (2006). I will distinguish four general aspects of this issue (for references see Jänig 2009d and Box 2.2).

Reactions of the Sympathetic Nervous System During Nociception and Pain

Acute and chronic tissue-damaging stimuli and stimuli that signal impending tissue damage affect the sympathetic nervous system involving generalized and specific reactions. The generalized reactions probably only occur in certain types of sympathetic system (e.g., muscle vasoconstrictor, visceral vasoconstrictor, sudomotor neurons, or sympathetic cardiomotor neurons) but are weak or absent in other systems (e.g., sympathetic systems to pelvic organs). They are organized in spinal cord, brain stem (medulla oblongata, mesencephalon), and hypothalamus, and can be conceptualized as component parts of the different patterns of defense behavior, such as 'confrontational defense', 'flight' or 'quiescence' that are organized in the periaqueductal gray (see below Coupling (cross-talk) from sympathetic postganglionic neurons to afferent neurons in the generation of pain, Fig. 2.14). These patterns of defense behavior

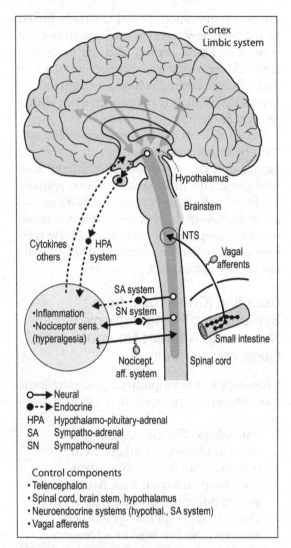

Figure 2.15 The spinal cord, brain stem, and hypothalamus contain neuronal circuits that control nociceptor sensitivity and inflammation in the periphery of the body via the sympathoadrenal (SA) and the hypothalamopituitary–adrenal (HPA) systems (shaded area). Feedback information from the peripheral inflammatory process occurs via nociceptive primary afferent neurons and cytokines. The central circuits linked to the SA system and the HPA system are modulated by activity in vagal afferents probably innervating the small intestine (and here the gut-associated lymphoid tissue). The telencephalon controls the inflammation and sensitivity of nociceptors via the circuits in the spinal cord, brain stem, and hypothalamus (see shaded double arrows). The sympathoneural (SN) system is also involved. (Modified from Jänig (2009d).)

are preprogrammed. They are closely linked to hypothalamic centers and are under the control of limbic centers and the prefrontal cortex. They are integral components of active and passive coping behaviors triggered by events threatening the organism from within or outside the body.

Spinal reflexes elicited in sympathetic systems by noxious stimuli of skin, deep somatic tissues, or viscera must also be considered to be protective. This includes the various spinally mediated reflexes in sympathetic systems that are at the base of the changes in referred zones in skin or deep somatic structures during noxious processes in the viscera or deep somatic tissues (see Spinal cord, pp. 28–35).

Coupling (Cross-Talk) from Sympathetic Postganglionic Neurons to Afferent Neurons in the Generation of Pain

Cross-talk from sympathetic postganglionic (noradrenergic) neurons may occur in several forms:

1. Physiologically, the postganglionic neurons of the sympathetic neural system are anatomically separate from the primary afferent neurons and do not communicate with them. Thus excitation of the sympathetic neurons does not lead to activation of afferent neurons (except perhaps under rather artificial experimental conditions). However, under pathophysiological conditions, such as trauma with or without nerve lesions, such communication may occur. Now activity in sympathetic postganglionic neurons may lead to activation or sensitization of afferent nociceptive fibers and lead to *sympathetically maintained pain*. This cross-talk between sympathetic postganglionic fibers and afferent neurons may be mediated by noradrenaline and α-adrenoceptors in the afferent neurons. It occurs in the peripheral tissues or even in the dorsal root ganglia (although I consider this latter type of coupling as unlikely to be an important peripheral mechanism underlying sympathetically maintained pain in patients [Jänig 2002, 2009d]). It may also occur indirectly via the vascular constriction generated by vasoconstrictor neurons and the ensuing changes in the affected tissue, or by other changes involving the sympathetic postganglionic fibers (possibly inflammatory processes).

2. Postganglionic axons and afferent nociceptive fibers may also be coupled independently of excitation of sympathetic neurons and noradrenaline release. This coupling has been shown to occur in animal experiments by using an intradermal injection of the inflammatory mediator bradykinin to elicit mechanical hyperalgesic behavior (Khasar et al. 1998a).

3. A further category of coupling in which the sympathetic–adrenal system may be involved is the effect of adrenaline on the sensitivity of nociceptors. Adrenaline released by the adrenal medulla may sensitize nociceptors for mechanical stimulation. This sensitization develops after exposing the nociceptive afferents to an increased concentration of adrenaline in the plasma over days (Khasar et al. 1998a,b, 2003).

Both methods of coupling between the sympathetic nervous system and the peripheral nociceptive afferent system mentioned above are new, and have so far only been shown to exist in animal experiments, using behavioral studies. Future experiments will show whether they are relevant in pathophysiological conditions.

Sympathetic nervous nystem and inflammation

The sympathetic nervous system may be involved in the expression and modulation of inflammatory processes beyond its role in controlling blood flow through these tissues

Box 2.2 Sympathetic nervous system and body protection: inflammation, pain and hyperalgesia (Modified from Jänig (2009d))

1. **Reactions of the sympathetic nervous system in nociception and pain**
   - Protective spinal reflexes
   - Fight, flight and quiescence organized at the level of the periaqueductal gray
   - Hyperalgesia and sympathetically mediated changes in referred zones during visceral pain

2. **Role of the sympathetic nervous system in the generation of pain**
   Sympathetic-afferent coupling in the periphery:
   - Coupling after nerve lesion (noradrenaline, α-adrenoceptors)
   - Coupling via the micromilieu of the nociceptor and the vascular bed
   - Sensitization of nociceptors mediated by sympathetic terminals independent of excitation and release of noradrenaline

   - Sensitization of nociceptors initiated by cytokines or nerve growth factor and mediated by sympathetic terminals
   - Sympathoadrenal system and nociceptor sensitization

3. **Sympathetic nervous system and central mechanisms**
   Control of inflammation and hyperalgesia by sympathetic and neuroendocrine mechanisms
   - Complex regional pain syndrome and sympathetic nervous system
   - Immune system and sympathetic nervous system
   - Rheumatic diseases and sympathetic nervous system
   - Persistent generalizing pain disorders (e.g., fibromyalgia, irritable bowel syndrome, other) and sympathetic nervous system

References:
For **1**: Bandler & Shipley (1994), Bandler et al. (2000), Jänig (1993, 2006)
For **2**: Green et al. (1997), Jänig (2002, 2005), Jänig & Häbler (2000b), Jänig & Levine (2006), Jänig et al. (2000), Khasar et al. (1998a,b), Miao et al. (1996a,b)
For **3**: Bradesi et al. (2009), Harden et al. (2001), Jänig & Baron (2002, 2003), Jänig & Häbler (2000a), Jänig & Levine (2006), Jänig & Stanton-Hicks (1996), Staud et al. (2009), Straub et al. (2005), Vierck (2006)

or other effector responses. This idea is closely linked to the question of whether the immune system is controlled by the brain via the sympathetic nervous system. Experiments in vivo on rats simulating acute inflammation generated by infusion of the inflammatory mediator bradykinin into the knee joint cavity and measuring synovial plasma extravasation rendered the following results, which highlight how important the sympathetic nervous system may be in this control:

1. Bradykinin-induced synovial venular plasma extravasation is largely dependent on the innervation of the synovia by postganglionic fibers, but surprisingly not on the activity in these fibers and not on release of noradrenaline. Thus the terminals of the postganglionic fibers seem to mediate this plasma extravasation (Green et al. 1997, Miao et al. 1996a,b).

2. Bradykinin-induced synovial plasma extravasation can be suppressed by activation of the hypothalamopituitary-adrenal (HPA) system and the release of corticosterone (Green et al. 1995). This fast inhibition of plasma extravasation via the HPA system, which can be elicited reflexly by noxious cutaneous stimuli, is dependent on the presence of the sympathetic innervation of the synovia and is absent in sympathetically denervated knee joints (Green et al. 1997), showing again that the sympathetic fibers mediate this effect by an as yet unknown mechanism.

3. Bradykinin-induced synovial plasma extravasation is also under the control of the sympathoadrenal system and its release of adrenaline. Noxious stimulation of skin or viscera activates the preganglionic neurons innervating the adrenal medulla, leading to release of adrenaline and depression of synovial plasma extravasation. The depression is not due to vasoconstriction in the synovia but is rather a β_2-adrenoceptor-mediated effect. This nociceptive–neuroendocrine reflex has a spinal and a spinobulbospinal component (Miao et al. 2000, 2001), is powerfully inhibited from the viscera via activity in vagal afferents (Miao et al. 1997a,b), and is probably under the control of supramedullary centers (Miao et al. 2003).

These animal experiments indicate that the sympathetic nervous system may have unprecedented functions in the context of protective (inflammatory) body reactions. These functions are regulated by the brain. Future experiments will have to show whether the conclusions made on the basis of these experimental data can be generalized.

Sympathetic nervous system, disease and central mechanisms

Based on observations made from patients and animal experimentation, it is likely that activity in sympathetic noradrenergic neurons and in the sympathoadrenal system, both generated in the brain, contributes directly or indirectly to modulation of nociceptors and inflammatory processes. This includes the reactions of the sympathetic nervous system during nociception and pain, various forms of sympathetic–afferent coupling (see Coupling (cross-talk) from sympathetic postganglionic neurons to afferent neurons in the generation of pain, p. 45, and Box 2.2) and the role of the sympathetic nervous system in the modulation of inflammation as well as the immune system. It

addresses the question in which way is the sympathetic nervous system involved in inflammation and hyperalgesia during rheumatoid diseases, during persistent generalizing pain disorders (such as fibromyalgia, chronic fatigue syndrome, irritable bowel syndrome, non-ulcer dyspepsia, chronic low back pain, complex regional pain syndromes, etc. [Bradesi et al. 2009, Clauw & Chrousos 1997, Henningsen et al. 2007, Jänig & Baron 2003, Staud 2009]) and in the modulation of the immune system during various diseases. These chronic diseases characterized by pain, hyperalgesia, and inflammation cannot be reduced to one of the involved peripheral processes (e.g., sensitization of nociceptors, sympathetic–afferent coupling, cellular processes of inflammation, etc.). I hypothesize that the key to the understanding of the mechanisms underlying these diseases is to be found in the brain and its reciprocal communication with the peripheral tissues of the body (see Figs 2.1, 2.13, and 2.15). The neural programs in the telencephalon representing the environment of the body as well as the different body domains are action systems that regulate at any moment the protective cellular machineries in the body. Changes (up- or down-regulation) or breakdown of this ongoing integrative action of the autonomic and endocrine systems orchestrated by the brain in response to changes in the environment of the body or within the body may lead to functional diseases. If this is the case we have to look into the brain to understand the mechanisms underlying these functional diseases (for detailed discussion see Jänig 2009a; Mayer & Bushnell 2009).

Conclusions

In healthy conditions tissue-damaging stimuli lead to concerted actions of the CNS involving the nociceptive system, the central endogenous control systems, and the somatic, autonomic, and endocrine motor systems. The sympathetic nervous system plays an important role in these concerted actions in the protection of the body tissues in health and disease. It is active during fast defense (fight and flight) and slow defense (recuperation, healing), both being organized in the hypothalamomesencephalic system. In pathophysiological conditions the sympathetic outflow to the affected peripheral part of the body may be actively involved in the generation of pain and inflammation by way of positive feedback loops.

1. Stimuli which normally are non-painful may now elicit painful reactions that are dependent on an intact sympathetic innervation. Several pathophysiological mechanisms may be involved in this process: (a) abnormal coupling of noradrenergic postganglionic fibers to primary afferent neurons; (b) alterations of the micromilieu of afferent receptors by changes of neurovascular transmission and by development of hyperreactivity of blood vessels; (c) alterations of the micromilieu of nociceptors by interference of noradrenergic fibers with non-neural inflammatory and immune-competent cells; (d) changes of the impulse pattern in neurons of the sympathetic outflow, possibly as a consequence of the central changes.

2. Novel mechanisms of involvement of sympathetic postganglionic neurons in the sensitization of nociceptors and in mechanical hyperalgesic behavior have only been studied in rats. Terminals of sympathetic neurons may mediate sensitization of nociceptors involving nerve growth factor, cytokines or bradykinin, independent of their excitability and release of noradrenaline. Adrenaline released by the adrenal medulla sensitizes nociceptors for mechanical stimulation, taking 1–2 weeks to develop.

3. Acute experimental inflammation (e.g., in the knee joint) is dependent on innervation by sympathetic postganglionic fibers, and this inflammation is controlled by the brain via the sympathoadrenal and hypothalamopituitary–adrenal systems. These observations are in line with the hypothesis that the sympathetic nervous system controls the immune system.

Synopsis

1. Behavior, defined as purposeful motor action of the organism in the environment, is generated by coordinated activation of the somatic, autonomic, and neuroendocrine motor systems. The internal milieu of the organism is actively prepared and adjusted by the brain via the autonomic and neuroendocrine systems.

2. The autonomic nervous system is involved in many regulations to adapt the organs and tissues to the internal and external demands on the body. The peripheral building blocks of these regulations are the autonomic pathways, consisting of populations of pre- and postganglionic neurons that are functionally defined according to the effector cells they supply (vascular smooth muscle cells, non-vascular smooth muscle cells, secretory epithelia, endocrine cells, etc.).

3. Each group of target cells is innervated (and regulated) by one (rarely two) autonomic peripheral pathways. Neurons of a functionally defined autonomic pathway exhibit a typical discharge pattern which is the result of integrative processes in distinct neural circuits of the spinal cord, brain stem, hypothalamus, and telencephalon.

4. Impulse activity in preganglionic neurons is transmitted in the autonomic ganglia to postganglionic neurons of the same functional type. There is no communication between functionally different autonomic pathways in the ganglia. Activity in postganglionic axons

is transmitted to most effector cells via anatomically and functionally defined neuroeffector junctions.

5. Spinal cord, brain stem, and hypothalamus contain functionally distinct neural circuits that are connected to the final autonomic pathways. Only a few of these central circuits have been explored and can be described in detail. The lowest level of central integration occurs in the spinal cord for spinal autonomic systems and in the brain stem for cranial parasympathetic systems. The basic reflex circuit is the spinal autonomic reflex or the equivalent reflex pathway in the brain stem between primary afferent neurons and preganglionic neurons. These basic autonomic reflex circuits are integrated in every regulation mediated by the autonomic pathways.

6. The lower brain stem (pons and medulla oblongata) contains the neural circuits involved in (a) homeostatic cardiovascular regulation and its integration with the regulation of respiration; (b) body core temperature; (c) pelvic organs; and (d) gastrointestinal tract (including regulation of food intake and metabolism).

7. Neural circuits in the spinal cord and lower brain stem, which represent the different types of homeostatic regulation, are integral components of complex regulations represented in the hypothalamus and mesencephalon. These complex regulations include neuroendocrine systems and somatomotor systems, and constitute elementary behaviors. They are related to regulation of body temperature, reproduction, fluid homeostasis, metabolism and nutrition, body protection, and circadian rhythm. The telencephalon (neocortex and limbic system) adapts these functions to the external state of the organism.

8. The sympathetic nervous system is involved in the regulation of protection of body tissues against external and internal threats. This function is closely related to the neural control of the immune system. During fast defense (confrontational defense [fight] or flight when threat is escapable; quiescence, immobility or decreased responsiveness when threat is inescapable) the body is prepared for protection, and during slow defense, characterized by a behavioral pattern during inescapable threat, the organism switches to recuperation. Both involve the sympathoneural systems and the sympathoadrenal system, and are related to the neural control of inflammation and sensitivity of nociceptors. The sympathetically mediated protective functions are controlled by neural circuits in the spinal cord, lower and upper brain stem (in particular the periaqueductal gray), and hypothalamus. These in turn are potentially under telencephalic control.

References

Araki, T., Hamamoto, T., Kurosawa, M., Sato, A., 1980. Response of adrenal efferent nerve activity to noxious stimulation of the skin. Neurosci. Lett. 17, 131–135.

Araki, T., Ito, K., Kurosawa, M., Sato, A., 1984. Responses of adrenal sympathetic nerve activity and catecholamine secretion to cutaneous stimulation in anesthetized rats. Neuroscience 12, 289–299.

Bahr, R., Bartel, B., Blumberg, H., Jänig, W., 1986. Functional characterization of preganglionic neurons projecting in the lumbar splanchnic nerves: neurons regulating motility. J. Auton. Nerv. Syst. 15, 109–130.

Bandler, R., Shipley, M.T., 1994. Columnar organization in the midbrain periaqueductal gray: modules for emotional expression? Trends Neurosci. 17, 379–389.

Bandler, R., Price, J.L., Keay, K.A., 2000a. Brain mediation of active and passive emotional coping. Prog. Brain Res. 122, 333–349.

Bandler, R., Keay, K.A., Floyd, N., Price, J., 2000b. Central circuits mediating patterned autonomic activity during active vs. passive emotional coping. Brain Res. Bull. 53, 95–104.

Baron, R., Jänig, W., McLachlan, E.M., 1985. The afferent and sympathetic components of the lumbar spinal outflow to the colon and pelvic organs in the cat. III. The colonic nerves, incorporating an analysis of all components of the lumbar prevertebral outflow. J. Comp. Neurol. 238, 158–168.

Baron, R., Jänig, W., With, H., 1995. Sympathetic and afferent neurones projecting into forelimb and trunk nerves and the anatomical organization of the thoracic sympathetic outflow of the rat. J. Auton. Nerv. Syst. 53, 205–214.

Bartel, B., Blumberg, H., Jänig, W., 1986. Discharge patterns of motility-regulating neurons projecting in the lumbar splanchnic nerves to visceral stimuli in spinal cats. J. Auton. Nerv. Syst. 15, 153–163.

Beal, M.C., 1983. Palpatory testing for somatic dysfunction in patients with cardiovascular disease. J. Am. Osteopath. Assoc. 82, 822–831.

Beal, M.C., 1985. Viscerosomatic reflexes: a review. J. Am. Osteopath. Assoc. 85, 786–801.

Besedovsky, H.O., del Rey, A., 1995. Immune–neuroendocrine interactions: facts and hypotheses. Endocr. Rev. 17, 64–102.

Boczek-Funcke, A., Dembowsky, K., Häbler, H.J., Jänig, W., McAllen, R., Michaelis, M., 1992. Classification of preganglionic neurones projecting into the cat cervical sympathetic trunk. J. Physiol. 453, 319–339.

Bradesi, S., Mayer, E.A., Schwetz, I., 2009. Irritable bowel syndrome. In: Basbaum, A.I., Bushnell, M.C. (Eds.), Science of Pain. Academic Press, San Diego, pp. 571–578.

Brown, A.G., 1981. Organization of the Spinal Cord. Springer-Verlag, Berlin.

Canning, B.J., Mazzone, S.B., 2005. Reflexes initiated by activation of the vagal afferent nerves innervating the airways and lung. In: Undem, B.J., Weinreich, D. (Eds.), Advances in Vagal Afferent Neurobiology. CRC, Taylor & Francis, Boca Raton, pp. 403–430.

Cannon, W.B., 1929. Organization for physiological homeostasis. Physiol. Rev. 9, 399–431.

Cannon, W.B., 1939. The Wisdom of the Body, second ed. Norton, New York.

Card, J.P., Swanson, L.W., Moore, R.Y., 2008. The hypothalamus: an overview of regulatory systems. In: Squire, L.R., Bloom, F.E., Spitzer, N.C., du Lac, S., Ghosh, A., Berg, D. (Eds.), Fundamental Neuroscience, third ed. Academic Press, San Diego, pp. 795–807.

Cervero, F., 1994. Sensory innervation of the viscera: peripheral basis of visceral pain. Physiol. Rev. 74, 95–138.

Clauw, D.J., Chrousos, G.P., 1997. Chronic pain and fatigue syndromes: overlapping clinical and neuroendocrine features and potential pathogenic mechanisms. Neuroimmunomodulation 4, 134–153.

Cox, J.M., Gorbis, S., Dick, L.M., Rogers, J.C., Rogers, F.J., 1983. Palpable musculoskeletal findings in coronary artery disease: results of a double-blind study. J. Am. Osteopath. Assoc. 82, 832–836.

Craig, A.D., 2002. How do you feel? Interoception: the sense of the physiological condition of the body. Nat. Rev. Neurosci. 3, 655–666.

Craig, A.D., 2003a. Interoception: the sense of the physiological condition of the body. Curr. Opin. Neurobiol. 13, 500–505.

Craig, A.D., 2003b. A new view of pain as a homeostatic emotion. Trends Neurosci. 26, 303–307.

Craig, A.D., 2003c. Pain mechanisms: labeled lines versus convergence in central processing. Annu. Rev. Neurosci. 26, 1–30.

Damasio, A., 1999. The feeling of what happens. Body and emotion in the making of consciousness. Harcourt Brace, New York.

Damasio, A., 2003. Looking for Spinoza. Joy, Sorrow, and the Feeling Brain. Harcourt, Inc, Orlando.

Dampney, R.A., 1994. Functional organization of central pathways regulating the cardiovascular system. Physiol. Rev. 74, 323–364.

De Groat, W.C., 2002. Neural control of the urinary bladder and sexual organs. In: Mathias, C.J., Bannister, R. (Eds.), Autonomic Failure. Oxford University Press, New York, pp. 151–165.

DeLeo, J.A., Sorkin, L.S., Watkins, L.R., 2007. Immune and Glial Regulation of Pain. IASP Press, Seattle.

Elenkov, I.J., 2008. Effects of catecholamines on the immune response. In: del Rey, A., Chrousos, G.P., Besedovsky, H.O. (Eds.), The Hypothalamo-Pituitary-Adrenal System, vol. 7. NeuroImmune Biology (ed. by Berci I & Szentivanyi A). Elsevier, Amsterdam, pp. 189–206.

Ellsworth, P.C., 1994. William James and emotion: is a century of fame worth a century of misunderstanding? Psychol. Rev. 101, 222–229.

Fields, H.L., Basbaum, A.I., Heinricher, M.M., 2006. Central nervous system mechanisms of pain modulation. In: McMahon, S.B., Koltzenburg, M. (Eds.), Wall and Melzack's Textbook of Pain, fifth ed. Elsevier, Edinburgh, pp. 125–142.

Fowler, C.J., Griffiths, D., De Groat, W.C., 2008. The neural control of micturition. Nat. Rev. Neurosci. 9, 453–466.

Furness, J.B., 2006. The Enteric Nervous System. Blackwell Science, Oxford.

Furness, J.B., Morris, J.L., Gibbins, I.L., Costa, M., 1989. Chemical coding of neurons and plurichemical transmission. Annu. Rev. Pharmacol. Toxicol. 29, 289–306.

Geis, G.S., Wurster, R.D., 1980. Cardiac responses during stimulation of the dorsal motor nucleus and nucleus ambiguus in the cat. Circ. Res. 46, 606–611.

Gibbins, I.L., 1995. Chemical neuroanatomy of sympathetic ganglia. In: McLachlan, E.M. (Ed.), Ganglia, Autonomic. Harwood Academic Publishers, Luxembourg, pp. 73–122.

Gibbins, I.L., 2004. Peripheral autonomic pathways. In: Paxinos, G., Mai, J.K. (Eds.), The Human Nervous System, second ed. Elsevier, Amsterdam, pp. 134–189.

Gibbins, I.L., Jobling, P., Morris, J.L., 2003. Functional organization of peripheral vasomotor pathways. Acta Physiol. Scand. 177, 237–245.

Green, P.G., Miao, F.J., Jänig, W., Levine, J.D., 1995. Negative feedback neuroendocrine control of the inflammatory response in rats. J. Neurosci. 15, 4678–4686.

Green, P.G., Jänig, W., Levine, J.D., 1997. Sympathetic terminal: target for negative feedback neuroendocrine control of inflammatory response in the rat. J. Neurosci. 17, 3234–3238.

Grewe, J., Jänig, W., Kümmel, H., 1995. Effects of hypothalamic thermal stimuli on sympathetic neurones innervating skin and skeletal muscle of the cat hindlimb. J. Physiol. 488, 139–152.

Grosse, M., Jänig, W., 1976. Vasoconstrictor and pilomotor fibres in skin nerves to the cat's tail. Pflügers Arch. 361, 221–229.

Guyenet, P.G., 1990. Role of the ventral medulla oblongata in blood pressure regulation. In: Loewy, A.D., Spyer, K.M. (Eds.), Central Regulation of Autonomic Functions. Oxford University Press, New York, pp. 145–167.

Guyenet, P.G., 2000. Neural structures that mediate sympathoexcitation during hypoxia. Respir. Physiol. 121, 147–162.

Guyenet, P.G., 2006. The sympathetic control of blood pressure. Nat. Rev. Neurosci. 7, 335–346.

Häbler, H.J., Hilbers, K., Jänig, W., Koltzenburg, M., Kümmel, H., Lobenberg-Khosravi, M., 1992. Viscero-sympathetic reflexes responses to mechanical stimulation of pelvic viscera in the cat. J. Auton. Nerv. Syst. 38, 147–158.

Häbler, H.J., Jänig, W., Michaelis, M., 1994. Respiratory modulation of activity in sympathetic neurones. Prog. Neurobiol. 43, 567–606.

Harden, R.N., Baron, R., Jänig, W., 2001. Complex Regional Pain Syndrome. IASP Press, Seattle.

Heinricher, M.M., Ingram, S.L., 2009. The brain stem and nociceptive modulation. In: Basbaum, A.I., Bushnell, M.C. (Eds.), Science of Pain. Academic Press, San Diego, pp. 593–626.

Henningsen, P., Zipfel, S., Herzog, W., 2007. Management of functional somatic syndromes. Lancet 369, 946–955.

Hirst, G.D.S., Bramich, N.J., Edwards, F.R., Klemm, M., 1992. Transmission at autonomic neuroeffector junctions. Trends Neurosci. 15, 40–46.

Hirst, G.D., Choate, J.K., Cousins, H.M., Edwards, F.R., Klemm, M.F., 1996. Transmission by post-ganglionic axons of the autonomic nervous system: the importance of the specialized neuroeffector junction. Neuroscience 73, 7–23.

Horeyseck, G., Jänig, W., 1974a. Reflexes in postganglionic fibres within skin and muscle nerves after mechanical non-noxious stimulation of skin. Exp. Brain Res. 20, 115–123.

Horeyseck, G., Jänig, W., 1974b. Reflex activity in postganglionic fibres within skin and muscle nerves elicited by somatic stimuli in chronic spinal cats. Exp. Brain Res. 21, 155–168.

Hori, T., Katafuchi, T., Take, S., Shimizu, N., Niijima, A., 1995. The autonomic nervous system as a communication channel between the brain and the immune system. Neuroimmunomodulation 2, 203–215.

James, W., 1884. What is an emotion? Mind 9, 188–205.

James, W., 1994. The physical bases of emotion. 1894. Psychol. Rev. 101, 205–210.

Jänig, W., 1975. Central organization of somatosympathetic reflexes in vasoconstrictor neurones. Brain Res. 87, 305–312.

Jänig, W., 1985. Organization of the lumbar sympathetic outflow to skeletal muscle and skin of the cat hindlimb and tail. Rev. Physiol. Biochem. Pharmacol. 102, 119–213.

Jänig, W., 1993. Spinal visceral afferents, sympathetic nervous system and referred pain. In: Vecchiet, L., Albe-Fessard, D., Lindblom, U., Giamberardino, M.A. (Eds.), New Trends in Referred Pain and Hyperalgesia, Pain Research and Clinical Management, vol. 7. Elsevier, Amsterdam, pp. 83–92.

Jänig, W., 1996. Spinal cord reflex organization of sympathetic systems. Prog. Brain Res. 107, 43–77.

Jänig, W., 2002. Pain in the sympathetic nervous system: pathophysiological mechanisms. In: Mathias, C.J., Bannister, R. (Eds.), Autonomic Failure, fourth ed. Oxford University Press, New York, pp. 99–108.

Jänig, W., 2005. Vagal afferents and visceral pain. In: Undem, B., Weinreich, D. (Eds.), Advances in Vagal Afferent Neurobiology. CRC Press, Boca Raton, pp. 465–493.

Jänig, W., 2006. The Integrative Action of the Autonomic Nervous System. Neurobiology of Homeostasis. Cambridge University Press, Cambridge.

Jänig, W., 2009a. Autonomic nervous system dysfunction. In: Mayer, A.E., Bushnell, M.C. (Eds.), Functional pain syndromes: Presentation and pathophysiology. IASP Press, Seattle, pp. 265–300.

Jänig, W., 2009b. Autonomic reflexes. In: Binder, M.D., Hirokawa, N., Windhorst, U. (Eds.), Encyclopedia of Neuroscience. Springer, Heidelberg, pp. 272–281.

Jänig, W., 2009c. Autonomic nervous system: Central control of the gastrointestinal tract. In: Squire, L.R. (Ed.), Encyclopedia of Neuroscience, vol 1. Academic Press, Oxford, pp. 871–881.

Jänig, W., 2009d. Autonomic nervous system and pain. In: Basbaum, A.I., Bushnell, M.C. (Eds.), Science of Pain. Academic Press, San Diego, pp. 193–225.

Jänig, W., Baron, R., 2002. Complex regional pain syndrome is a disease of the central nervous system. Clin. Auton. Res. 12, 150–164.

Jänig, W., Baron, R., 2003. Complex regional pain syndrome: mystery explained? Lancet Neurol. 2, 687–697.

Jänig, W., Häbler, H.J., 1995. Visceral-autonomic integration. In: Gebhart, G.F. (Ed.), Visceral Pain. IASP Press, Seattle, pp. 311–348.

Jänig, W., Häbler, H.J., 2000a. Specificity in the organization of the autonomic nervous system: a basis for precise neural regulation of homeostatic and protective body functions. Prog. Brain Res. 122, 351–367.

Jänig, W., Häbler, H.J., 2000b. Sympathetic nervous system: contribution to chronic pain. Prog. Brain Res. 129, 451–468.

Jänig, W., Häbler, H.J., 2003. Neurophysiological analysis of target-related sympathetic pathways – from animal to human: similarities and differences. Acta Physiol. Scand. 177, 255–274.

Jänig, W., Koltzenburg, M., 1993. Pain arising from the urogenital tract. In: Burnstock, G. (Ed.), The Autonomic Nervous System. Harwood, Chur, Switzerland, pp. 523–576.

Jänig, W., Kümmel, H., 1981. Organization of the sympathetic innervation supplying the hairless skin of the cat's paw. J. Auton. Nerv. Syst. 3, 215–230.

Jänig, W., Levine, J.D., 2006. Autonomic-neuroendocrine-immune responses in acute and chronic pain. In: McMahon, S.B., Koltzenburg, M. (Eds.), Wall & Melzack's Textbook of Pain, fifth ed. Elsevier, Edinburgh, pp. 205–218.

Jänig, W., McLachlan, E.M., 1987. Organization of lumbar spinal outflow to distal colon and pelvic organs. Physiol. Rev. 67, 1332–1404.

Jänig, W., McLachlan, E.M., 1992. Characteristics of function-specific pathways in the sympathetic nervous system. Trends Neurosci. 15, 475–481.

Jänig, W., McLachlan, E.M., 2002. Neurobiology of the autonomic nervous system. In: Mathias, C.J., Bannister, R. (Eds.), Autonomic failure. fourth ed. Oxford University Press, New York, pp. 3–15.

Jänig, W., Spilok, N., 1978. Functional organization of the sympathetic innervation supplying the hairless skin of the hindpaws in chronic spinal cats. Pflügers Arch. 377, 25–31.

Jänig, W., Stanton-Hicks, M. (Eds.), 1996. Reflex Sympathetic Dystrophy – a Reappraisal. IASP Press, Seattle.

Jänig, W., Khasar, S.G., Levine, J.D., Miao, F.J.P., 2000. The role of vagal visceral afferents in the control of nociception. Prog. Brain Res. 122, 273–287.

Jansen, A.S., Loewy, A.D., 1997. Neurons lying in the white matter of the upper cervical spinal cord project to the intermediolateral cell column. Neuroscience 77, 889–898.

Jansen, A.S., Wessendorf, M.W., Loewy, A.D., 1995. Transneuronal labeling of CNS neuropeptide and monoamine neurons after pseudorabies virus injections into the stellate ganglion. Brain Res. 683, 1–24.

Joyner, M.J., Halliwill, J.R., 2000. Sympathetic vasodilatation in human limbs. J. Physiol. 526, 471–480.

Keast, J.R., 1995. Pelvic ganglia. In: McLachlan, E.M. (Ed.), Autonomic Ganglia. Vol 6 of The Autonomic Nervous System (ed. by G. Burnstock). Harwood Academic, London, pp. 445–479.

Keay, K.A., Bandler, R., 2004. Periaqueductal gray. In: Paxinos, G. (Ed.), The rat nervous system, third ed. Academic Press, San Diego, pp. 243–257.

Keay, K., Bandler, R., 2009. Emotional and behavioral significance of the pain signal and the role of the midbrain periaqueductal gray (PAG). In: Basbaum, A.I., Bushnell, M.C. (Eds.), Science of Pain. Academic Press, San Diego, pp. 627–634.

Khasar, S.G., Miao, F.J.P., Jänig, W., Levine, J.D., 1998a. Modulation of bradykinin-induced mechanical hyperalgesia in the rat skin by activity in the abdominal vagal afferents. Eur. J. NeuroSci. 10, 435–444.

Khasar, S.G., Miao, F.J.P., Jänig, W., Levine, J.D., 1998b. Vagotomy-induced enhancement of mechanical hyperalgesia in the rat is sympathoadrenal-mediated. J. Neurosci. 18, 3043–3049.

Khasar, S.G., Green, P.G., Miao, F.J., Levine, J.D., 2003. Vagal modulation of nociception is mediated by adrenomedullary epinephrine in the rat. Eur. J. NeuroSci. 17, 909–915.

Kimura, A., Ohsawa, H., Sato, A., Sato, Y., 1995. Somatocardiovascular reflexes in anesthetized rats with the central nervous system intact or acutely spinalized at the cervical level. Neurosci. Res. 22, 297–305.

Kümmel, H., 1983. Activity in sympathetic neurons supplying skin and skeletal muscle in spinal cats. J. Auton. Nerv. Syst. 7, 319–327.

Lange, C.G., 1922. The emotions (W. James & I.A. Haupt, Trans.)[Über Gemüthsbewegungen. Ein psycho-physiologische Studie (H. Kurella, transl.) 1987]. Williams & Wilkins, Baltimore.

Langley, J.N., 1921. The Autonomic Nervous System. Part I. W. Heffer, Cambridge.

Madden, K.S., Felten, D.L., 1995. Experimental basis for neural–immune interactions. Physiol. Rev. 75, 77–106.

Madden, K.S., Sanders, K., Felten, D.L., 1995. Catecholamine influences and sympathetic modulation of immune responsiveness. Reviews of Pharmacology and Toxicology 35, 417–448.

Maier, S.F., Watkins, L.R., 1998. Cytokines for psychologists: implications of bidirectional immune-to-brain communication for understanding behavior, mood, and cognition. Psychol. Rev. 105, 83–107.

Mason, P., 2001. Contributions of the medullary raphe and ventromedial reticular region to pain modulation and other homeostatic functions. Annu. Rev. Neurosci. 24, 737–777.

Mason, P., 2005a. Ventromedial medulla: pain modulation and beyond. J. Comp. Neurol. 493, 2–8.

Mason, P., 2005b. Deconstructing endogenous pain modulations. J. Neurophysiol. 94, 1659–1663.

Mayer, E.M., Bushnell, M.C. (Eds.), 2009. Functional Pain Syndromes: Presentation and Pathophysiology. IASP Press, Seattle.

McLachlan, E.M. (Ed.), 1995. Autonomic Ganglia. Vol 6 of The Autonomic Nervous System (ed. by G. Burnstock). Harwood Academic, Luxembourg.

McLachlan, E.M., Davies, P.J., Häbler, H.J., Jamieson, J., 1997. On-going and reflex synaptic events in rat superior cervical ganglion cells. J. Physiol. 501, 165–181.

McLachlan, E.M., Häbler, H.J., Jamieson, J., Davies, P.J., 1998. Analysis of the periodicity of synaptic events in neurones in the superior cervical ganglion of anaesthetized rats. J. Physiol. 511, 461–478.

Miao, F.J.P., Green, P.G., Coderre, T.J., Jänig, W., Levine, J.D., 1996a. Sympathetic-dependence in bradykinin-induced synovial plasma extravasation is dose-related. Neurosci. Lett. 205, 165–168.

Miao, F.J.P., Jänig, W., Levine, J.D., 1996b. Role of sympathetic postganglionic neurons in synovial plasma extravasation induced by bradykinin. J. Neurophysiol. 75, 715–724.

Miao, F.J.P., Jänig, W., Levine, J.D., 1997a. Vagal branches involved in inhibition of bradykinin-induced synovial plasma extravasation by intrathecal nicotine and noxious stimulation in the rat. J. Physiol. 498, 473–481.

Miao, F.J.P., Jänig, W., Green, P.G., Levine, J.D., 1997b. Inhibition of bradykinin-induced plasma extravasation produced by noxious cutaneous and visceral stimuli and its modulation by vagal activity. J. Neurophysiol. 78, 1285–1292.

Miao, F.J.P., Jänig, W., Levine, J.D., 2000. Nociceptive-neuroendocrine negative feedback control of neurogenic inflammation activated by capsaicin in the skin: role of the adrenal medulla. J. Physiol. 527, 601–610.

Miao, F.J.P., Jänig, W., Jasmin, L., Levine, J.D., 2001. Spino-bulbo-spinal pathway mediating vagal modulation of nociceptive-neuroendocrine control of inflammation in the rat. J. Physiol. 532, 811–822.

Miao, F.J.P., Jänig, W., Jasmin, L., Levine, J.D., 2003. Blockade of nociceptive inhibition of plasma extravasation by opioid stimulation of the periaqueductal gray and its interaction with vagus-induced inhibition in the rat. Neuroscience 119, 875–885.

Morris, J.L., Gibbins, I.L., 1992. Co-transmission and neuromodulation. In: Burnstock, G., Hoyle, C.H.V. (Eds.), Autonomic Neuroeffector Mechanisms. Vol. 1 of The Autonomic Nervous System (ed. by G. Burnstock). Harwood, Chur, Switzerland, pp. 33–119.

Morrison, S.F., 1999. RVLM and raphe differentially regulate sympathetic outflows to splanchnic and brown adipose tissue. Am. J. Physiol. 276, R962–R973.

Morrison, S.F., 2001. Differential control of sympathetic outflow. Am. J. Physiol. 281, R683–R698.

Morrison, S.F., Cao, W.H., 2000. Different adrenal sympathetic preganglionic neurons regulate epinephrine and norepinephrine secretion. Am. J. Physiol. 279, R1763–R1775.

Nicholas, A.S., Debias, D.A., Ehrenfeuchter, W., England, K.M., England, R.W., Greene, C.H., Heilig, D., Kirschbaum, M., 1985. A somatic component to myocardial infarction. Br. Med. J. 291, 13–17.

Paxinos, G., Watson, C., 2007. The Rat Brain in Stereotaxic Coordinates, sixth ed. Elsevier, San Diego.

Rathner, J.A., Owens, N.C., McAllen, R.M., 2001. Cold-activated raphe-spinal neurons in rats. J. Physiol. 535, 841–854.

Rekling, J.C., Feldman, J.L., 1998. PreBotzinger complex and pacemaker neurons: hypothesized site and kernel for respiratory rhythm generation. Annu. Rev. Physiol. 60, 385–405.

Sato, A., Schmidt, R.F., 1971. Spinal and supraspinal components of the reflex discharges into lumbar and thoracic white rami. J. Physiol. 212, 839–850.

Sato, A., Schmidt, R.F., 1973. Somatosympathetic reflexes: afferent fibers, central pathways, discharge characteristics. Physiol. Rev. 53, 916–947.

Sato, A., Sato, Y., Suzuki, A., 1992. Mechanism of the reflex inhibition of micturition contractions of the urinary bladder elicited by acupuncture-like stimulation in anesthetized rats. Neurosci. Res. 15, 189–198.

Sato, A., Sato, Y., Suzuki, A., Uchida, S., 1993. Neural mechanisms of the reflex inhibition and excitation of gastric motility elicited by acupuncture-like stimulation in anesthetized rats. Neurosci. Res. 18, 53–62.

Sato, A., Sato, Y., Suzuki, A., Uchida, S., 1996. Reflex modulation of catecholamine secretion and adrenal sympathetic nerve activity by acupuncture-like stimulation in anesthetized rat. Jpn. J. Physiol. 46, 411–421.

Sato, A., Sato, Y., Schmidt, R.F., 1997. The impact of somatosensory input on autonomic functions. Rev. Physiol. Biochem. Pharmacol. 130, 1–328.

Shefchyk, S.J., 2001. Sacral spinal interneurones and the control of urinary bladder and urethral striated sphincter muscle function. J. Physiol. 533, 57–63.

Shenker, N., Haigh, R., Roberts, E., Mapp, P., Harris, N., Blake, D., 2003. A review of contralateral responses to a unilateral inflammatory lesion. Rheumatology (Oxford) 42, 1279–1286.

Shenker, N.G., Haigh, R.C., Mapp, P.I., Harris, N., Blake, D.R., 2008. Contralateral hyperalgesia and allodynia following intradermal capsaicin injection in man. Rheumatology (Oxford) 47, 1417–1421.

Sherrington, C.S., 1900. Cutaneous sensation. In: Schäfer, E.A. (Ed.), Textbook of Physiology, vol. 2. Young J. Pentland, Edinburgh, pp. 920–1001.

Spyer, K.M., 1994. Central nervous mechanisms contributing to cardiovascular control. J. Physiol. 474, 1–19.

Staud, R., 2009. Fibromyalgia. In: Basbaum, A.I., Bushnell, M.C. (Eds.), Science of Pain. Academic Press, San Diego, pp. 775–782.

Strack, A.M., Sawyer, W.B., Hughes, J.H., Platt, K.B., Loewy, A.D., 1989a. A general pattern of CNS innervation of the sympathetic outflow demonstrated by transneuronal pseudorabies viral infections. Brain Res. 491, 156–162.

Strack, A.M., Sawyer, W.B., Platt, K.B., Loewy, A.D., 1989b. CNS cell groups regulating the sympathetic outflow to adrenal gland as revealed by transneuronal cell body labeling with pseudorabies virus. Brain Res. 491, 274–296.

Straub, R.H., Baerwald, C.G., Wahle, M., Jänig, W., 2005. Autonomic dysfunction in rheumatic diseases. Rheum. Dis. Clin. North Am. 31, 61–75.

Sugiura, Y., Terui, N., Hosoa, Y., 1989. Differences in the distribution of central terminals between visceral and somatic unmyelinated primary afferent fibers. J. Neurophysiol. 62, 834–847.

Swanson, L.W., 2000. Cerebral hemisphere regulation of motivated behavior. Brain Res. 886, 113–164.

Swanson, L.W., 2008. Basic plan of the nervous system. In: Squire, L.R., Bloom, F.E., Spitzer, N.C., du Lac, S., Ghosh, A., Berg, D. (Eds.), Fundamental Neuroscience. third ed. Academic Press, San Diego, pp. 15–40.

Travagli, R.A., Hermann, G.E., Browning, K.N., Rogers, R.C., 2006. Brain stem circuits regulating gastric function. Annu. Rev. Physiol. 68, 279–305.

Undem, B., Weinreich, D. (Eds.), 2005. Advances in Vagal Afferent Neurobiology. CRC Press, Boca Raton.

Vierck Jr., C.J., 2006. Mechanisms underlying development of spatially distributed chronic pain (fibromyalgia). Pain 124, 242–263.

Wallin, B.G., 2002. Intraneural recordings of normal and abnormal sympathetic activity in humans. In: Mathias, C.J., Bannister, R. (Eds.), Autonomic Failure. fourth ed. Oxford University Press, Oxford, pp. 224–231.

Watkins, L.R., Maier, S.F., 2000. The pain of being sick: implications of immune-to-brain communication for understanding pain. Annu. Rev. Psychol. 51, 29–57.

Willis, W.D., Coggeshall, R.E., 2004. Sensory Mechanisms of the Spinal Cord. Primary Afferent Neurons and the Spinal Dorsal Horn, third ed., vol. 1. Kluwer Academic, New York, London.

Somatosympathetic reflex mechanisms

Joel G Pickar • Michael J Kenney • Charles N R Henderson • M Ram Gudavalli

Acknowledgements

This work was supported by NIH/NCCAM grants U19AT001701 and U19AT002006. Some work was conducted in a facility constructed with support from Research Facilities Improvement Grant Number C06 RR15433 from the National Center for Research Resources.

Introduction

Healthcare professions whose patient care includes manual therapy, such as chiropractic, osteopathy, and massage, are most commonly recognized for their beneficial effects on the musculoskeletal system. All use some form of manipulation or mobilization of joints, muscles, and other soft tissues. The osteopathic and chiropractic professions in particular have diagnostic algorithms for determining dysfunctional areas of the musculoskeletal system to manipulate or mobilize. These algorithms are remarkably similar. In osteopathic medicine, the acronym TART denotes four signs and symptoms that identify a somatic dysfunction (Kuchera & Kappler 2003): abnormal tissue Texture, positional Asymmetry of hard or soft tissue landmarks, Restricted motion between jointed segments, and tissue Tenderness. Criteria used by chiropractors have been adopted by the Health Care Financing Administration and are embodied in the acronym *PART* (Sportelli & Tarola 2005): *P*ain and tenderness, segmental or regional *A*symmetry or misalignment, abnormal *R*ange of motion, change in soft tissue *T*one. Changes in the biomechanical and chemical environment of the tissues are thought to underlie these signs and symptoms. The practitioner's goal in manipulating, mobilizing, or massaging these areas is to restore normal motion and normalize the physiology of the neuromusculoskeletal system.

Disturbances in somatic tissues may have consequences that extend beyond the neuromusculoskeletal system and involve visceral function. Many clinicians who practice manual therapy consider the signs and symptoms elicited by TART and PART procedures as representing a combination of altered sensory signaling from the local tissues and altered central neural processing of those signals (Korr 1978, Pickar 2002). All of the chapters in this book demonstrate in some way the biological roles played by the autonomic nervous system, including control of visceral function, homeostatic regulation, promotion of healing, and contributions to the feeling of well-being. Evidence from both clinical experience and experimental studies indicate that mechanical treatment of the musculoskeletal system can indeed provide benefits beyond the neuromusculoskeletal system (Haldeman 1978, Masarsky & Todres-Masarsky 2001).

To better understand the mechanisms that might underlie interactions between the clinical application of manual therapy and visceral function, this chapter addresses the effects that mechano- and chemosensory stimuli in somatic tissues have on the sympathetic part of the autonomic nervous system. Because many manual therapists, osteopaths, and chiropractors in particular focus their treatment on the spinal column, evidence concerning the relationship of somatosensory changes in paraspinal tissues to the sympathetic nervous system is emphasized.

A type of neural circuit that functionally links the biomechanical and chemical environment of musculoskeletal tissues with non-musculoskeletal tissue is the somatovisceral reflex. Our heuristic definition of this reflex is a neural circuit comprising three parts: 1) a sensory arm or pathway from musculoskeletal tissues (the somato- portion of the feedback circuit) consisting of primary afferent neurons whose receptive endings transduce mechanical, chemical, and thermal stimuli into neuronal activity, 2) which is integrated within the central nervous system, and 3) changes neuronal activity in the motor arm or pathway to a solid or hollow visceral organ (the visceral portion of the circuit). Motor pathways to the viscera are the sympathetic and parasympathetic portions of the autonomic nervous system. Somatovisceral reflexes are studied in two ways. Neural activity in sympathetic and parasympathetic neurons or modification of end-organ function can be studied in response to controlled changes in the mechanical or chemical environment of a somatic tissue. This chapter focuses on neural activity in sympathetic neurons. It begins with a broad discussion of somatosympathetic interactions from limb tissues, and then focuses on studies in the spinal column.

Stimulation of somatic afferents innervating limbs

Substantial evidence demonstrates that somatic afferents from non-paraspinal tissues can reflexly affect the sympathetic nervous system. Neural recordings from white rami of the sympathetic chain reveal three reflex components of efferent sympathetic discharge in response to electrical stimulation of a peripheral nerve in anesthetized cats and rats (Sato & Schmidt 1971). The A-reflex, so-called because it is elicited by stimulation of $A\beta$ and $A\delta$ primary somatic afferents, has two components: early and late. The early A-reflex has a short latency (25–50 ms) and arises from stimulation of low-threshold $A\beta$ fibers. The early component is integrated segmentally requiring only an intact spinal cord. The late A-reflex has a long latency (80–120 ms) and arises from stimulation of low-threshold $A\beta$ and high-threshold $A\delta$ fibers. The late component requires medullary integration in the brainstem (Sato et al. 1969). If an experimental preparation is lightly anesthetized, a very late A-reflex can be recorded which requires an intact nervous system rostral to the pons (Sato 1972).

The fibers mediating this very late component are unknown. The third reflex component, the C-reflex, was first described by Fedina et al. (1966), and Schmidt and Weller (1970) coined the name. The C-reflex has a long latency (250–500 ms) and arises from stimulation of the smallest-diameter unmyelinated primary afferents, the C fibers. By electrically stimulating a peripheral nerve, Schmidt and Weller (1970) identified the stimulation parameters necessary to consistently evoke the C-reflex.

The A- and C- somatosympathetic reflexes have been recorded in efferent sympathetic nerves in the cat and the rat. For example, electrical stimulation of a peripheral nerve evokes early and late A-reflexes in cardiac, renal, splanchnic, and adrenal sympathetic nerves (Araki et al. 1981, Coote & Downman 1966, Iwamura et al. 1969, Katunsky & Khayutin 1968, Kirchner et al. 1971, Miyamoto & Alanis 1970, Sato et al. 1969). In addition, electrical stimulation at strengths that recruit unmyelinated somatic afferents elicits the C-reflex in cardiac, renal, splanchnic, and adrenal sympathetic nerves (Araki et al. 1981, Fedina et al. 1966, Kimura et al. 1996, Nosaka et al. 1980, Sato et al. 1985). These reflex discharges were often evident only after cardiac- and respiratory-related bursts of sympathetic nerve activity were eliminated by baroreceptor denervation.

The elicitation of somatosympathetic reflexes by electrically stimulating a peripheral nerve convincingly demonstrates the presence of neural circuitry by which somatic afferent input can affect efferent sympathetic output. However, electrical stimulation of a peripheral nerve is probably non-physiological, in that somatic afferents are activated synchronously and with discharge patterns that are probably unnatural. A number of studies have used relatively natural stimuli to determine the influence of somatic inputs on the sympathetic nervous system. These studies confirm that somatic afferents can reflexly affect the sympathetic nervous system. Somatosympathetic reflexes elicited by relatively natural stimuli to peripheral muscles and joints are presented below. Although stimulation of the skin can also elicit somatosympathetic reflexes (see Sato et al. 1997 for a review), these reflexes are not described here.

Contraction of skeletal muscle activates the sympathetic nervous system via a reflex whose afferent arm consists of small-diameter thinly myelinated (Aδ or group III) and unmyelinated (C or group IV) fibers (Kaufman & Forster 1996). For example, group III afferents discharge rapidly and vigorously to maintained and intermittent tetanic contractions as well as to twitch contractions (Hayward et al. 1991, Kaufman et al. 1983, Mense & Stahnke 1983, Paintal 1960). These types of muscle contraction have been shown to reflexly increase renal, adrenal, cardiac, and hindlimb sympathetic nerve discharge (SND) in both anesthetized and decerebrate cats (Gelsema et al. 1985, Hill et al. 1996, Matsukawa et al. 1990, McMahon & McWilliam 1992, Victor et al. 1989, Vissing et al. 1994). In addition to muscle contraction, muscle stretch also increases renal SND (Wilson et al. 1994). These somatosympathetic reflexes elicited by small-diameter afferents in skeletal muscle increase blood pressure, heart rate, and ventilation, and are thought to contribute to cardiovascular and respiratory adjustments during exercise (Coote et al. 1971, McCloskey & Mitchell 1972).

Somatosensory input from synovial joints also contributes to sympathetic nerve regulation via a reflex whose afferent arm is comprised of three types of sensory fibers innervating the joint capsule: Aβ, Aδ, and C-fibers (Langford & Schmidt 1983). Sato et al. (1985) recorded from the inferior cardiac nerve while applying passive movements to the knee joint of the cat. Joint movements in the normal working range of the knee typically did not influence activity in the cardiac sympathetic nerve unless the joint was inflamed. In the uninflamed joint, cardiac sympathetic nerve activity increased when the knee was rotated beyond the physiological range. These results indicate that high-threshold Aδ and C fibers from the knee joint directly affect cardiac sympathetic nerve outflow. However, Sato et al. (1983) showed that A-reflexes could be elicited when electrical stimulation of the articular nerve to the knee was at a strength that primarily activated Aβ fibers. Thus low-threshold input from synovial joints may provide input to sympathetic preganglionic neurons and influence somatosympathetic reflexes by summation of their subthreshold inputs.

Stimulation of afferents innervating axial/paraspinal tissues

To specifically identify somatosympathetic reflexes initiated by receptive nerve endings in axial tissues of the vertebral column, we will label them vertebrosympathetic reflexes. Substantially fewer studies have investigated these reflexes, with only four found in the published literature that directly measured sympathetic nerve discharge (SND) in response to mechanical or chemical stimulation of axial tissues.

In 1984, Sato and Swenson (1984) were the first to investigate vertebrosympathetic reflexes. They studied the effect of vertebral movement (mechanosensory stimulation) on adrenal and lumbar SND. Figure 3.1 is a schematic of their preparation. In chloralose/urethane-anesthetized rats, thoracic and lumbar vertebrae were isolated by surgical exposure and by removing their attached muscles. Lateral bending moments were induced between T11 and T12 or L3 and L4. Forces ranged between 0.5 and 3.0 kg. With removal of the musculature, somatic input was probably derived from facet joint tissues, intervertebral discs and/or intervertebral ligaments. Nerves to the kidney and adrenal gland were exposed and whole nerve recordings obtained. SND was quantified by threshold crossings of the electrical

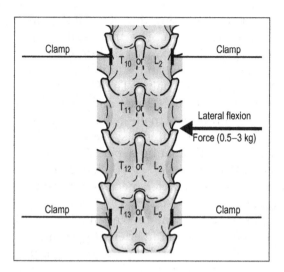

Figure 3.1 Schematic of the experimental approach used by Sato and Swenson (1984) to mechanically evoke vertebrosympathetic reflexes in the chloralose-anesthetized rat.

discharge. Crossings were counted as impulses and placed into 5-second bins.

Vertebral movement was short in duration, lasting approximately 30 s. Lateral bending of the thoracic and lumbar spinal column reduced mean renal SND (Fig. 3.2, left panel). In the adrenal nerve, bending initially reduced mean SND, which was followed by a longer-lasting increase (Fig. 3.2, right panel). All decreases were 25–40% of baseline and appeared to attenuate rapidly. Maximal responses were found with 2.0 kg loads (19.6 N). A depressor response accompanied the changes in SND; both arterial blood pressure and heart rate decreased. This raised the possibility that the baroreflex had mediated the changes in SND. This possibility was assessed by cutting the carotid sinus and vagus nerves. Neither the decreases in renal nor adrenal SND were affected, but the denervation abolished the late increase in adrenal SND, indicating that the latter was baroreflex mediated as a result of baroreceptor unloading during the decrease in blood pressure (Fig. 3.2, both panels). Sato and Swenson further demonstrated that the decreased adrenal and renal SND was mediated reflexly. Cutting

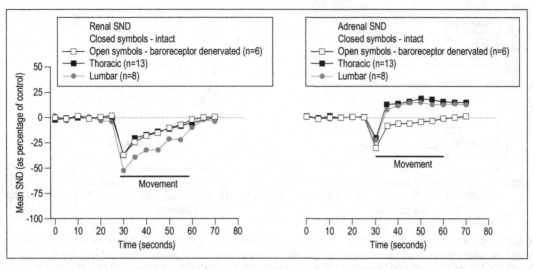

Figure 3.2 Changes in mean renal and adrenal sympathetic nerve discharge (SND) activity during lateral bending movement of thoracic or lumbar vertebra. Note that only thoracic movement was tested following baroreceptor denervation. SND was quantified by threshold crossings of the electrical activity. Crossings were counted as impulses and placed into 5-second bins, each bin being identified by a symbol. (Redrawn from data in Sato and Swenson (1984).)

the lower thoracic and upper lumbar dorsal roots abolished the decreases, whereas cutting the dorsal roots at lower lumbar levels had no effect. Whereas the overall vertebrosympathetic response was inhibitory, the segmental portion of the reflex appeared excitatory because cutting the spinal cord between the upper two cervical vertebrae transformed the decreased SND into a 40% increase. The descending inhibitory supraspinal input could have been tonic, or initiated by the lateral bending itself.

In this study, the 0.5–3 kg applied loads were considered innocuous. However, this may need to be reconsidered. Loads in this range are 1.7–10 times greater than a rat's body weight (assuming an average adult weight of 300 g), and it is not known whether the resulting strains approach the injury or failure limits of paraspinal tissues. In a previous study of the rabbit lumbar spine, axial loads five times body weight were considered noxious (Avramov et al. 1992).

Nearly 10 years after Sato and Swenson's study, Budgell et al. (1997b) continued investigating vertebrosympathetic reflexes in Sato's laboratory. In contrast to the previous

study of mechanosensory effects, they investigated chemosensory effects in the form of a noxious algesic chemical, namely capsaicin. Stimulation was applied to the interspinous tissues of the thoracic and lumbar vertebral column, and adrenal nerve activity was recorded. In urethane-anesthetized rats, 20 μL of physiological saline or capsaicin (10 mM) was injected in the midline, at the cephalad margin of the caudal spinous process from T8 to T13 and from L3 to S1. Threshold crossings of adrenal nerve activity were counted as impulses and placed into 5-second bins.

Saline injected into either the thoracic or the lumbar interspinous tissues had no effect, whereas capsaicin injection increased adrenal SND by ~80% (Fig. 3.3). Upper cervical spinal cord transection did not affect capsaicin-induced excitation in the thoracic spine and slightly reduced the excitation (to ~50%) in the lumbar spine. The responses were considered reflexive in origin, based on adrenal nerve responses to electrical stimulation of the L2 medial branch of the dorsal ramus. This nerve innervates midline tissues in the rat vertebral column (Budgell et al. 1997a). Different

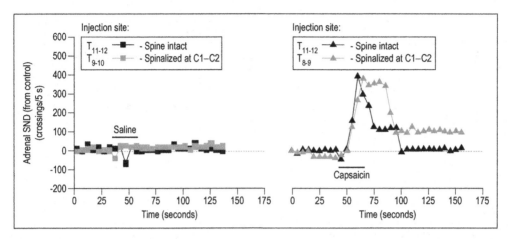

Figure 3.3 Changes in adrenal sympathetic nerve activity during noxious chemical stimulation of interspinous tissues in the thoracic vertebral column of a chloralose-anesthetized rat. Threshold crossings of adrenal nerve activity were counted as impulses and placed into 5-second bins, each bin being identified by a symbol. (Redrawn from data in Budgell et al. (1997b).)

somatic sensory fibers were recruited as stimulating parameters were increased. Adrenal nerve responses were considered reflexive because repetitive electrical stimulation of the L2 medial branch of the dorsal ramus evoked a C wave in the adrenal nerve (Fig. 3.4). The excitatory response persisted after spinalization similar to that after capsaicin; however, the C-fiber latency was shortened after spinalization, for reasons not discussed in the study. Thus, as in the mechanical studies of Sato and Swenson, noxious chemosensory stimulation produced an excitatory vertebrosympathetic reflex in the adrenal nerve. This response was thought to be mediated segmentally and, unlike the response to mechanical stimulation, may have little or no supraspinal component, but further work is necessary to confirm this owing to the change in latencies after spinalization.

Studies of vertebrosympathetic reflexes in the rat have been extended to the cat (Kang et al. 2003). This study had a threefold purpose. The first was to determine whether mechanosensory input from lumbar vertebral movement reflexly alters SND to the kidney or spleen. The second was to determine whether inflammatory input from lumbar paraspinal muscles reflexly

alters SND to these organs, and the third was to determine the interaction between these two types of stimuli. To move the L3 vertebra, forceps were rigidly attached to its spinous process. A feedback-controlled motor actuated the vertebra ventrally until it was loaded with 100% of the cat's body weight. Small volumes of the inflammatory agent and C-fiber stimulant mustard oil (Hu et al. 1992, Woolf & Wall 1986) were injected into the lumbar multifidus muscles at three segmental levels. Figure 3.5 shows the location of vertebral movement and sites of mustard oil injection. SND was rectified and integrated ($\tau = 10$ ms) and placed in 25-second bins. At the end of the experiment, postganglionic sympathetic activity in the renal and splenic nerves was confirmed using the ganglionic blocker hexamethonium (30 mg/kg, IV). This residual activity was subtracted from SND.

In chloralose-anesthetized cats vertebral movement did not affect either renal or splenic SND (Fig. 3.6A), in contrast to Sato and Swenson's findings in the rat (see above). However, mustard oil increased splenic SND by 60% and renal SND by 30% (Fig. 3.6B). This increase to a C-fiber stimulant is similar to Budgell et al.'s findings in the rat (see above). Together, these

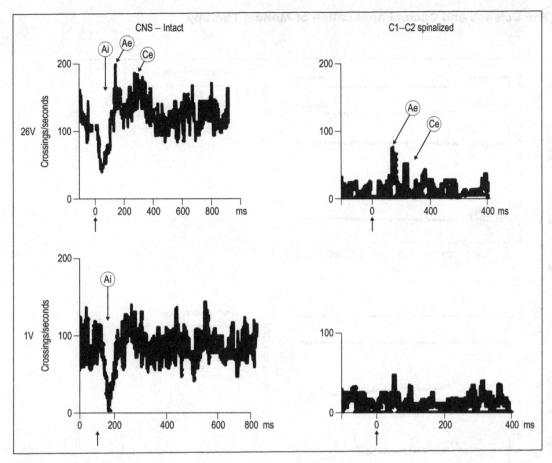

Figure 3.4 Neural activity in the adrenal nerve during graded electrical stimulation of the L2 medial branch of the dorsal ramus. This branch innervates medial tissues in the rat spine. Mild electrical stimulation (1 volt, lower panel), which presumably recruited the larger myelinated Aβ fibers, reflexly produced an inhibitory response in the adrenal nerve (A_i). The stronger electrical stimulation (26 V, upper panel), also recruited smaller myelinated Aδ and unmyelinated C-fibers, both of which induced reflex excitatory responses in the adrenal nerve (A_e and C_e, respectively). Spinal cord transection abolished only the A_i response. Tracings represent the summation of 60 stimulus trains, each train being given at 2-second intervals in a single rat. Each train lasted 20 ms and consisted of four 500 μs square wave pulses. (Redrawn from data in Budgell et al. (1997b).)

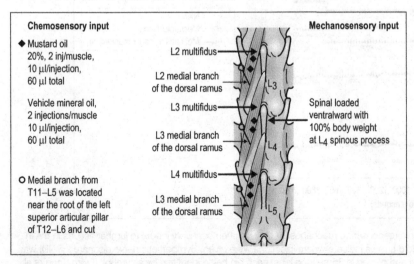

Figure 3.5 Schematic summarizing the locations of mustard oil injection and the site where mechanical load was applied. (From Kang et al. (2003), with permission of the American Physiological Society.)

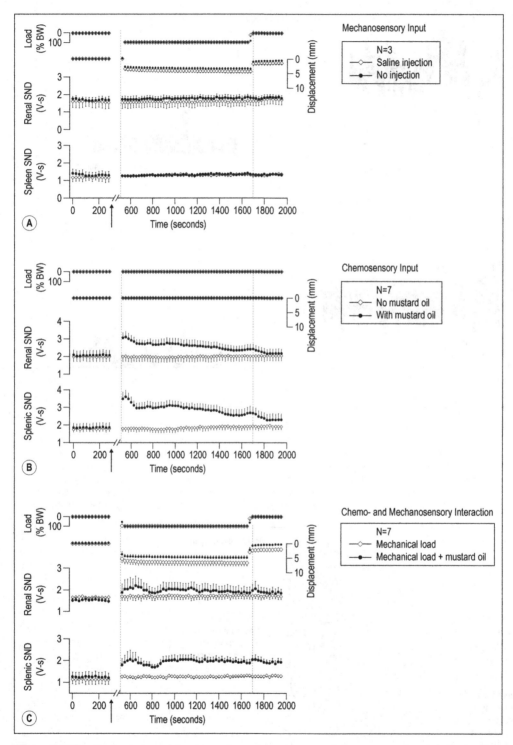

Figure 3.6 Renal and splenic nerve responses to mechanosensory and chemosensory inputs to lumbar tissues in the in the chloralose-anesthetized cat. Bold arrows indicate where injections were given. Sympathetic nerve discharge (SND) was rectified and integrated ($\tau = 10$ ms) and placed in 25-second bins, each bin being identified by a symbol. (From Kang et al. (2003), with permission of the American Physiological Society.)

combined forms of stimulation increased splenic SND by 55% and renal SND by 16% (Fig. 3.6C). The pattern of SND during the 20 minutes following mustard oil injection, combined with mechanical stimulation, was significantly different from that during the inflammatory stimulus alone: the inflammatory-induced increase in SND persisted throughout the 20-minute mechanical stimulation (Fig, 3.6C compared with 3.6B between the dashed lines). These sympathetic responses were mediated by a reflex whose afferent arm traveled in the medial branch of the dorsal ramus, because cutting this nerve totally abolished the increases (not shown). This nerve is known to innervate the medial-most lumbar paraspinal tissues (Bogduk 1976). The reflex required supraspinal integration from the upper cervical cord or higher, because spinal cord transection between the second and third cervical vertebrae abolished the increases in SND (not shown). Together, the data led the authors to conclude that, when accompanied by inflammation of paraspinal tissues, biomechanical changes in the lumbar spine help sustain reflex increases in renal and splenic sympathetic nerve activity caused by the inflammation.

The clinical relevance of these findings was considered from several perspectives, with the data providing some support for the idea that sensory feedback from paraspinal tissues reflexly affects adaptive and homeostatic mechanisms requiring autonomic regulation. Comorbidities often accompany spinal disorders (Fanuele et al. 2000) and could be influenced by vertebrosympathetic reflexes. Sympathetic outflow to the kidney affects numerous physiological responses. Increases in renal sympathetic discharge will reduce renal blood flow and increase salt and water retention by the renal tubules (DiBona 1994, Koepke & DiBona 1985). Sympathetic outflow to the spleen provides a link between the central nervous system and the immune system, in that increased splenic SND has

suppressive effects on cellular immune responses, including reduced natural killer cell cytotoxicity (Katafuchi et al. 1993). A vertebrosympathetic reflex initiated by injury-induced inflammation and sustained by biomechanical loading of lumbar tissues may provide a restraint upon the immune system's response to the internal injury.

Further examination of afferent impact on peripheral tissues

Recently, the authors sought to obtain preliminary data in rats that could confirm and extend the results described above. The goal was to apply a mechanical stimulus, characterized biomechanically, in order to grade the stimulus from innocuous to noxious. To accomplish this, force–displacement curves were obtained from a control group of anesthetized rats. Small clamps (Fig. 3.7A) were attached to the spinous process of two contiguous lumbar vertebrae (L5 and L6) so that they could be distracted in the horizontal plane (Fig. 3.7B and C) using a feedback-controlled motor. The caudal vertebra was held in a fixed position and the cranial vertebra was actuated cranially under displacement control. The motor's control unit allowed the resistive force to be measured. Force–displacement curves are shown in Fig. 3.7D. Mechanical loading was considered innocuous in the less stiff toe region (<4 mm) and considered noxious in the stiffer region towards failure (>6 mm).

In the experimental group of chloralose/urethane-anesthetized rats, controlled ramp-and-hold displacements of 2, 5, and 8 mm were applied (Fig. 3.8, lower tracings in each panel), and activities in the adrenal, splenic, lumbar, and renal nerves were recorded (Fig. 3.8, upper tracings in each panel). SND was confirmed at the end of the experiment using ganglionic blockade or nerve crush. Nerve activity was integrated and rectified and the level of activity quantified as volts times seconds. None of the mechanical loads produced large

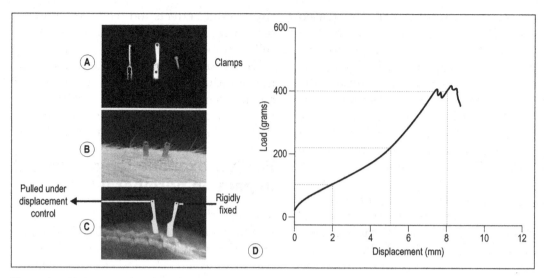

Figure 3.7 Method used for loading the spine. **A–C:** clamps used to load the spine. **D:** mean force–displacement curve for ventralward loading of 13 rat lumbar spines at the L3 vertebra.

changes in SND in any of the four nerves (Fig. 3.8). Changes appeared subtle and inconsistent. Mechanical loading of the lumbar spine tended to inhibit renal and lumbar SND, consistent with findings from Sato and Swenson prior to spinalization (see above). Specifically for the lumbar nerve, following the intermediate (5 mm) level of mechanical stimulation, SND was inhibited ~10% compared to controls. Compared to the time control (identical conditions but no displacement) lumbar and renal SND decreased ~10–15%. This decrease was not graded with the level of vertebral distraction. For the adrenal nerve, noxious mechanical stimulation (8 mm) increased SND during and after its application, a finding consistent with Sato and Swenson in the spinalized rat (see above). For the splenic nerve, noxious mechanical loading (8 mm) of the lumbar spine increased SND ~20% compared with controls. Overall, the small effect that innocuous mechanical loading of paraspinal tissues had on sympathetic nerve discharge in this rat model was similar to the lack of effect found in the model of Kang et al. (2003) to mechanical loading of a lumbar vertebra in the cat (see Fig. 3.6A).

All the studies previously described were performed in the thoracic and lumbar portions of the vertebral column. A recent study investigated vertebrosympathetic reflexes from the cervical spine. Bolton et al. (2006) determined whether mechanical changes in the neck affect SND to the adrenal gland (Fig. 3.9). Using chloralose-anesthetized rats, passive rotation of the C2 (axis) vertebra was controlled. The axis was rotated 2°, 6°, 12°, 20°, 25°, and 30° using slow ramp (12°/s) and hold (2 s) rotations. The head was fixed in position to abolish vestibulosympathetic reflexes. Rotations could both increase and reduce adrenal SND. The changes in SND were small during mild rotations and increased in magnitude during 7% of the trials as rotations began to produce observably coupled motions at C3 (at 12° and 20°). The changes became greatest at rotations that engaged the T1 vertebra (25–30°).

Summary

In the spinal column, soft tissue pain and tenderness, altered soft tissue tone, and regional asymmetry or intersegmental malalignment accompanied by an abnormal

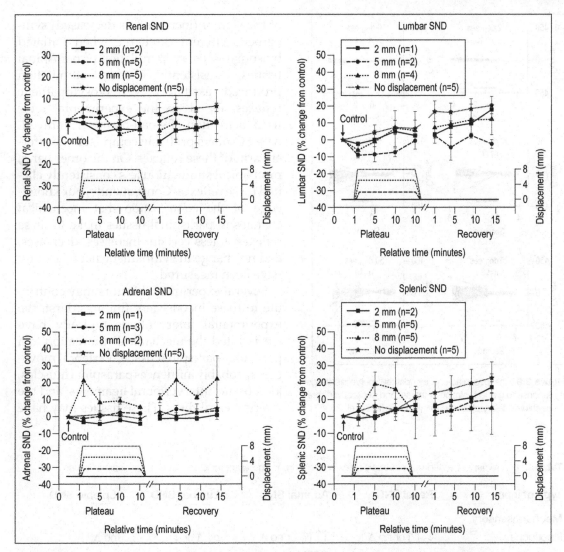

Figure 3.8 Changes in sympathetic nerve discharge (SND) during ramp and hold distraction of the L4 vertebra relative to the L5 vertebra in the chloralose-anesthetized rat. Nerve activity was integrated and rectified and the level of activity quantified as volts × seconds. Error bars are 1 standard error (SD). The first symbol in each panel (control) represents the mean value obtained over 5 minutes prior to the onset of the ramp. The ramp-and-hold load was not applied to the 'time control' group.

range of motion often accompany clinical presentations of neuromuscular and visceral complaints. These signs and symptoms are thought to represent a combination of altered signaling from the paraspinal tissues themselves, and altered central neural processing of those signals. This somatosensory input from paraspinal tissues may evoke reflex responses in the sympathetic portion of the autonomic nervous system and hence the viscera innervated by the sympathetic efferents. As a number of chapters in this book discuss, changes in sympathetic tone can have important consequences for physiological and biological function. Reduction or removal of reflex changes through the mechanical actions of spinal mobilization or manipulation provides a putative mechanism for explaining clinical experiences.

Table 3.1 summarizes the findings from the experimental animal studies described above and represents our current understanding

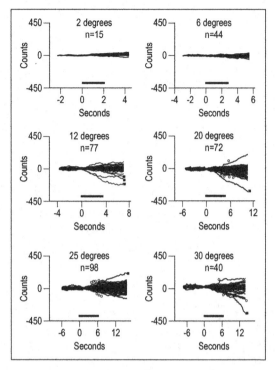

Figure 3.9 Changes in adrenal sympathetic nerve discharge in response to graded rotation of the second cervical vertebra in the chloralose-anesthetized rat. (From Bolton et al. 2006.)

of the sign of (increased vs decreased) sympathetic efferent discharge when initiated by somatosensory stimulation of paraspinal tissues. Consistently, chemical stimulation produced excitatory vertebrosympathetic reflexes. Based on the experimental tools used, activation of small-diameter unmyelinated C-fibers probably comprised the afferent arm of these reflexes. On the other hand, mechanical stimulation less consistently elicited these reflexes. Consequently, our knowledge of the contribution that mechanical changes in paraspinal tissues make to these reflexes is less certain. Increases, decreases, and no change in sympathetic nerve activity have been measured.

Several experimental factors may contribute to these inconsistent findings. First, the experimental interventions typically have not isolated the mechanical stimulation to a particular paraspinal tissue. Vertebral movement probably influences paraspinal muscles, joint tissue, intervertebral ligaments, and the intervertebral discs. These tissues may have

Table 3.1 Summary of vertebrosympathetic reflex changes from lumbar thoracic and cervical paraspinal tissues

Type of input	Renal SND	Adrenal SND	Lumbar SND	Splenic SND
Mechanosensory				
Innocuous	↓↓(?) or no Δ	↑↑ (?) or no Δ *CERVICAL* no Δ	no Δ or ↓	no Δ
Noxious	↓↓ or no Δ	↓↓†, ↑↑‡ *CERVICAL* 1) Mostly no Δ 2) ↑ and ↓	↓	↑
Chemosensory				
Capsaicin	–	↑↑, ↑↑‡	–	–
Mustard oil	↑↑	–	–	↑↑
Interaction	Prolongs the ↑↑			Prolongs the ↑↑
Mustard oil + mechano				

† Baroreceptor denervated, ‡ Spinal cord transected, ? Suggests a possibility. Single arrow = small change, double arrow = relatively greater change.
SND, sympathetic nerve discharge.

contrasting effects on vertebrosympathetic reflexes and may even cancel each other out. Resolving this issue is not without technical difficulties in isolating specific paraspinal tissues. Second, contributions from the baroreflex, as well as competing influences from segmental and suprasegmental reflexes, may affect the final sign of the reflex. Third, vertebrosympathetic reflexes may be segmentally organized such that the magnitude of reflex SND will be experimentally related to the relationship between the spinal cord level at which the paraspinal sensory input arrives and the spinal cord level giving rise to preganglionic, sympathetic motor neurons for a given viscera. Fourth, the animal studies described above investigated vertebrosympathetic responses over relatively short timescales. The longest mechanical stimulation lasted 30 minutes, during which sympathetic nerve discharge was evaluated. Clinical experience suggests that spinal column alterations associated with autonomic disturbances have been present longer than this. Although the natural history of these conditions has not been investigated, in human volunteers patterns of segmental paraspinal tissue abnormalities have been shown to persist over a period of months (Denslow 1944, Denslow et al. 1947, Denslow & Hassett 1942). Paraspinal muscles with firm palpatory texture that accompany postural abnormalities show patterns of electromyographic (EMG) activity different from those in muscles with normal texture (Denslow 1944). In addition, patterns of reflex erector spinae muscle activity evoked by pressure applied to paraspinal tissues correlate with sensory pain thresholds (Denslow 1944). The patterns were interpreted to mean that spinal cord neurons can remain in a facilitated state when sensory input from paraspinal structures persists (Denslow & Hassett 1942). Thus, experimental models that seek to understand conditions giving rise to vertebrosympathetic reflexes may need to consider somatosensory stimulation under chronic conditions where abnormal mechanosensory input is prolonged.

These considerations may help provide a basis for the design of future basic science experiments. In addition, future clinical studies should clearly identify the anatomical loci identified with the TART or PART analysis. These loci are presumably the source of aberrant somatic input adversely affecting visceral function. With this additional information, clinical findings may translate to the laboratory and aid in experimental designs to provide a better understanding of the mechanisms by which spinal dysfunction influences visceral function.

References

Araki, T., Ito, K., Kurosawa, M., Sato, A., 1981. The somato-adrenal medullary reflexes in rat. J. Auton. Nerv. Syst. 3, 161–170.

Avramov, A.I., Cavanaugh, J.M., Getchell, T.V., King, A.I., 1992. The effects of controlled mechanical loading on group II, III, and IV afferent units from the lumbar facet joint and surrounding tissue. J. Bone. Joint. Surg. 74-A (10), 1464–1471.

Bogduk, N., 1976. The lumbosacral dorsal rami of the cat. J. Anat. 122, 653–662.

Bolton, P., Budgell, B., Kimpton, A., 2006. Influence of innocuous cervical vertebral movement on the efferent innervation of the adrenal gland in the rat. Auton. Neurosci. 124, 103–111.

Budgell, B., Noda, K., Sato, A., 1997a. Innervation of posterior structures in the lumbar spine of the rat. J. Manipulative Physiol. Ther. 20, 359–368.

Budgell, B., Sato, A., Suzuki, A., Uchida, S., 1997b. Responses of adrenal function to stimulation of lumbar and thoracic interspinous tissues in the rat. Neurosci. Res. 28, 33–40.

Coote, J.H., Downman, C.B.B., 1966. Central pathways of some autonomic reflex discharges. J. Physiol. 183, 714–729.

Coote, J.H., Hilton, S.M., Perez-Gonzalez, J.F., 1971. The reflex nature of the pressor response to muscular exercise. J. Physiol. 215, 789–804.

Denslow, J.S., 1944. An analysis of the variability of spinal reflex thresholds. J. Neurophysiol. 7, 207–215.

Denslow, J.S., Hassett, C.C., 1942. The central excitatory state associated with postural abnormalities. J. Neurophysiol. 5, 393–401.

Denslow, J.S., Korr, I.M., Krems, A.D., 1947. Quantitative studies of chronic facilitation in human motoneuron pools. Am. J. Physiol. 150, 229–238.

DiBona, G.F., 1994. Neural control of renal function in health and disease. Clin. Auton. Res. 4, 69–74.

Fanuele, J.C., Birkmeyer, N.J.O., Abdu, W.A., Tosteson, T.D., Weinstein, J., 2000. The impact of spinal problems on the health status of patients: have we underestimated the effects. Spine 25, 1509–1514.

Fedina, L., Katunskii, A.Y., Khayutin, V.M., Mitsanyi, A., 1966. Responses of renal sympathetic nerves to stimulation of afferent A and C fibres of tibial and mesenteric nerves. Acta Physiol. Acad. Sci. Hung. 29, 157–175.

Gelsema, A.J., Bouman, L.N., Karemaker, J.M., 1985. Short-latency tachycardia evoked by stimulation of muscle and cutaneous afferents. Am. J. Physiol. 248, R426–R433.

Haldeman, S., 1978. The clinical basis for discussion of mechanisms of manipulative therapy. In: Korr, I.M. (Ed.), The Neurobiologic Mechanisms in Manipulative Therapy. Plenum, NY, pp. 53–75.

Hayward, L., Wesselmann, U., Rymer, W.Z., 1991. Effects of muscle fatigue on mechanically sensitive afferents of slow conduction velocity in the cat triceps surae. J. Neurophysiol. 65, 360–370.

Hill, J.M., Adreani, C.M., Kaufman, M.P., 1996. Muscle reflex stimulates sympathetic postganglionic efferents innervating triceps surae muscles of cats. Am. J. Physiol. 271, H38–H43.

Hu, J.W., Sessle, B.J., Raboisson, P., Dallel, R., Woda, A., 1992. Stimulation of craniofacial muscle afferents induces prolonged facilitatory effects in trigeminal nociceptive brain-stem neurones. Pain 48, 53–60.

Iwamura, Y., Uchino, Y., Ozawa, S., Kudo, N., 1969. Excitatory and inhibitory components of somato-sympathetic reflexes. Brain Res. 16, 351–358.

Kang, Y.M., Kenney, M.J., Spratt, K., Pickar, J.G., 2003. Somatosympathetic reflexes from the low back in the anesthetized cat. J. Neurophysiol. 90, 2548–2559.

Katafuchi, T., Take, S., Hori, T., 1993. Roles of sympathetic nervous system in the suppression of cytotoxicity of splenic natural killer cells in the rat. J. Physiol. 465, 343–357.

Katunsky, A.Y., Khayutin, V.M., 1968. The reflex latency and the level of mediation of spinal afferent impulses to the cardiovascular sympathetic neurones. Pflügers Arch. 298, 294–304.

Kaufman, M.P., Forster, H.V., 1996. Reflexes controlling circulation, ventilatory and airway responses to exercise. In: Handbook of Physiology. Exercise: Regulation and Integration of Multiple Systems. American Physiological Society, Bethesda, MD, pp. 381–447.

Kaufman, M.P., Longhurst, J.C., Rybicki, K.J., Wallach, J.H., Mitchell, J.H., 1983. Effects of static muscular contraction on impulse activity of groups III and IV afferents in cats. J. Appl. Physiol. 55 (1), 105–112.

Kimura, A., Sato, A., Sato, Y., Suzuki, H., 1996. A- and C-reflexes elicited in cardiac sympathetic nerves by single shock to a somatic afferent nerve includes spinal and supraspinal components in anesthetized rats. Neurosci. Res. 25, 91–96.

Kirchner, R., Sato, A., Weidinger, H., 1971. Bulbar inhibition of spinal and supraspinal sympathetic reflex discharges. Pflügers Arch. 326, 324–333.

Koepke, J.P., DiBona, G.F., 1985. Functions of the renal nerves. Physiologist 28, 47–52.

Korr, I.M., 1978. Sustained sympathicotonia as a factor in disease. In: Korr, I.M. (Ed.), The Neurobiologic Mechanisms in Manipulative Therapy. Plenum Press, New York, pp. 269–288.

Kuchera, W.A., Kappler, R.E., 2003. Musculoskeletal examination for somatic dysfunction. In: Ward, R.C. (Ed.), Foundations for Osteopathic Medicine. Lippincott Williams & Wilkins, pp. 633–659.

Langford, L.A., Schmidt, R.F., 1983. Afferent and efferent axons in the medial and posterior articular nerves of the cat. Anat. Rec. 206, 71–78.

Masarsky, C.S., Todres-Masarsky, C., 2001. Somatovisceral Aspects of Chiropractic: An Evidence-based Approach. Churchill Livingstone, New York.

Matsukawa, K., Wall, P.T., Wilson, L.B., Mitchell, J.H., 1990. Reflex responses of renal nerve activity during isometric muscle contraction in cats. Am. J. Physiol. 259, H1380–H1388.

McCloskey, D.I., Mitchell, J.H., 1972. Reflex cardiovascular and respiratory responses originating in exercising muscle. J. Physiol. 224, 173–186.

McMahon, S.E., McWilliam, P.N., 1992. Changes in R-R interval at the start of muscle contraction in the decerebrate cat. J. Physiol. 447, 549–562.

Mense, S., Stahnke, M., 1983. Responses in muscle afferent fibers of slow conduction velocity to contractions and ischaemia in the cat. J. Physiol. 342, 383–397.

Miyamoto, Y., Alanis, J., 1970. Reflex sympathetic responses produced by activation of vibrational receptors. Jpn. J. Physiol. 20, 725–740.

Nosaka, S., Sato, A., Shimada, F., 1980. Somatosplanchnic reflex discharges in rats. J. Auton. Nerv. Syst. 2, 94–104.

Paintal, A.S., 1960. Functional analysis of group III afferent fibers of mammalian muscles. J. Physiol. 152, 250–270.

Pickar, J.G., 2002. Neurophysiological effects of spinal manipulation. Spine J. 2, 357–371.

Sato, A., 1972. Somato-sympathetic reflex discharges evoked through supramedullary pathways. Pflügers Arch. 332, 117–126.

Sato, A., Kaufman, A., Koizumi, K., Brooks, C.M., 1969. Afferent nerve groups and sympathetic reflex pathways. Brain Res. 14, 575–587.

Sato, A., Schmidt, R.F., 1971. Spinal and supraspinal components of the reflex discharges into lumbar and thoracic white rami. J. Physiol. 212, 839–850.

Sato, A., Swenson, R.S., 1984. Sympathetic nervous system response to mechanical stress of the spinal column in rats. J. Manipulative Physiol. Ther. 7, 141–147.

Sato, Y., Schaible, H.G., Schmidt, R.F., 1983. Types of afferents from the knee joint evoking sympathethic reflexes in cat inferior cardiac nerves. Neurosci. Lett. 39, 71–75.

Sato, Y., Schaible, H.G., Schmidt, R.F., 1985. Reaction of cardiac postganglionic sympathetic neurons to movements of normal and inflamed knee joints. J. Auton. Nerv. Syst. 12, 1–13.

Sato, A., Sato, Y., Schmidt, R.F., 1997. The impact of somatosensory input on autonomic functions. In: Blaustein, M.P., Grunicke, H., Pette, D., Schultz, G., Schweiger (Eds.), Reviews of Physiology, Biochemistry and Pharmacology, vol. 130. M. Springer, Tokyo.

Schmidt, R.F., Weller, E., 1970. Reflex activity in the cervical and lumbar sympathetic trunk induced by unmyelinated somatic afferents. Brain Res. 24, 207–218.

Sportelli, L., Tarola, G., 2005. Documentation and record keeping. In: Haldeman, S., Dagenais, S., Budgell, B., Grunnet-Nilsson, N., Hooper, P.D., Meeker, W.C., Triano, J. (Eds.), Principles and Practice of Chiropractic. McGraw-Hill, NY, pp. 725–741.

Victor, R.G., Rotto, D.M., Pryor, S.L., Kaufman, M.P., 1989. Stimulation of renal sympathetic activity by static contraction: evidence for mechanoreceptor-induced reflexes from skeletal muscle. Circ. Res. 64, 592–599.

Vissing, J., Iwamoto, G.A., Fuchs, I.E., Galbo, H., Mitchell, J.H., 1994. Reflex control of glucoregulatory exercise responses by group III and IV muscle afferents. Am. J. Physiol. 266, R824–R830.

Wilson, L.B., Wall, P.T., Pawelczyk, J.A., Matsukawa, K., 1994. Cardiorespiratory and phrenic nerve responses to graded muscle stretch in anesthetized cats. Respir. Physiol. 98, 251–266.

Woolf, C.J., Wall, P.D., 1986. Relative effectiveness of C primary afferent fibers of different origins in evoking a prolonged facilitation of the flexor reflex in the rat. J. Neurosci. 6, 1433–1442.

Modulation of visceral function by somatic stimulation

Brian S Budgell

Introduction

This chapter will discuss somatovisceral reflexes, addressing whole organ and system responses to natural somatic stimuli, especially those with clinical relevance. We will examine the effects of noxious somatic stimuli, as many of our patients suffer from somatic pain, and the mechanical stimuli characteristic of physical treatments. Relevant observations will be drawn from the clinic and the laboratory.

At the most superficial level, we may ask how somatic stimuli produce effects on visceral function. In fact, various practices, such as osteopathy and chiropractic, have gravitated towards an attractive explanation for this phenomenon: reflex neurological mechanisms, especially those involving the autonomic nervous system. This collective, intuitive evolution in thinking is addressed by a number of authors elsewhere in this book. We may also ask how it is that, as observed by practitioners of various disciplines, stimulation at a particular somatic site reliably produces physiological responses at a specific distant visceral site. This topographical mapping of stimulation points onto target viscera is most systematized in acupuncture, but is also seen in chiropractic and osteopathy, wherein some practitioners have related chiropractic subluxation or somatic lesion at one level of the spine to symptoms in specific organs as discussed in Chapter 12.

Thus, this chapter will first define and examine somatovisceral reflexes, drawing primarily on work involving anesthetized animals. We will proceed to look in more detail at somatovisceral reflexes evoked by stimulation of musculoskeletal structures, and then consider a specific subclass of somatovisceral reflexes, the spinovisceral reflexes. For convenience, we have focused on cardiovascular effects. However, the underlying principles can be applied equally to other organ systems (Fig. 4.1; see also Chapter 1).

Somatovisceral reflexes

A somatovisceral reflex is a reflex elicited by stimulation of the somatic tissues, that is, the tissues of the musculoskeletal system

or skin, and manifesting as alterations in the functions of visceral organs. Somatovisceral reflexes are often mediated by way of the autonomic nervous system. However, other mechanisms exist, including non-autonomic neural mechanisms such as the axon reflex, and the various humoral responses to somatic stimulation, such as those triggered by nursing pathways. A spinovisceral reflex is a subclass of somatovisceral reflex initiated by stimulation of the somatic tissues associated with the spine: the vertebrae, associated connective tissues, and paraspinal muscles.

Quantitative descriptions of somato-autonomic and somatovisceral reflexes are numerous. A review published by Sato et al. in 1997 cited approximately 800 original data articles. Many studies in a variety of species have documented increases in heart rate and blood pressure following

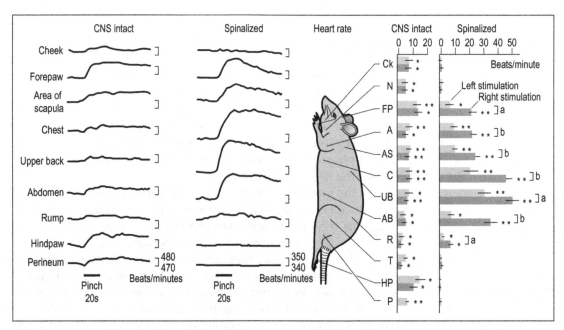

Figure 4.1 Responses of heart rate in urethane-anesthetized rats following pinching of various skin areas. Panels on the left show sample recordings from a single animal. Panels on the right show pooled results of all trials (n=6). In central nervous system-intact (CNS-intact) animals, pinching virtually anywhere produced some response and there was no clear segmental tendency. In spinalized animals only certain areas elicited a response, and there was a clear segmental organization and even a laterality: pinching on the right gave a greater response than pinching on the left side of the animal. Ck, cheek; N, neck; A, arm; AS, area of scapula; C, chest; UB, upper back; Ab, abdomen; R, rump; T, thigh; HP, hindpaw; P, perineum. (From Kimura A, Ohsawa H, Sato A, Sato Y 1995 Somatocardiovascular reflexes in anesthetized rats with the central nervous system intact or acutely spinalized at the cervical level. Neuroscience Research 22: 297–305.)

noxious somatosensory stimulation. Cutting the peripheral afferent nerves or the dorsal spinal roots serving the stimulated tissues invariably abolishes the reflex. Similarly, drugs that inhibit autonomic transmission attenuate or eliminate reflex responses. Thus, lesioning experiments and pharmacological blockade consistently indicate that these autonomic and visceral responses to somatic stimulation are mediated at the spinal and/or supraspinal level; that the afferent arm of the reflex involves somatic sensory nerves; and that the efferent arm consists predominantly of autonomic motor neurons. Reflex effects vary depending upon the nature and depth of anesthesia, and the physiological condition of the animal, for example body temperature and levels of blood gases. From the point of view of clinical relevance, it is important to note that innocuous somatic stimulation most often produces weak and inconsistent responses in anesthetized animals, whereas noxious stimulation generally produces substantial reflex responses.

An excellent paper which demonstrates many of the cardinal features of somatovisceral reflexes (Kimura et al. 1995) examined blood pressure and heart rate responses to noxious mechanical cutaneous stimulation (pinching) applied to different dermatomes in the anesthetized rat (Fig. 4.1). Noxious stimulation resulted in changes in sympathetic motor neuron activity which corresponded to the magnitudes of the effects on blood pressure and heart rate. More specifically, pinching induced increases in heart rate which were matched by increases in cardiac sympathetic nerve activity. Similarly, increases in blood pressure were accompanied by corresponding increases in renal sympathetic nerve activity. In central nervous system-intact (CNS-intact) animals the segmental organization of these reflexes was not well resolved. However, in spinalized animals – animals whose cervical spinal cords had been cut – it was immediately apparent that much more profound effects were achieved

when stimulation was applied at or immediately adjacent to the segmental levels of sympathetic outflow to the target end-organs. In fact, with heart rate there was even a clear laterality to the response, with stimulation to the right side of the animal producing significantly larger effects than stimulation to the left. Thus, with noxious cutaneous stimulation, at least in the spinalized animal, the somatotopic relationships between site of stimulation and end-organ response are well established and well accounted for by somato-autonomic reflex mechanisms.

Somatovisceral reflexes elicited by stimulation of musculoskeletal tissues

Of equal or greater relevance to the somatic therapies are studies involving stimulation – particularly innocuous mechanical stimulation – of musculoskeletal structures. Earlier studies examined responses to limb muscle stimulation where results are likely to be less precisely defined. Nonetheless, we have studies demonstrating cardiovascular responses to innocuous stimulation (stretch and compression) of limb muscles in anesthetized animals (Tallarida et al. 1981). Several studies have demonstrated the effects of massage and pressure-point therapy on autonomic tone and cardiovascular function in healthy volunteers and patients (Delaney et al. 2002, Mok & Woo 2004, Wang & Keck 2004). Similar effects have also been achieved with acupuncture (Lin et al. 2003, Nishijo et al. 1997), although results vary quantitatively and qualitatively according to the acupuncture point used and the parameters of stimulation.

Effects on heart rate and blood pressure are easily monitored and of considerable clinical interest. However, we also have demonstrations in animal models of innocuous somatosensory stimulation influencing muscle, nerve, skin, gastric and hepatic blood flow, as well as gastric, duodenal and jejunal motility, urinary bladder motility, adrenal and pancreatic secretion, and immune functions of various sorts (see Sato et al. 1997).

Thus we observe that under laboratory and clinical conditions somatic stimulation, including innocuous stimulation, induces changes in the activity of autonomic motor neurons and hence changes in the physiology of the dependent end-organs. Occasionally in CNS-intact animals, and often in spinalized animals, there is a clear somatotopic relationship between the site of stimulation and the end-organ that is principally affected. In spinalized animals, stimulation is likely to produce its most vigorous responses in end-organs whose autonomic innervation originates at or very close to the spinal segment receiving the sensory input. As increasing numbers of patients are surviving spinal cord injuries, parallel investigations may soon be practical in humans. The phenomenon of sympathetic dysreflexia seen in patients with high spinal cord injuries provides an unfortunate demonstration that spinally mediated somatosympathetic reflexes do indeed exist in humans. It remains to be seen whether a segmental organization to these reflexes can be demonstrated in patients with chronic spinal cord injuries (but see Burton et al. 2008).

Spinovisceral reflexes

Spinovisceral reflexes are a subclass of somatovisceral reflex wherein stimulation delivered to paraspinal or spinal tissues evokes changes in visceral function. A familiar example of a spinovisceral reflex would be paralytic ileus – the loss of bowel motility that accompanies significant injury to the lower spinal column. Spinovisceral reflexes have particular significance in the disciplines of osteopathy and chiropractic. Historically – albeit less so today – practitioners of these disciplines have maintained that a biomechanical lesion at a particular level of the spinal column is most likely to produce

symptoms in a specific visceral organ, especially an organ that receives autonomic innervation from the same level of the spine as the lesion (Burns et al. 1948).

The appeal of putative somato-autonomic reflex mechanisms is largely due to the clear segmental organization of the peripheral sympathetic nerves: something that is obvious even to those with no more than a textbook acquaintance with human anatomy. This anatomical feature is seen as providing a scientific rationale for the clinical observation of reliable topographical relationships between site of somatic dysfunction and visceral disorder (see Chapter 1, Fig. 4.1 and Chapter 12). The internal structure of the spinal cord, where the autonomic motor neurons originate, also has a clear segmental organization. The motor neurons of the spinal sympathetic nuclei are not distributed in continuous columns (Cabot 1990), but rather are arranged as linked nests in the thoracic and upper lumbar spinal cord (Fig. 4.2). Axons from each nest of sympathetic preganglionic neurons (SPNs) exit the spinal cord mainly through the nerve roots originating at their level and project to discrete peripheral targets (Oldfield & McLachlan 1981). Hence, in the rat, more than 95% of SPNs projecting to the middle cervical ganglion originate between the T1 and T5 spinal segments, whereas more than 95% of SPNs to the adrenal medulla originate between T5 and T11 (Strack et al. 1988). Studies in other species and using different labeling methods have shown even more restricted viscerotopic clustering of SPNs (Rubin & Purves 1980). Upper thoracic SPNs project to the heart, particularly the ventricles, via the middle cervical ganglion and stellate ganglion. In the cat, preganglionic neurons to the cervical sympathetic trunk originate almost exclusively in the upper five thoracic segments of the spinal cord (Oldfield & McLachlan 1981).

The cell bodies of postganglionic neurons within the stellate ganglion are also arranged in a somatotopic fashion so that, in

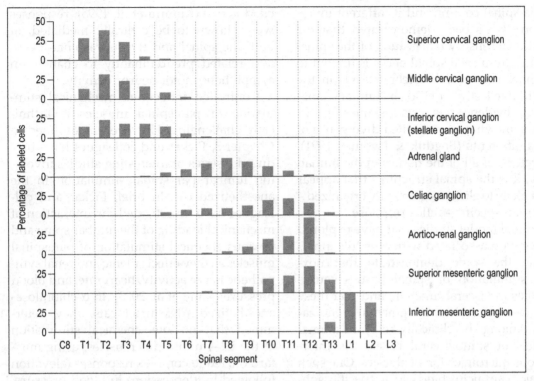

Figure 4.2 The segmental levels of origin of spinal (preganglionic) sympathetic neurons projecting to peripheral ganglia and the adrenal medulla. (From: Strack AM, Sawyer WB, Marubio LM, Loewy AD 1988 Spinal origin of sympathetic preganglionic neurons in the rat. Brain Research 455: 187–191.)

the cat, neurons projecting to the heart are clustered in the middle part of the ganglion (Masliukov et al. 2000). These cells are morphologically distinct from stellate ganglion cells projecting to other organs such as the sternocleidomastoid muscle. The size and number of stellate ganglion cells to the heart increases shortly after birth, but by 1 month the number of neurons to the heart begins to decrease as cells that have failed to make functional connections undergo apoptosis (Masliukov et al. 2000).

Therefore, from animal studies one could understand that stimuli entering the spinal cord at a given level are likely to elicit the strongest somato-autonomic reflex responses via local autonomic motor neurons which have a limited distribution to specific visceral organs. Additionally, peripheral events, such as compression or irritation of paravertebral sympathetic

ganglia, are most likely to produce effects limited to a few visceral organs.

In humans it is also apparent that spinal preganglionic neurons and paravertebral ganglia have specific projections, and changes in output of particular peripheral autonomic nerves are associated with specific changes in peripheral organ function (Armour 1972, Hageman 1973, Haws & Burgess 1978, Schwartz et al. 1976). Hence, the gross anatomy and fine structure of the autonomic nervous system, and physiological investigations, support the concept of a segmental and even lateral organization to somatovisceral reflexes, stimuli at particular sites preferentially affecting specific organs.

So far, we have concentrated on the efferent arm of the somato-autonomic reflex. However, the segmental anatomy of the sympathetic nervous system is mirrored to a degree by the obviously segmental anatomy of the spinal column and its afferent innervation. It has been demonstrated that the functional sensory innervation of the spinal column from each spinal nerve is limited to no more than three vertebral levels in the rat (Budgell et al. 1997a). In humans, anatomical evidence suggests a similar or perhaps somewhat more limited divergence of spinal afferents (Bogduk & Twomey 1991). Therefore, of all of the tissues in the human body, it is the spinal structures that appear most likely to elicit a segmentally organized – i.e. organ-specific – reflex response.

Animal model studies that have explored nociception associated with afferents innervating the spine demonstrate that noxious stimulation of spinal tissues causes changes in visceral function, and that these responses often show a segmental organization. Among the clinically relevant animal models of spinovisceral reflexes is interspinous microinjection of algesics. One such algesic, capsaicin, binds to a specific subclass of polymodal nociceptors (primarily TRPV1-receptor) and produces an intense noxious stimulation which may last for 20–30 minutes. In anesthetized rats, capsaicin has been injected into the interspinous tissues (also called the interspinous ligament) at specific spinal levels, and effects have been observed in sympathetic nerve activity and visceral function. This model has been used to demonstrate spinovisceral reflex effects on cardiac function and sciatic nerve blood flow (Budgell et al. 1995), adrenal nerve activity and catecholamine secretion (Budgell et al. 1997b), urinary bladder motility (Budgell et al. 1998), and gastric motility (Budgell & Suzuki 2000). Especially in spinalized animals, the reflex response is apparently facilitated when stimulation is applied to afferents entering the spinal cord at or close to the level of sympathetic efferent output to the target organ. Responses to vehicle injection alone were insignificant, confirming that the reflex responses were particularly elicited by the noxious stimulation of the algesic. As with Kimura's work, as

cited above (Kimura et al. 1995), responses were shown to be centrally mediated, at both the spinal and the supraspinal levels, and related predominantly to changes in sympathetic motor neuron activity.

Controlled innocuous mechanical stimulation of paraspinal muscles is technically challenging. However, as outlined in Chapter 3, Pickar and colleagues have produced a series of interesting studies involving lumbar paraspinal stimulation in the anesthetized cat. In brief, Pickar and colleagues have investigated the interaction of mechanical loading of the lumbar spine and noxious chemical stimulation of paraspinal muscles as they effect splenic and renal sympathetic nerve activity, heart rate, and blood pressure (Kang et al. 2003). In α-chloralose-anesthetized CNS-intact cats, they determined that noxious chemical stimulation of the L2–4 multifidus muscles, using mustard oil, led to complex responses (elevation followed by depression) in blood pressure, with concomitant and sustained increases in heart rate, and splenic and renal sympathetic nerve activity. These responses were mediated at the supraspinal level and were modified by loading the L3 spinous process with a force equivalent to 100% of the animal's body weight directed from posterior to anterior. The magnitudes of splenic and renal sympathetic nerve reflex responses were somewhat attenuated, but remained elevated longer in the presence of mechanical loading. However, mechanically loading the spine in the absence of noxious stimulation produced no significant changes in the parameters measured. These results suggest that, within this experimental system, relatively forceful but innocuous mechanical loading of the spine is ineffective in eliciting somato-autonomic reflexes. These results are consistent with the majority of laboratory observations to date, noting generally clear and reproducible reflex autonomic responses to noxious stimulation, but weak and inconsistent responses to innocuous mechanical stimulation.

Interactions of vestibular and somatic stimulation

Whereas Pickar's work deals primarily with the lumbar spine, Bolton developed an animal model to measure the effects of innocuous somatosensory input from cervical muscles (Bolton & Holland 1998). This system employs precise manipulations of the upper cervical vertebrae while the skull is immobilized, thereby permitting differentiation between the effects of vestibular and cervical input. Using this model in anesthetized cats, Bolton and colleagues have provided strong evidence that somatic input from the upper cervical region interacts with vestibular information to modulate the activity of the splanchnic sympathetic nerves (Fig. 4.3) (Bolton et al. 1998).

Note that in the upper panels of Fig. 4.3, when both the vestibular system and cervical afferents are intact, head movement (either a sinusoidal or a ramp-and-hold displacement) produces no apparent change in splanchnic or abdominal nerve activity, but some alteration in hypoglossal nerve activity. Furthermore, in cats, the splanchnic nerve helps to regulate blood pressure through constriction of mesenteric blood vessels, and the abdominal nerve is only an auxiliary respiratory nerve. It is logical that these functions would not change with a simple head tilt in a stationary animal. The hypoglossal nerve response to head movement probably represents a reflex designed to prevent the tongue from blocking the airway when the cat's nose is raised.

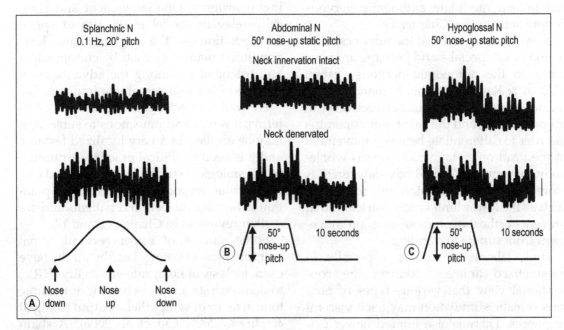

Figure 4.3 Responses in the anesthetized cat of sympathetic (splanchnic) and respiratory (abdominal and hypoglossal) nerves to head rotation before and after sectioning of the C1–C3 dorsal roots in order to eliminate sensory input from the upper cervical region. Note particularly that with neck innervation intact (upper panels) splanchnic nerve activity does not respond to head movement. However, in the absence of input from cervical afferents (lower panel) there is a substantial response in the splanchnic nerve. These data suggest that normally vestibular and cervical afferent input produce opposite and balanced effects on the splanchnic nerve when the head moves on a stationary body – essentially, vestibular and cervical input cancel each other's effects. Tracings beneath nerve recordings indicate sinusoidal and ramp-and-hold displacements of the head. (From Bolton PS, Kerman IA, Woodring SF, Yates BJ 1998 Influences of neck afferents on sympathetic and respiratory nerve activity. Brain Research Bulletin 47(5): 41.)

Note further that, as shown in the lower panels, when cervical afferents are transected, head movement (and so vestibular stimulation in the absence of cervical stimulation) produces quite pronounced responses in splanchnic, abdominal, and hypoglossal nerves. These responses suggest that innocuous somatosensory input from neck muscles normally cancels out reflex responses to vestibular stimulation when the head moves on a stationary body.

In the anesthetized rat, again using fixation of the head to eliminate vestibular input, movement of the C2 vertebra within the physiological range of motion has been shown to modulate (both increase and reduce) the activity of a small subpopulation of adrenal sympathetic nerves (Bolton et al. 2006). These observations in animal models demonstrate that, contrary to previous opinion, innocuous somatic stimulation can indeed modulate autonomic nervous system activity (see Chapter 1).

It has been argued that the upper cervical region has a special – and perhaps unique – input to the autonomic nervous system (Bolton & Ray 2000). This is mandated by the necessity for interaction between cervical proprioceptors and the vestibular apparatus in order to differentiate between movement of the head on a static body versus whole-body movement. Whole-body movement is more likely to require autonomic responses, such as the lower limb vasoconstriction that prevents orthostatic hypotension on movement from supine to standing.

Thus, laboratory studies, especially in anesthetized animals, confirm the conventional view that various types of noxious somatic stimulation may elicit visceral responses. There is also limited newer evidence of autonomic responses to innocuous mechanical stimulation of the spine. These responses are centrally mediated, at both spinal and supraspinal levels, virtually exclusively as a result of somatic afferent nerve stimulation, and manifest primarily through the autonomic efferents.

Importantly, in spinalized animals the segmental organization (and even the laterality) of reflex responses to noxious stimulation becomes fully manifested. Responses mediated at the spinal level tend to be excitatory in nature, even in response to stimuli which are apparently innocuous. Apparently in CNS-intact animals, supraspinal influences tend to dampen the excitatory spinal reflexes and mask their segmental organization. These results suggest mechanisms by which somatic insult might result in visceral symptomatology, and, conversely, mechanisms by which somatic therapies might ameliorate visceral complaints.

Spinovisceral studies in humans

Physiological studies in conscious humans are less prevalent, but still provide meaningful insights. One convenient and clinically relevant model is the use of spinal manipulation – the high-velocity low-amplitude maneuver used by chiropractors and osteopaths. Among the advantages of this model are that spinal manipulation has been well characterized in biomechanical terms; it is safe and innocuous to subjects; it may be applied in a very localized fashion; and it is used in clinical practice. A number of physiological studies have examined cardiovascular responses to spinal manipulation in healthy subjects and patients and are further reviewed in Chapters 5 and 12.

Some studies of upper cervical spinal manipulation in young, healthy adults have used analysis of heart rate variability (HRV) to demonstrate a shift in cardiac autonomic tone in favor of sympathetic output (Budgell & Hirano 2001, Cui et al. 2006). A sham manipulation produced no effects on autonomic output to the heart, suggesting that the effects achieved with spinal manipulation were due to input from cervical afferents rather than vestibular stimulation. Similar results were also obtained with prone upper thoracic spinal manipulation, again implicating input from spinal or paraspinal proprioceptors (Budgell & Polus 2006). These studies therefore provide strong evidence of spinovisceral reflexes, specifically spinocardiovascular reflexes, in healthy conscious humans.

Several case studies and a larger controlled trial have demonstrated clinically significant changes in cardiovascular function in response to spinal manipulation. One interesting case study (Budgell & Igarashi 2001) documented the virtually instantaneous resolution of a longstanding arrhythmia coincident with a single upper cervical manipulation (Fig. 4.4). Although case studies normally cannot provide strong evidence of cause and effect, the temporal relationship between treatment and resolution in this case essentially precludes alternative explanations. More recently, a randomized controlled clinical trial convincingly demonstrated relief of hypertension in response to upper cervical spinal manipulation (Bakris et al. 2007). Both systolic and diastolic blood pressure declined significantly over the 8-week trial in

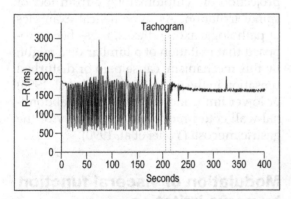

Figure 4.4 A tachogram (heart rate) recording from a patient undergoing a single upper cervical manipulation between the cursor markings at approximately 205–215 seconds. Note that prior to the manipulation the patient displayed a trigeminal rhythm, with the R–R (beat-to-beat) interval alternating between approximately 600 ms and almost 2000 ms. Following the manipulation, the R–R interval stabilized considerably at somewhat less than 2000 ms, and the patient displayed a fixed bradycardia. (From Budgell BS, Igarashi Y 2001 Response of arrhythmia to spinal manipulation: monitoring by ECG with analysis of heart-rate variability. Journal of the Neuromusculoskeletal System 9: 97–102.)

those patients receiving only manipulation directed to the upper cervical vertebrae. The control group showed no such benefits.

Thus, studies in humans confirm that apparently innocuous somatosensory stimulation is capable of inducing alterations in autonomic and visceral function, and that sometimes these changes can be quite dramatic. Segmental organization of such responses has not been demonstrated in cohorts of apparently well subjects. This is not surprising, as the animal studies discussed previously suggested that, when the spinal cord is intact, descending supraspinal influences tend to mask the segmental organization of spinal somato-autonomic reflexes. Investigations of somato-autonomic reflexes in subjects with frank spinal injuries are currently focused primarily on autonomic dysreflexia. Nonetheless, studies pursuing the phenomenon of segmental organization are practical (see Brown et al. 2007).

Vestibulosympathetic reflexes

Apart from somato-autonomic reflexes, a number of other mechanisms may be involved in spinovisceral reflexes. These include the vestibulosympathetic reflex, which is particularly relevant to studies of cervical mobilization and manipulation. The intention of the authentic cervical manipulation is to impart motion to a vertebra while the head is stabilized. Visual observation confirms only low-amplitude head movement during cervical manipulation. However, no scrupulous studies have been undertaken to calculate acceleration of the head, which could provide considerable vestibular stimulation despite the small amplitude of movement. In both humans and animals vestibular stimulation may elicit cardiovascular reflexes (for example, see Yates et al. 1991). In animal studies, it has been shown that many of the neurons in the ventrolateral medulla which respond to vestibular nerve stimulation also respond to stimulation of the carotid sinus nerve. In animals with a mid-cervical spinal transection, to eliminate input from visceral receptors, vertical and horizontal movements of the head were shown to affect rostral ventrolateral medullary cells, which received inputs principally from the otolith organ (Yates et al. 1993). Thus, brain stem centers involved in regulation of cardiovascular function are receiving vestibular information. Renal sympathetic nerve activity has also been shown to be modulated by stimulation of the utricular and saccular nerves in cats (Zakir et al. 2000). Additionally, low-amplitude accelerations of the head have been shown to produce short-latency responses in heart rate in humans, with the latency of the response prolonged in subjects with vestibular dysfunction (Radtke et al. 2000).

Therefore, we see that studies in both animals and humans implicate the vestibular apparatus in modulating regulation of cardiovascular function, and this makes sense from an adaptive point of view: regional blood flow must adapt to the demands of changing posture and acceleration of the body (Bolton et al. 1998). Besides modulating cardiac autonomic output, some forms of vestibular stimulation affect muscle sympathetic nerve activity (see, however, Bolton et al. 2004) and hence blood pressure (Cui et al. 1999). This mechanism is recruited when we move from lying down to the upright position: contraction of blood vessels in the leg muscles prevents pooling of blood in the lower limbs, and thereby prevents orthostatic hypotension.

The axon reflex

Apart from vestibulosympathetic reflexes, there is another neurological mechanism which may be involved in segmental responses to spinal stimulation: the axon reflex. The axon reflex produces the local vasodilation that appears after minor trauma to the skin. The explanation for this vascular phenomenon is that when superficial nociceptors are excited, the action potential is transmitted not only to the spinal cord but also to arborizations to local blood vessels (within proximity of the stimulated nociceptor). Vasoactive substances such as substance P and CGRP are released, causing vasodilation and the characteristic reddening of the skin that appears within a minute of the skin being scratched.

It is now apparent that much more widespread dichotomization occurs (Dawson et al. 1992, McCarthy et al. 1995, Pierau et al. 1984). That is to say, a single C-fiber may divide and send branches to different organs, both somatic and visceral, which are quite distant from one another. The implied interaction is self-evident in, for example, cardiovascular responses to pain. It has also been suggested that the axon reflex, projected through such divergent dichotomizations, might provide one mechanism of referred pain. Thus, ischemia in the heart might induce not just perceived pain in the arm, but real physiological changes. Conversely, pain in a musculoskeletal structure could by the same mechanism provoke symptomatology in the viscera. This would include projection of symptomatology from foci of spinal irritation. As hypothetical examples of pathologic axon reflexes, it has been proposed that irritation of a lumbar disc might, by this mechanism, cause pain or disturbed sensation in the groin (Takahashi et al. 1993) or lower limb, and that pain in the abdominal wall could modulate the activity of the gastric mucosa (Yonei et al. 1990).

Modulation of visceral function by nerve irritation

An early hypothesis which was quick to find wide acceptance among practitioners of spinal manipulation was that irritation of nerves at the intervertebral foramen or more peripherally would alter output to dependent organs and thereby compromise visceral function (see, for example Burchett 1968, Johnston 1981). Postmortem studies in animals and humans have been said to reveal correlations between compressed or distorted autonomic ganglia and pathological changes in dependent organs, and even symptomatology prior to death (Nathan 1968). Studies of this design cannot provide strong evidence of cause and effect, and so theories of nerve impingement causing visceral disease have largely been abandoned. Nonetheless, recent physiological evidence from the laboratory of Geoffrey Bove may breathe new life into these theories. Bove has demonstrated that inflammation of peripheral sympathetic nerves does indeed impede nerve activity (Bove 2008). It remains to be seen whether nerve impingement, for example by osteophytes or herniated disc material, could cause physiologically significant alterations in peripheral autonomic activity. However, such a chain of events would provide an alternative or supplementary explanation for the putative somatotopic relationships between biomechanical problems of the spine and visceral dysfunction.

Conclusions

This chapter began by identifying two important questions concerning the somatic

therapies: how somatic stimulation produces changes in visceral function, and why it is that particular sites of stimulation appear to be functionally linked to particular target organs. In answer to the first question, we have seen that somato-autonomic reflexes provide a likely mechanism for many somatovisceral interactions. However, other mechanisms are also probably in play, including vestibular reflexes, the axon reflex, and direct effects of physical and chemical stimuli on the behavior of autonomic motor neurons. The partitioning of preganglionic motor neurons into nests within the spinal cord, and the limited distributions of individual peripheral autonomic nerves, may help to explain the somatotopic relationships between stimuli and effects. However, the clear segmental organization of spinally mediated somato-autonomic (and therefore somatovisceral) reflexes is normally masked by descending supraspinal influences. That is to say (Fig. 4.5), when the spinal cord is intact, the net response to somatic stimulation is governed by the interaction of spinally mediated and supraspinally mediated somato-autonomic reflexes, perhaps with

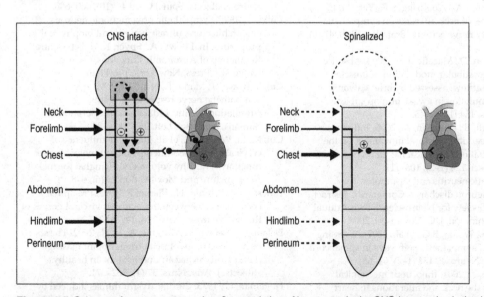

Figure 4.5 Schema of somato-autonomic reflex regulation of heart rate. In the CNS-intact animal stimulation from any segmental level may affect heart rate via reflex centers in both brain and spinal cord. In the spinalized animal, however, only thoracolumbar stimulation affects heart rate via spinal reflex centers. (From Kimura et al. 1995 Somatocardiovascular reflexes in anesthetized rats with the central nervous system intact or acutely spinalized at the cervical level. Neuroscience Research 22: 297–305.)

some minor contributions by other mechanisms (for example, see Hotta et al. 1996). When the cervical spinal cord is cut, or when some other mechanism blocks descending supraspinal influences, spinally mediated somato-autonomic reflexes are unmasked. Spinally mediated somato-autonomic reflexes are generally excitatory in nature, and often display a segmental organization.

References

Armour, J., 1972. Arrhythmias induced by local cardiac nerve stimulation. Am. J. Physiol. 223, 1068–1075.

Bakris, G., Dickholtz Sr., M., Meyer, P.M., et al., 2007. Atlas vertebra realignment and achievement of arterial pressure goal in hypertensive patients: a pilot study. J. Hum. Hypertens. 21 (5), 347–352.

Bogduk, N., Twomey, L.C., 1991. In: Bogduk, N., Twomey, L. (Eds.), Clinical anatomy of the lumbar spine, second ed. Churchill-Livingstone, Melbourne, pp. 113–114.

Bolton, P.S., Holland, C.T., 1998. An in vivo method for studying afferent fibre activity from cervical paravertebral tissue during vertebral motion in anaesthetised cats. J. Neurosci. Methods 85, 211–218.

Bolton, P.S., Ray, C.A., 2000. Neck afferent involvement in cardiovascular control during movement. Brain Res. Bull. 53 (1), 45–49.

Bolton, P.S., Kerman, I.A., Woodring, S.F., Yates, B.J., 1998. Influences of neck afferents on sympathetic and respiratory nerve activity. Brain Res. Bull. 47 (5), 413–419.

Bolton, P., Wardman, D., Macefield, V., 2004. Absence of short-term vestibular modulation of muscle sympathetic outflow, assessed by brief galvanic vestibular stimulation in awake human subjects. Exp. Brain Res. 154 (1), 39–43.

Bolton, P.S., Budgell, B., Kimpton, A., 2006. Influence of innocuous cervical vertebral movement on the efferent innervation of the adrenal gland of the rat. Auton. Neurosci. 124 (1–2), 103–111.

Bove, G., 2008. Sciatic neuritis and vasomotor sympathetic neuron discharge. Conference abstract presented at: Society for Neuroscience 38th Anuual Meeting, Washington, DC. Nov 15-19, 2008.

Brown, R., Engel, S., Wallin, B.G., et al., 2007. Assessing the integrity of sympathetic pathways in spinal cord injury. Auton. Neurosci. 134 (1–2), 61–68.

Budgell, B., Hirano, F., 2001. Innocuous mechanical stimulation of the neck and alterations in heart rate variability in healthy young adults. Auton. Neurosci. 91, 96–99.

Budgell, B., Igarashi, Y., 2001. Case study: response of arrhythmia to upper cervical adjustment; monitoring by ECG with analysis of heart-rate variability. Journal of the Neuromusculoskeletal System 9, 97–103.

Budgell, B., Polus, B., 2006. The effects of thoracic manipulation on heart rate variability: a controlled crossover trial. J. Manipulative Physiol. Ther. 29, 603–610.

Budgell, B., Suzuki, A., 2000. Inhibition of gastric motility by noxious chemical stimulation of interspinous tissues in the rat. J. Auton. Nerv. Syst. 80, 162–168.

Budgell, B., Hotta, H., Sato, A., 1995. Spinovisceral reflexes evoked by noxious and innocuous stimulation of the lumbar spine. Journal of the Neuromusculoskeletal System 3 (3), 122–131.

Budgell, B., Noda, K., Sato, A., 1997a. Innervation of posterior structures in the lumbar spine of the rat. J. Manipulative Physiol. Ther. 20 (6), 1–10.

Budgell, B., Sato, A., Suzuki, A., et al., 1997b. Responses of adrenal function to stimulation of lumbar and thoracic interspinous tissues in the rat. Neurosci. Res. 28, 33–40.

Budgell, B., Hotta, H., Sato, A., 1998. Reflex responses of bladder motility after stimulation of interspinous tissues in the anesthetized rat. J. Manipulative Physiol. Ther. 21, 593–599.

Burchett, G.D., 1968. Segmental spinal osteophytosis in visceral disease. J. Am. Osteopath. Assoc. 67 (6), 675–678.

Burns, L., Chandler, L., Rice, R., 1948. Pathogenesis of Visceral Disease Following Vertebral Lesions. American Osteopathic Association, Chicago.

Burton, A.R., Brown, R., Macefield, V.G., 2008. Selective activation of muscle and skin nociceptors does not trigger exaggerated sympathetic responses in spinal-injured subjects. Spinal Cord 46 (10), 660–665.

Cabot, J., 1990. Sympathetic preganglionic neurons: cytoarchitecture, ultrastructure, and biophysical properties. In: Loewy, A., Spyer, K. (Eds.), Central Regulation of Autonomic Functions. Oxford University Press, New York, pp. 44–67.

Cui, J., Iwase, S., Mano, T., et al., 1999. Muscle sympathetic nerve response to vestibular stimulation by sinusoidal linear acceleration in humans. Neurosci. Lett. 267, 181–184.

Cui, K., Li, W., Liu, X., et al., 2006. The influence of cervical spine massotherapy on autonomic nerve function in healthy volunteers. Shanghai Journal of Acupuncture and Moxibustion 25 (6), 6–8.

Dawson, N., Schmid, H., Pierau, F., 1992. Pre-spinal convergence between thoracic and visceral nerves of the rat. Neurosci. Lett. 138, 149–152.

Delaney, J., Leong, K., Watkins, A., et al., 2002. The short-term effects of myofascial trigger point massage therapy on cardiac autonomic tone in healthy subjects. J. Adv. Nurs. 37 (4), 362–371.

Hageman, G., 1973. Cardiac dysrhythmias induced by autonomic nerve stimulation. Am. J. Cardiol. 32, 823–830.

Haws, C., Burgess, M., 1978. Effects of bilateral and unilateral stellate stimulation on canine ventricular refractory periods at sites of overlapping innervation. Circ. Res. 42 (2), 195–198.

Hotta, H., Sato, A., Sato, Y., 1996. Stimulation of the saphenous afferent nerve produces vasodilatation of the vasa nervorum via axon reflex-like mechanism in the sciatic nerve of the anesthetized rat. Neurosci. Res. 24, 305–308.

Johnston, R.J., 1981. Vertebrogenic autonomic dysfunction – subjective symptoms: a prospective study. Journal of the Canadian Chiropractic Association 25 (2), 51–57.

Kang, Y.M., Kenney, M.J., Spratt, K.F., et al., 2003. Somatosympathetic reflexes from the low back in the anesthetized cat. J. Neurophysiol. 90 (4), 2548–2559.

Kimura, A., Ohsawa, H., Sato, A., et al., 1995. Somatocardiovascular reflexes in anesthetized rats with the central nervous system intact or acutely spinalized at the cervical level. Neurosci. Res. 22, 297–305.

Lin, C., Liao, J., Tsai, S., et al., 2003. Depressor effect on blood pressure and flow elicited by electroacupuncture in normal subjects. Auton. Neurosci. 107, 60–64.

Masliukov, P., Pankov, V., Strelkov, A., 2000. Morphological features of neurons innervating different viscera in the cat stellate ganglion in postnatal ontogenesis. Auton. Neurosci. 84, 169–175.

McCarthy, P., Prabhakar, E., Lawson, S., 1995. Evidence to support the peripheral branching of primary afferent C-fibres in the rat: an in vitro intracellular electrophysiological study. Brain Res. 704, 79–84.

Mok, E., Woo, C.P., 2004. The effects of slow-stroke back massage on anxiety and shoulder pain in elderly stroke patients. Complement. Ther. Nurs. Midwifery 10 (4), 209–216.

Nathan, H., 1968. Compression of the sympathetic trunk by osteophytes of the vertebral column in the abdomen: an anatomical study with pathological and clinical considerations.

Nishijo, K., Mori, H., Yosikawa, K., 1997. Decreased heart rate by acupuncture stimulation in humans via facilitation of cardiac vagal activity and suppression of cardiac sympathetic activity. Neurosci. Lett. 227, 165–168.

Oldfield, B., McLachlan, E., 1981. An analysis of the sympathetic preganglionic neurons projecting from the upper thoracic spinal roots of the cat. J. Comp. Neurol. 196, 329–345.

Pierau, F., Fellmer, G., Taylor, D., 1984. Somato-visceral convergence in cat dorsal root ganglion neurones demonstrated by double-labeling with fluorescent tracers. Brain Res. 321, 63–70.

Radtke, A., Popov, K., Bronstein, A., 2000. Evidence for a vestibulo-cardiac reflex in man. Lancet 356, 736–737.

Rubin, E., Purves, D., 1980. Segmental organization of sympathetic preganglionic neurons in the mammalian spinal cord. J. Comp. Neurol. 192, 163–174.

Sato, A., Sato, Y., Schmidt, R., 1997. The impact of somatosensory input on autonomic functions. Rev. Physiol. Biochem. Pharmacol. 130, 1–328.

Schwartz, P., Stone, H., Brown, A., 1976. Effects of unilateral stellate ganglion blockade on the arrhythmias associated with coronary occlusion. Am. Heart J 92 (5), 589–599.

Strack, A., Sawyer, W., Loewy, A., 1988. Spinal origin of sympathetic preganglionic neurons in the rat. Brain Res. 455, 187–191.

Takahashi, H., Nakajima, Y., Sakamoto, T., 1993. Capsaicin applied to rat lumbar intervertebral disc causes extravasation in the groin skin: a possible mechanism of referred pain of the intervertebral disc. Neurosci. Lett. 161 (1–3).

Tallarida, G., Baldoni, F., Peruzzi, G., 1981. Cardiovascular and respiratory reflexes from muscles during dynamic and static exercise. J. Appl. Physiol. 50, 784–791.

Wang, H.L., Keck, J.F., 2004. Foot and hand massage as an intervention for postoperative pain. Pain Manag. Nurs. 5 (2), 59–65.

Yates, B., Yamagata, Y., Bolton, P., 1991. The ventrolateral medulla of the cat mediates vestibulosympathetic reflexes. Brain Res. 552, 265–272.

Yates, B., Goto, T., Bolton, P., 1993. Responses of neurons in the rostral ventrolateral medulla of the cat to natural vestibular stimulation. Brain Res. 601, 255–264.

Yonei, Y., Holzer, P., Guth, P.H., 1990. Laparotomy-induced gastric protection against ethanol injury is mediated by capsaicin-sensitive sensory neurons. Gastroenterology 99, 3–9.

Zakir, M., Ono, S., Meng, H., 2000. Saccular and utricular influences on sympathetic nerve activities in cats. Exp. Brain Res. 134, 402–406.

Manual medicine and the autonomic nervous system: assessing autonomic function in humans

Michael L Smith • Kari Guinn Clark • Xiangrong Shi

Introduction

There is ample evidence for somatovisceral and viscerosomatic interactions throughout the body. Many of these structural and functional relationships are described in this book (see Chapters 1–4, 7, 8, 10, 12). There is now a growing body of evidence to support that these structural relationships can often translate into functional effects, and it is likely that these effects are manifested through neural and humoral mechanisms. The autonomic nervous system is the primary neural mediator of these interactions between the visceral and somatic systems; therefore, it is important to be able to assess autonomic activity and control in order to measure somatovisceral effects, whether these are evoked by naturally occurring conditions (injury, subluxation, or somatic dysfunction) or modulated by manual medicine or other medical interventions. This chapter reviews the methods by which autonomic function can be assessed in humans and the associated limitations of these tools, and summarizes the results of the limited studies of manual medicine and autonomic function.

Theories of autonomic modulation by manual medicine

That the autonomic nervous system can be affected by manual therapies and treatments has been a tenet of the major disciplines of manual medicine for over a century. In osteopathic medicine, Still first hypothesized in 1899 that the autonomic nervous system could be altered by manual pressure applied to the paravertebral muscles approximating the sympathetic chain ganglia (Still 1899). In the development of osteopathic manipulative treatment (OMT) techniques, many have been described to influence the autonomic nervous system (Chapters 1 and 12). In chiropractic medicine, organic or visceral dysfunction has been attributed to subluxation of vertebral segments, and an imbalance within the autonomic nervous system has been a focus of chiropractic management of disease processes (Plaugher & Lopes 1993). Similarly, massage therapists also hypothesize that massage aids in interrupting physiopathological reflex arcs that may be set up in the body, thereby helping to re-establish 'equilibrium' (Salvo 2003). Collectively, these theories espouse both direct and indirect benefits of manual medicine on visceral function by modulation of the autonomic nervous system. The systematic determination of the benefits of manual medicine and the role that autonomic, endocrine, or autocrine mechanisms play in achieving the benefits is beginning to evolve (see Chapter 10). Therefore, effective assessment of autonomic activity, function, and control is essential to determine the potential impact of somatovisceral effects accompanying manual therapies and treatments. The primary tools for assessing autonomic function are reviewed below, as are the limitations for investigation of manual medicine.

It is important to recognize that the two branches of the autonomic nervous system (ANS) do not always behave as a single unit, and that there can be selective changes within one branch of the system to mediate a given response. In addition, although the basal activity of either branch of the ANS is often presumed to reflect a given state or condition, the relative activity and how the ANS responds to a subsequent stress is often the more important outcome. Thus, we emphasize that the control of the autonomic nervous system appears to have the most significant impact on the outcome of a treatment or disease state in many cases.

Methods for assessing ANS function in humans

Circulating blood levels of catecholamines

The original standard for measuring sympathetic activity involved the measurement of circulating catecholamines. Epinephrine serves as a measure of sympathoadrenal activation, but since epinephrine functions primarily as a hormone circulating throughout the cardiovascular system to have wide-ranging effects at multiple sites, it does not serve well as a measure of sympathetic neural activity. Norepinephrine (NE) is the primary neurotransmitter at sympathetic nerve terminals and is released in proportion to the neural activity. Deactivation of norepinephrine primarily involves reuptake into nerve terminals and other non-neuronal cells in the region; however, a portion of the norepinephrine released at sympathetic nerve terminals spills over into the vascular bed and determines the circulating concentration within the plasma. Therefore, venous samples of norepinephrine from a given vein represent the global sympathetic activity specific to the tissues from that vein, combined with the background level of overall sympathetic activity within the system. Consequently, it is at best a 'ball park' measure of sympathetic activity.

Nevertheless, changes in peripheral venous norepinephrine concentrations do reflect changes associated with changes in sympathetic activation accompanying physical or mental stress, pain, reflex responses, and other modulatory inputs (Esler et al. 1990, Goldstein 1995). Alternatively, a central venous sample from a great vein (superior or inferior vena cava or right atrium) provides a true mixed venous sample representing activity throughout the system. This is a better measure than a peripheral venous sample, but it is also more invasive and lacks specificity with respect to the target tissues. A peripheral arterial sample provides a similar measure of general sympathetic activity under most circumstances; however, it requires arterial cannulation and the associated increased risk and discomfort.

An alternative measure of sympathetic activity from plasma samples is the norepinephrine spillover technique (Goldstein 1995). This involves the infusion of a known amount of tritiated norepinephrine into a peripheral artery and sampling from the associated regional vein. Assessment of the ratio of tritiated to non-tritiated NE and blood flow rate allows an estimation of the spillover rate of NE from the nerve terminals in this particular vascular bed. This is a more accurate measure of regional sympathetic activity than a venous sample.

Using blood samples to assess the effects of manual medicine on sympathetic activity is a practical option if the goal is to determine the longer-term (minutes to hours) steady-state effects of a given therapy. It can also have some value when making comparisons across days if care is taken to establish a basal state when the measures are obtained. Mixed venous samples are preferred; however, peripheral samples from the arm can be used with most applications as long as the arm is not stressed (e.g., exercise or temperature fluxes). If the effect of a treatment on a regional tissue is to be studied, the norepinephrine spillover

can be used if venous and arterial sampling can be achieved for that region.

Skin physiology

Several different techniques can be used to assess skin physiology based on measuring changes in either skin blood flow or sweat rate (Lima & Bakker 2005, Rossi et al. 2006). The traditional measurement of a galvanic skin response or skin conductance is reflective of sweat gland activity and the associated sympathetic nerve activity controlling these sweat responses (Rossi et al. 2006). The standard measurement of skin blood flow uses laser Doppler technology and is very sensitive to small changes in superficial blood flow (Lima & Bakker 2005, Rossi et al. 2006). Each of these measures is limited by the fact that basal quantization cannot be readily compared across measurement sites or between individuals. Therefore, they are used primarily to assess responses to a given intervention. Although these measures have been used in manual medicine research as noted below, for most applications their utility is limited by the physiological nature of the responses. Changes in skin blood flow and sweat rate are predominantly under the control of thermoregulatory mechanisms or as part of a psychological response. In some regions of the body there may be local reflex responses; however, the physiological purposes of these responses are unclear and thus, the utility of these measurements is equally uncertain. Further investigations into the meaning and utility of changes in skin conductance or blood flow associated with regional manipulative treatments merits consideration.

Microneurography (directly measured sympathetic activity)

Directly measured efferent sympathetic nerve activity can be obtained for sympathetic nerves that innervate either the skin or muscle vascular beds of the leg or arm

(Grassi & Esler 1999, Mancia & Grassi 1991, Wallin 1984). These measures are most commonly obtained at the peroneal nerve (at either the fibular head or the popliteal fossa), but are also obtained from the radial or ulnar nerves. The recordings are from unmyelinated fibers that have burst patterns which are distinctive for the skin efferent and muscle efferent nerves; thus, recordings can be obtained that are specific to the type of fiber that is desired. The nerve is identified via surface stimulation and then a microelectrode similar to an acupuncture needle is inserted percutaneously into the nerve and advanced and adjusted until an acceptable recording is obtained. The integrated activity and frequency of sympathetic bursts are used to quantify the sympathetic activity from a given recording. The recording is a multiunit recording (multiple postganglionic axons), therefore, all quantization involving the activity must be normalized to either a maximum response (such as during a cold pressor stimulus) or a controlled baseline period.

The measurement of skin sympathetic activity is limited for the same reasons as those described for the measures of skin blood flow and sweat rate: it is responsive primarily to thermoregulatory and emotional stimuli. On the other hand, muscle sympathetic nerve activity tends to respond in parallel to other branches of the sympathetic nervous system, such as cardiac and renal, when provoked by stressors. Thus, it can be used as a 'global' index of sympathetic activity.

The use of microneurography for investigations involving manual medicine can be quite limited owing to the sensitivity of the recording to movement. The subject or patient must remain relatively still and cannot move the limb from which the recording is obtained. Thus, the types of manipulative intervention that can be assessed are limited. One approach to circumvent this limitation is to obtain recordings before and after a treatment; however, this is also limited by the inherent challenges of obtaining a recording. If this approach is used, only the burst frequency can be used to quantify the sympathetic activity, because the signal from different recording sites cannot be compared owing to the differing 'quality' of the multiunit recordings from different sites. Similarly, if a recording is lost and then re-obtained, only the burst frequency can be compared, or the change in total activity in response to an intervention.

Heart rate variability (HRV) for assessment of autonomic function

Heart rate fluctuations can be analyzed in both the time-domain and the frequency-domain. In each case, a beat-to-beat heart rate signal is continuously monitored within a defined period, ranging from 1 minute up to 24 hours (using an electrocardiogram or Holter monitor). These continuous heart rate fluctuations are primarily determined by alterations in cardiac autonomic tone and thus can be used as an index of autonomic control of heart rate (American Heart Association 1996, Appel et al. 1989). Most frequently, cardiac cycle length or RR interval (in ms) is preferentially selected and used for data analysis.

Time-domain or time-series measures use statistical or geometrical methods. The statistical methods are mainly used to examine HRV using the variance and standard deviation of the normal-to-normal (consecutive sinus rhythm heart beats) RR intervals (RRI), whereas the geometrical methods are used to assess the sample density distribution of the R–R intervals. The simplest variable to compute RRI variability is the standard deviation, along with the mean, of the normal-to-normal (NN) RR intervals (SDNN), usually over 24-hour ECG recording; or the mean and the standard deviation of the mean of the RR intervals for each 5-minute period (SDANN) of the 24-hour ECG recording. As the variance of RR intervals varies with sample size, the duration of the ECG recording for an SDNN estimation should be standardized. Other statistical methods for time-domain analyses are based on the difference between adjacent RR intervals. These measurements include 1) calculating the root mean square of successive differences (RMSSD), where each difference is squared, summed, and the result is averaged and then the square root is obtained; and 2) the number of interval differences of successive RR intervals > 50 ms (NN50) or the proportion derived by dividing NN50 by the total number of RR intervals (pNN50). Each of these measures is more specific to beat-to-beat fluctuations and is less affected by random shifts in the RR interval. Table 5.1 summarizes the primary time-domain measures.

The short-term (≤5 min) measures in the time-domain, and particularly the RMSSD

Table 5.1 Definitions for Time-Domain Measures of RRI Variability

Variable	Units	Definition
SDNN	ms	Standard deviation of all normal RR intervals in the entire 24 hour ECG recording (also referred also as SDRR)
SDANN	ms	Standard deviation of the mean of normal RR intervals for each 5-min period of the 24-hour ECG recording
RMSSD	ms	The square root of the mean of the sum of the squares of differences between adjacent RR intervals
pNN50	%	Percent of difference between adjacent normal RR intervals that are > 50 ms
Counts	beats	The number of times that the difference between adjacent normal RR intervals is > 50 ms

and pNN50, are predominantly influenced by the parasympathetic nervous system, and thus are indices of parasympathetic control, whereas the longer-term measures are also predominantly influenced by the parasympathetic neural control but are also affected by sympathetic control. The time-domain measures should be cautiously interpreted as an index of autonomic control.

Frequency-domain analysis of HRV determines how power spectral density (PSD) or variance of the RR intervals distributes as a function of frequency. The traditional spectral analysis requires ≥256 HR beats or ≥5 minutes of stationary or steady-state ECG data. A commonly applied frequency-domain analysis is based on the fast Fourier transform (FFT). The expression of the PSD as a function of the frequency, $P(f)$, can be directly obtained from the time series $y(k)$, where k is the discrete time index, by using the periodogram expression:

$$P(f) = \frac{1}{N\Delta t}\left|\Delta t\sum_{k=0}^{N-1} y(k)e^{-j2\pi fk\Delta t}\right|^2 = \frac{1}{N\Delta t}|Y(f)|^2$$

where Δt is the sampling period, N is the number of samples, $y(f)$ is the discrete time Fourier transform of $y(k)$, and the PSD unit is ms^2 (i.e., the area under the curve). This efficient classic PSD analysis decomposes time-series data (time-domain) into components of different frequencies (frequency-domain). Programs for this frequency-domain analysis have been embedded in many commercial software programs. Different optional filters or methods are also available, which may enhance the curve smoothness of a PSD; however, with the filtering there can be a trade-off of the curve resolution.

In general, PSD analyses provide three main spectral components, i.e., very-low-frequency (VLF), low-frequency (LF), and high-frequency (HF) components. Table 5.2 defines the different power spectral density.

The interpretation of these different spectra is as follows. First, the VLF power, the spectrum ≤0.04 Hz, is believed to be modulated

Table 5.2 Definitions for frequency–domain measures of RRI variability

Variable	Units	Definition
VLF power	ms^2	PSD <0.04 Hz
LF power	ms^2	PSD between 0.04 and 0.15 Hz
HF power	ms^2	PSD between 0.15 and 0.40 Hz
5-min total power	ms^2	PSD ≤0.40 Hz or ≤RRI variance over the 5-min segment
LF norm	nu	100x LF/(LF + HF), normalized LF power
HF norm	nu	100x HF/(LF + HF), normalized HF power
LF/HF	ratio	Ratio LF (ms^2)/HF (ms^2)

by the renin–angiotensin hormone and thermal regulations. The LF power spectrum, range 0.04–0.15 Hz, has a rhythm centered around 0.1 Hz, which is not affected by normal breathing. The physiological interpretation remains controversial. An augmentation of LF power density has been observed during postural maneuvers, hemorrhage, or mental stress (American Heart Association 1996, Appel 1989). Therefore, it has been considered a marker of sympathetic nerve activity. However, pharmacological intervention has shown that the parasympathetic antagonist atropine almost vanishes total power and the sympathetic antagonist atenolol markedly increases both LF and HF power (Bigger et al. 1992). The prevailing view is that LF power is modulated by both sympathetic and parasympathetic nerve activity, and changes in LF or normalized LF PSD accompanying an intervention are commonly associated with activation of sympathetic nerve activity. The HF power spectrum, range 0.15–0.40 Hz, is an accepted marker of parasympathetic neural modulation of the heart. Greater HF PSD is a good indication of augmented parasympathetic nerve influences. The HF PSD

usually peaks at the respiratory frequency (typically between 0.2 and 0.3 Hz), which is tonically synchronous with the breathing-related alterations of intrathoracic pressure and volume. Finally, the LF/HF ratio can be calculated and has been used as an index of sympathetic–parasympathetic balance; however, this interpretation remains controversial.

Measures of HRV are often misrepresented as a measure of autonomic tone. It is important to recognize that the quantities obtained are a function of the effect of oscillations of autonomic tone on heart rate, and not a measure of the autonomic tone itself. It is also important to understand that, as autonomic tone increases, the effects that are measured will often also increase. This is particularly true for the parasympathetic control of heart rate. The interpretative value for assessment of sympathetic control is less clear, and must be made with caution. Consequently, the clearest interpretation from a power spectrum relates to the parasympathetic control that is imparted at the HF respiratory band. The most important use of HRV lies in its assessment when there is change associated with an intervention, and in the predictive value for certain disease outcomes (e.g. risk of sudden cardiac death).

Effects of manual medicine on autonomic function in humans

There has been a wealth of animal-based research and experimental work on humans that has demonstrated neural pathways to support the notion of these somatovisceral responses that can be mediated by the autonomic nervous system, and much of this work was reviewed by Sato (1992) and by Janig (2006) (see also Chapter 2). The focus of this chapter is on human measures of autonomic function.

A handful of human models have described the effects of cervical manipulation on the autonomic effects. Changes in skin conductance, skin temperature, heart rate, respiratory rate, systolic and diastolic blood pressure have been interpreted as increases in sympathetic activity accompanying high-velocity low-amplitude manipulation in the cervical region (Chiu & Wright 1996, McGuiness et al. 1997, Sterling 2001). A significant reduction in pain was also noted in those experiments that recruited subjects who were experiencing pain (Sterling et al 2001). In a related study, Vincenzino and colleagues (1998) used cervical spine lateral glide oscillatory manipulation and observed hypoalgesia and increased skin conductance suggestive of changes in skin sympathetic activity. More recently, Perry and Green (2008) used unilateral P-A mobilization of the left L4/5 zygopophyseal joint and reported significant side-specific changes in skin conductance in the lower limb. In each of these studies it is likely that the responses (particularly any heart rate changes) were mediated in part by changes of activity in parasympathetic neurons innervating the heart, and it is also likely that the skin responses were, at least in part, a function of emotional responses to the specific manipulative stimulus.

Using measures of heart rate variability, Budgell and Hirano (2001) demonstrated that innocuous mechanical stimulation of the cervical spine in healthy young adults produced significant alterations in heart rate and HRV as calculated by power spectral analysis. The most significant change being an increase in the LF/HF component of the spectral analysis (Budgell & Hirano 2001). This study thus supports previous theory regarding facilitated segments, in that it may create a situation of either enhanced vagal or sympathetic discharge (Leach 2004). In a study performed by Henley et al. (2008), the use of cervical myofascial release during a period of maximal sympathetic stimulation produced a vagal response that was strong enough to significantly overcome sympathetic tone. The LF component and the LF/HF component were both reduced, whereas the HF component was increased in comparison to the control and sham protocols (Henley et al. 2008).

Cranial manipulation, specifically the CV-4 technique, has been shown to alter blood flow velocity and the low-frequency Traube–Hering (TH) oscillation as recorded by LDF. This technique is reproducible with substantial inter- and intra-operator reliability (Nelson et al. 2006). However, the effect on the autonomic nervous system is uncertain. In a related study using microneurography to directly measure sympathetic activity, Cutler et al. (2004) demonstrated that the use of a CV-4 to treat the cranial field resulted in significant reductions in sympathetic nerve activity.

Collectively, these very limited studies demonstrate that a variety of manipulative interventions can affect both the parasympathetic and the sympathetic nervous systems. However, these studies have not been systematic, manipulative techniques vary considerably, and the primary outcomes have focused on the acute timeframe. Consequently, there is both a great need and an opportunity for further investigations into the autonomic effects of manual therapies and treatments. Equally important is the need for studies that follow patients beyond the acute period of treatment. If somatovisceral effects are to have important clinical outcomes, the long-term effect on autonomic function will be most important to determine. In conclusion, assessment of human autonomic function is feasible and the opportunities for future studies are broad in scope as it relates to the effect of manual medicine on clinical outcomes and the role that autonomic function may play in the benefits derived from manual medicine.

Summary

As discussed extensively throughout this book, the evidence for structural relationships and functional effects of somatovisceral interactions is clear. The primary mediator of most end-organ functional effects is probably the autonomic nervous system; however, there is a paucity of data in humans to support or refute the significance of these effects, particularly as they relate to the application of manual medicine. In this chapter we have reviewed several methods of assessing autonomic activity and control, and discussed the utility and limitations as they apply to assessing somatovisceral mechanisms of manual medicine. As noted, there is a growing body of evidence to support acute effects of manual therapies and treatments on autonomic activity and control. And despite many technical limitations of the methodologies, there is ample opportunity and feasibility for further investigation of the role that the autonomic nervous system plays in mediating the effects of manual medicine via somatovisceral mechanisms.

References

AHA, 1996. Heart rate variability: standards of measurement, physiological interpretation and clinical use. Task Force of the European Society of Cardiology and the North American Society of Pacing and Electrophysiology. Circulation 93 (5), 1043–1065.

Appel, M.L., et al., 1989. Beat to beat variability in cardiovascular variables: noise or music? J. Am. Coll. Cardiol. 14 (5), 1139–1148.

Bigger Jr., J.T., et al., 1992. Correlations among time and frequency domain measures of heart period variability two weeks after acute myocardial infarction. Am. J. Cardiol. 69 (9), 891–898.

Budgell, B., Hirano, F., 2001. Innocuous mechanical stimulation of the neck and alterations in heart-rate variability in healthy young adults. Auton. Neurosci. 91 (1–2), 96–99.

Chiu, T.W., Wright, A., 1996. To compare the effects of different rates of application of a cervical mobilisation technique on sympathetic outflow to the upper limb in normal subjects. Man. Ther. 1 (4), 198–203.

Cutler, M.J., et al., 2004. Periods of intermittent hypoxic apnea can alter chemoreflex control of sympathetic nerve activity in humans. Am. J. Physiol. Heart Circ. Physiol. 287 (5), H2054–H2060.

Esler, M., et al., 1990. Overflow of catecholamine neurotransmitters to the circulation: Source, fate and functions. Physiol. Rev. 70, 963–985.

Goldstein, D.S., 1995. Stress, Catecholamines, and Cardiovascular Disease. Oxford University Press, New York.

Grassi, G., Esler, M., 1999. How to assess sympathetic activity in humans. J. Hypertens. 17 (6), 719–734.

Henley, C.E., et al., 2008. Osteopathic manipulative treatment and its relationship to autonomic nervous system activity as demonstrated by heart rate variability: a repeated measures study. Osteopathic Medicine and Primary Care 2, 7.

Jänig, W., 2006. The Integrative Action of the Autonomic Nervous System. Neurobiology of Homeostasis. Cambridge University Press, Cambridge, New York.

Leach, R.A., 2004. The Chiropractic Theories: A Textbook of Scientific Research, fourth ed. Lippincott Williams & Wilkins, Philidelphia.

Lima, A., Bakker, J., 2005. Noninvasive monitoring of peripheral perfusion. Intensive Care Med. 31 (10), 1316–1326.

Mancia, G., Grassi, G., 1991. Assessment of sympathetic cardiovascular influences in man: haemodynamic and humoral markers versus microneurography. Clin. Auton. Res. 1 (3), 245–249.

McGuiness, J., Vicenzino, B., Wright, A., 1997. Influence of a cervical mobilization technique on respiratory and cardiovascular function. Man. Ther. 2 (4), 216–220.

Nelson, K.E., Sergueef, N., Glonek, T., 2006. The effect of an alternative medical procedure upon low-frequency oscillations in cutaneous blood flow velocity. J. Manipulative Physiol. Ther. 29 (8), 626–636.

Perry, J.A., Green, A., 2008. An investigation into the effects of a unilaterally applied lumbar mobilisation technique on peripheral sympathetic nervous system activity in the lower limbs. Man. Ther. 13 (6), 492–499.

Plaugher, G., Lopes, M.A. (Eds.), 1993. Textbook of Clinical Chiropractic: A Specific Biomechanical Approach. Williams & Wilkins, Baltimore.

Rossi, M., et al., 2006. The investigation of skin blood flow motion: a new approach to study the microcirculatory impairment in vascular diseases? Biomedical Pharmacotherapeutics 60 (8), 437–442.

Salvo, S.G., 2003. Massage Therapy: Principles and Practice, second ed. Saunders, St. Louis.

Sato, A., 1992. The reflex effects of spinal somatic nerve stimulation on visceral function. J. Manipulative Physiol. Ther. 15 (1), 57–61.

Sterling, M., Jull, G., Wright, A., 2001. Cervical mobilisation: concurrent effects on pain, sympathetic nervous system activity and motor activity. Man. Ther. 6 (2), 72–81.

Still, A.T., 1899. Philosophy of Osteopathy. Still, AT, Kirksville, MO.

Vicenzino, B., et al., 1998. An investigation of the interrelationship between manipulative therapy-induced hypoalgesia and sympathoexcitation. J. Manipulative Physiol. Ther. 21 (7), 448–453.

Wallin, B.G., 1984. Muscle sympathetic activity and plasma concentrations of noradrenaline. Acta Physiol. Scand. Suppl. 527, 21–24.

Survey of mechanotransduction disorders

John J Triano

Introduction

Living systems rely on complex biochemical interactions within the framework of a diverse biomechanical environment. Knowledge of the physical basis of health and disease has been underdeveloped even though clinical symptoms may result from altered tissue structure or mechanics. With the exception of the study of ergonomic factors in injury, only recently has attention been given to the regulatory role of external and internal forces on cell, tissue, and system behaviour. How tissues interact and respond to variations in mechanical force is critical in maintaining homeostasis (Yang et al. 1998). Well-recognized examples include the effects of large-scale environmental force modulation of development, as with bone compression, muscle exercise, and vascular pressures. Less clear is the influence of dispersed, microscale forces on all cells. A wide range of disorders have etiology and clinical presentation resulting from abnormal cell and tissue response to mechanical stress (Ingber 2003). Expanding appreciation of these mechanisms poses both a challenge and an opportunity for future care givers.

The use of mechanical, manual modes of treatment for human disorders is ancient and empirical. Scientific investigations into questions of validity and effectiveness for these approaches gained momentum in the late 20th century. As favorable clinical evidence has accumulated, research has accelerated with progress in new technologies and improved understanding of physiology. What has been clear from the outset is that the underlying lesions and mechanisms of action associated with manual therapies are complex and multifactorial.

As evidence-based medicine has come to dominate health policy, the preferred use of manual medicine procedures has shifted primarily to musculoskeletal (MSK) conditions, where the rationale and evidence are clearer. However, observations that nonmusculoskeletal conditions may respond to mechanically based treatments continue to be voiced. Based on systematic review (Hawk et al. 2007), evidence from controlled studies, and usual practice potentially supports the clinical encounter in chiropractic care as beneficial to patients with asthma, cervicogenic vertigo, and infantile colic. Specific therapeutic components that may be responsible remain to be clarified. Similarly, there is evidence of potential benefit for an ensemble of osteopathic manual procedures for children with otitis media and elderly patients with pneumonia (Degenhardt & Kuchera 2006; Noll et al 2008). Manipulation of the upper cervical spine has been associated with a reduction of blood pressure in mild to moderately hypertensive patients (Bakris et al. 2007). Treatment of these disorders remains controversial, partly because of the absence of clear theoretical foundations and mechanisms to guide both the selection of appropriate candidates for care and the identification of effective procedures. Are favorable results associated with specific mechanosensitive disorders or for special populations where there is a convergence of circumstances involving genetic and environmental factors? Are treatment effects purely mechanical, reflexive, or the complex interaction of neurohumoral and mechanical factors? How may the results of care be predicted and replicated? If more is understood about mechanotransduction in disease and

the treatments offered, appropriate strategies may be developed that bring the right treatment to the right patient at the right time.

Convergence of three lines in basic research – biomechanics, mechanobiology, and mechanotransduction – offers new opportunities to answer these questions. Biomechanics supplies knowledge of the quantity of extrinsic force, including therapeutic loads, acting on the body. With the development and application of new technologies, including theoretical and computational models, mechanobiology provides information on how forces are transmitted to and deform organs, tissues, and cell systems.

Mechanotransduction focuses on the mechanism by which physical and chemical signals interplay to control how individual cells alter their growth, differentiation, function, or death. Whereas a thorough description of the research in this area deals almost exclusively with peripheral phenomena, these phenomena may also be monitored and at times modified by higher-center activity. References, cited above, suggestive of an impact of manual therapy on vertigo and hypertension are examples where interactions between peripheral and higher-center activity may exist, a theme consistent throughout all the chapters of this book. However, it is obvious that we must better understand these peripheral, cellular phenomena in their own right, in order to understand how they may interact with central higher-center activity in health and disease.

Tissue infrastructure for loading

An organized web of connective tissue throughout the body provides structural support and integrity for all cells and organs. The plasticity of bony and fibrous connective tissue in response to immobility and exercise is commonly known. However, the influence of deformation on mechanosensation outside the nervous system and force distribution has only recently been recognized.

Body segments are constructed in a cross-sectional stratum of overlapping systems, organized in a functional hierarchy. Each system, whether an extremity, the torso or the head, is composed of different organs and tissues (Fig. 6.1). The organ parenchyma is divided by connective tissue partitions. The specialized cells are held together by an extracelluar matrix (ECM) that is continuous across the strata through a network of collagen, glycoprotein, and proteoglycans. Each cell is adherent to the ECM and its neighbors by specialized patches of the cellular membrane termed 'focal adhesions' (Katsumi et al. 2004). The membrane, an elastic proteolipid bilayer, deforms instantaneously, bending or stretching in proportion to the application and withdrawal of force. Membrane shape

is reinforced by a filamentous cytoskeleton (CSK) that connects to all intracellular organelles and the nucleus (Maniotis et al. 1997). Molecules important to cell function cluster about the focal adhesions and the CSK fibers. The extracellular and intracellular environments are connected through the membrane by specialized integrin proteins. In summary, the stratified structure creates a functional hierarchy where force acting on the tissues results in a coordinated deformation at various size scales that is transmitted through the system. Experts suggest (Suki et al. 2005) that collagen, in its several isoforms, is the key load-bearing component determining cellular health and response to injury.

The cross-sectional hierarchy is interconnected with the remainder of the body through its dense innervation by primary afferent neurons with Aδ- and C-fibers (among others) and cellular soluble messenger molecules that continuously monitor the states of the tissues. These afferent neurons and humoral factors signal local conditions to the spinal cord, brain, and endocrine organs. Return signals are integrated to coordinate tissue function within the overall needs of the system.

Biology of loading

The experience of mechanical stimulus surrounds us on a daily basis. Biological systems accommodate to steady-state inputs that allow decision-making processes to focus on signals of change. The adaptation of light touch to the presence of clothing, for example, is a common experience. The flexibility of the extracellular matrix (ECM) in the Pacinian mechanoreceptors rapidly adapts to steady pressure, contributing to a lack of conscious awareness (Ingber 2003). To appreciate this phenomenon, one has only to consider one's own state of awareness. Are you aware of the touch and weight of your clothing? Only when force changes sufficiently is a signal generated for conscious recognition. Mechanical signals within a healthy

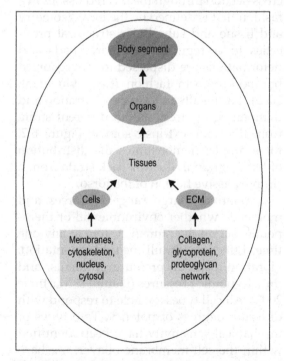

Figure 6.1 The majority of forces acting on the body are applied locally, having an effect across the layers of tissue that are organized in a nested hierarchy of organs, tissues, cells, extracellular matrix (ECM), cellular organelles and cytoskeleton. All are susceptible to deformation from environmental loads.

range foster function, stimulate growth, metabolic activity, and development. Low physical stress reduces physiologic fitness and increases the risk of heart disease, obesity, and diabetes, and excess exertion risks inflammation, apoptosis (Jaalouk & Lammerding 2009), tissue failure (Chaffin & Anderson 1984) or maladaptive remodelling (Lotz et al. 2004, Tavi et al. 2001). Health is bounded, from above and below, by a range of mechanical forces.

Clearly, mechanosensation is not the only mechanism of regulation. Complex interactions between neurological stimulation, soluble messenger molecules, and mechanical strain have been identified. Each has its own primary pathway to influence and regulate function as a balance of inputs. Regulation of function and response to the environment occurs at multiple levels: local (e.g., cellular balance of mechanical, neurotransmitter, and endocrine messengers), spinal (e.g., segmental reflexes) and central (e.g., efferent and afferent neural interactions and vascular delivery of circulating messengers). Combined, these processes continuously monitor the mechanical, thermal, and metabolic states of the tissues. The afferent neurons signal these states to the brain, some of them also having efferent functions back to the cell, where they are integrated with the humoral and mechanical messages to regulate function.

Tissues thrive in a state of mechanical homeostasis (Turner & Pavalko 1998), with cells responding to and interpreting biochemical signals within the context of mechanical forces to provide a structurally rational system. Cells sense mechanical forces which are then translated into modified intracellular biochemistry, structure, and gene expression. For example, it is well known that musculoskeletal tissues respond to exercise and use. What is less well recognized is that mechanical stress contributes to the development and clinical expression of a number of important diseases (Table 6.1) which are among the major sources of health costs internationally (Ingber 2003).

Table 6.1 Diseases that involve mechanotransduction error in their etiology or expression of symptoms

Musculoskeletal	Non-musculoskeletal
Ankylosing spondylitis	Asthma
Low back pain	Atherosclerosis
Carpal tunnel syndrome	Diabetes
Discopathy	Heart failure
Osteoporosis	Irritable bowel syndrome
Osteoarthritis	Migraine
	Stroke

Mechanisms of mechanotransduction

Mechanical regulation distinguishes function across nested structural systems within body regions (see Fig. 6.1). Force is transmitted in cross-section through the layered tissues in a fashion that is defined by the local geometry and tissue and subcellular structural properties to co-regulate behavior. Loads and deformations are dispersed in an organized but non-uniform fashion (Langevin et al. 2005) that results in local concentration and dampening of stress within different strata from the same extrinsic source. Figure 6.2, for example, demonstrates the distribution of tissue strain in the low back strata from a simple passive flexion of the torso.

A relatively large range of forces and moments, whether environmental or therapeutic, act on the human system at any one time. Effective stimuli include indentation, vibration, osmotic pressure gradients, and fluid dynamic pressures (Hamill & Martinac 2001). All cell types are able to respond with differing degrees of potency. Two types of mechanical sensitivity have been identified within the cell membrane bilayer: mechanically gated (MG) channels (Hamill & Martinac 2001, Huang et al. 2003) and transmembrane protein receptors (Jalali et al. 2001, Kamm & Kaazempur-Mofrad 2004). Shear tends to initiate stronger reaction than

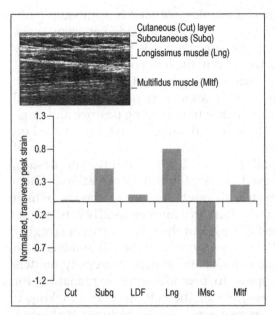

Figure 6.2 Strain in the transverse plane of the muscle at the L2–L3 level, observed during a 10° trunk flexion, normalized to the maximum strain observed. The inset shows the ultrasound scan image 2 cm parallel to the spine with layers identified. LDF, lumbodorsal fascia; IMsc, intramuscular septum.

does compression, with threshold levels that range from 30 to 200 piconewtons (pN).

MG channels sense membrane tension directly, being either ion selectively permeable nonspecific, exchanging fluid volumes (Hamill & Martinac 2001) or passing tension directly to the CSK. Calcium flux across the membrane, for example, is involved in the control of a number of important functions, including growth, differentiation, motility, synaptic transmission, apoptosis, and necrosis. Local membrane stretch opens (stretch activated) or closes (stretch inactivated) channels. Albeit similar to active membrane pump systems in that they transfer ions, MG channels are separate mechanisms that do not generate global electrical responses as seen with neurons.

The transmembrane receptors are composed of integrin proteins (Katsumi et al. 2004) that affect a physical coupling between fibronectin or vitronectin of the ECM and the CSK lattice (actin microtubules and

intermediate fibers). Integrin attachments are concentrated at focal adhesions of the membrane, where they provide mechanical stiffening and support to the tissue. The lattice extends deep into the cell, connecting to the nucleus (Maniotis et al. 1997) and other organelles. Shear force transmitted by the ECM tugs on integrin and, through it, is shared with the intracellular structural proteins (Fig. 6.3) and their associated molecular messengers (Burkholder 2007, Ingber 2003, Jalali et al. 2001, Kamm & Kaazempur-Mofrad 2004). The CSK is pre-stressed within the cell as a function of the cell type and the mechanical properties conferred by genetic regulation (Huang & Ingber 2005). The baseline pre-stress, focusing at the intermediate fiber attachments, provides shape control and intracellular tone. The evidence suggests that it is the change in shape of the integrin molecule and the intracellular microtubules that bring key enzymes and proteins together, promoting up- or downregulation of biochemical and nuclear activity. The specific responses to mechanical sensitivity are based on cell type, stimulus type, and the time frame of operation.

There are no available data that explore the relationship between the dosage of exposure

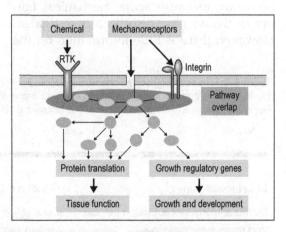

Figure 6.3 Cell membrane demonstrating the overlap of chemical and mechanical sensing systems that co-regulate biochemical reactions, gene expression, and shape. Curved structures represent intracellular enzymes and secondary messenger molecules.

(time or amplitude) of tissue layers to extrinsic load and mechanotransduction outcomes. However, the evidence on mechanochemical transduction itself shows effects from ligand triggering that can extend across multiple time periods (Table 6.2). Local mediation appears to require the activation of chemical substrates and enzymes that are already present and available within the cytosol. The interactions occur within seconds to minutes after stimulation. Genetic regulation with protein transcription and translation can begin within minutes to hours of stimulus onset, whereas structural modification is seen within days. These longer-term effects were demonstrated recently when local motion limitation was surgically induced to the rat lumbar spine (Henderson et al. 2007a,b). Lost motion produced local joint adhesions within the articulations and was followed within 8 weeks by osteophytic growth formation off the articular process (Personal communication, Henderson et al. 2007b).

Mechanobiology

Much has been learned about the mechanosensitivity of cells and the mechanisms by which cell structure and function are influenced by force application. Loads necessary to cause acute mechanical failure of tissues have also been investigated. However, there is little information on the mechanobiology of load transmission pathways, the sharing of loads between layers, and the effective loads that are biologically active within the homeostatic range.

Load sharing is most studied in the area of the myofascial networks. Various clinical approaches to managing posture and musculoskeletal disorders have been based on the assumption of a kinetic chain or 'lines of pull' (Mayers 2009) within the soft tissues, based on anatomical observations, interpreted through tensegrity theory, which states that force applied locally is transmitted throughout the whole structure (Ingber 1997). Clearly, within the cell and based on the cytoskeletal matrix, tensegrity models appear to provide some explanation for pre-stress of the cell structure, making it responsive as a whole to loads that reach it. Within the organ and tissue layers, however, the evidence suggests that the transmission pathways may be more complex. At the very least, the load distributions that occur within the tissues do not appear to be linear (Triano et al. 2009a, 2009b) and are not evenly distributed (Langevin et al. 2005). Loads acting between and within organ structures, at least in the case of muscle, are highly influenced by the geometry of the dense connective tissue attachments. Epimuscular connective tissue separates muscles and muscle compartments, and encases the neurovascular

Table 6.2 Timeframe of mechanochemical response from cells triggered by stretch-sensitive channels or ligand transmembrane proteins. Local mediation relies on a cache of enzymes, messengers, and ions available at the membrane. Genetic regulation and structural modifications require the transcription and protein synthesis

Seconds	Minutes	Hours	Days

Local mediation→	Genetic regulation→	Structural modification
Membrane channel activation (K$^+$, Ca^{2+})	Gene up- & downregulation	Cytoskeleton changes
2nd messenger cascades	Protein synthesis	Remodeling of focal adhesions and extracellular matrix
Enzyme activations	Endocytosis (cellular ingestion)	
Signal damping & modulation	Cell replication	Cell morphology & behavioral change

bundles entering them. The percentage of total load transferred by these mechanisms is as high as 50%, depending on joint angle and direction (Yucesoy et al. 2008). Load sharing across and within tissues has four important observations, particularly for the softer myofascial systems (Huijing 2007):

1. Muscular force is transmitted both through the intramuscular organization of muscle fiber, endomysium, perimysium, and epimysium, and through the extramuscular organization of interconnecting fascia.

2. Intramuscular force transmission is non-uniform, showing differences across the muscle diameter and along its length.

3. Force is transmitted between compartments by neurovascular bundles which reinforce and protect these structures, but which also convey significant tensile force.

4. Transmission of both intramuscular and epimuscular forces is altered by the relative position of the joints they surround.

Recent work with porcine psoas shows that the organ response to passive tissue stretch is neither linear nor uniform (Sovak & Triano 2009, Triano et al. 2009a). Using excised and clamped skeletal muscle with intact perimysium, an elongation load was applied while monitoring change in muscle shape externally and displacements of tissue internally using ultrasound elastography. The regions of the muscle beneath the surface aponeurosis, at its surface appearance and more centrally, were compared. Aponeurosis accounts for two-fifths of the dense connective tissue in cross-section, whereas deeper fascial septa were sparse and homogeneous along the length of the muscle. Contrary to expectations, the muscle mass showed a highly asymmetrical response to lengthening. In cross-section, the muscle became narrower in one direction while expanding in the perpendicular direction. Deeper muscle tissue was strained less in length than were superficial muscle fibers. Finally, sectioning (2 mm depth) of the aponeurosis at its distal end near the clamp relaxed all of the longitudinal differential lengthening effects. Similar longitudinal differences in load sharing between the proximal and distal ends of muscle have been shown by others (Rijkelijkhuizen et al. 2007).

Force applied extrinsically or generated intrinsically by muscle activation deforms the tissue and causes a redistribution of load to adjacent muscles by epimuscular force transmission. In a series of studies on the intact crural muscles in the rat, the phenomenon of epimuscular force transmission was established (Rijkelijkhuizen et al. 2007). Using a fixed joint angle, the tendons of select muscles about the ankle were tensioned by Kevlar thread attachments. In addition to altering load sharing within an agonist group of muscles, antagonist tension was reduced (Huijing et al. 2007). Lengthening of the peroneal group reduced the tibial complex muscle force by 25%. In the reverse direction, the peroneal force reduction was 30%.

Langevin and co-workers (Langevin et al. 2005), using transcutaneous needle perturbation of muscle, have demonstrated that local perturbation is not transmitted uniformly through the tissues. As a robotically controlled acupuncture needle was oscillated in the tissue, elastograms revealed that while the needle was being moved in one direction, the tissue strain experienced at different depths along the needle was stratified in alternating layers of compression and distraction.

Whether a tensegrity model is adequate to describe load transmission behavior over the whole of integrated connective tissue systems is sufficient, what is clear is that a potent form of kinetic chain does exist.

Biomechanics

At the macroscopic level, the influence of physical activity (Table 6.3) on health is frequently reported (McGill 2007, Shaw et al. 2009, Triano 2008). Issues related to injury

Table 6.3 Environmental load factors contributing to mechanical homeostasis within the system and the possible negative effects when they are experienced out of normal range

Low exposure risk	Physiologically relevant factor	High exposure risk
	Acceleration/ speed	
Low cardiovascular reserve		Impact injury Strain/fatigue
	Amplitude	
Disuse atrophy		Excess force
Osteopenia		Overuse/strain
	Distribution	
Low flexibility		Local stress concentration Extreme joint position
	Duration	
Low endurance		Prolonged static posture/ fatigue
	Frequency	
Low endurance		High repetition

with tissue failure are repeated throughout the literature. The central focus is on six biomechanical features, including: 1) the load's amplitude in proportion to tissue ultimate strength; 2) effects of velocity of loading; 3) potentiation of injury by repetition; 4) concentration of local stress; 5) effects of unexpected sudden loading; and 6) fatigue with reduction in optimal motor control and coordination. Gravitational effects on body weight and external loads are amplified by movement and posture. For example, relaxed standing positions exert a force of one-half body weight on the lumbosacral disc. The compressive stress is increased to twice body weight with walking at a normal pace, but by up to a factor of 4 when running or walking in high heels. The mechanical deformation of whole systems of tissues results in structural rearrangements on multiple scales (Ingber 2003). High repetition, or prolonged static activity at extremes of joint position, concentrate stress in cartilage, ligament, tendon, and muscle. The local connecting elements undergo creep deformity and lose elastic reserve until they are sufficiently rested. Excessive forces to tissues arise from highly accelerated loading, for example with impact, or catching a suddenly dropped weight; from carrying heavy loads; or from using relatively weak muscle groups to accomplish tasks. Stress concentration occurs from tissue intrusion when holding tools, sitting on furniture, and leaning on structures. Rapid, short movements, awkward/extreme postures, and prolonged static positions often focus the effect of physical effort or posture to local within a body segment.

The central question, yet to be explained, is why persons performing the same work or activity may persist with no adverse effects whereas others begin to experience a range of symptoms (Triano 2001, Triano 2005a,b). Physically and mentally challenging environments foster higher levels of illness than others. The evidence on the psychosocial model of illness is well established, but does not adequately account for all of the problems of a population of individuals and their disorders (Shaw et al. 2009), as mechanical interactions remain important.

Biomechanics of manipulable lesions

The common feature of all types of manual therapy is the application of extrinsic load to the body segments in an effort to moderate symptoms and encourage recovery of injured tissues (Kimberly 2006, Triano 2001). Objective identification of the specific lesion or lesions amenable to manual treatment has remained elusive, causing investigations of clinical outcomes to rely on nonspecific measures. A number of theoretical mechanisms have been proposed that, in general, are tissue specific, e.g., disc, nerve, joint capsule, etc. In each case, empirical explanations for why the application of loading to the spine should be beneficial are incomplete, being unable to fully account for the observed characteristics of patients.

A new biomechanical model steps away from the tissue-based classifications to explain clinical musculoskeletal complaints as an epiphenomenon. In this model, the tissue structure that has become symptomatic is a consequence of a common etiologic factor. The factor itself is amenable to change through the application of force or moment (e.g., a physical intervention) to the structure. The biomechanical epiphenomenon is a form of structural instability defined as 'buckling'. The buckling phenomenon, in a multijoint, multimuscle system, is a sudden deformation or bending within the linkage that increases the local tissue strain. The deformation is a disproportionate response to the task being performed and/or a traumatic overload. Details of the buckling event in the case of joint structures (e.g., wrist and spine) are given elsewhere (McGill 2007, Preuss & Fung 2005, Triano 2001).

Stability, particularly in a multijoint system, is a measure of the effectiveness of motor-control strategies over posture and movement. In its most simple form, a buckling event can arise when the motor-control mechanisms are overwhelmed by a single catastrophic event, or are out of sequence and mistimed with respect to the amplitude of a load acting through the joint. The work of several investigators (for example Bergmark 1989, Wilder et al. 1989, Ogon et al. 1997; Howarth et al. 2004, McGill 2007, Solomonow et al. 2008, Youssef et al. 2008) has provided characteristics of the underlying circumstances thought to contribute to buckling events. They occur at loads far lower than those required for disruption of the tissues. Prolonged postures that are perturbed by sudden loads, or repetitive movement with fatigue of the coordinated muscles may both yield an event. Buckling is facilitated by higher rate loads well within the

capacity of normal activities (500 lb/s), and vibrating environments (Wilder 1993) may lower the threshold and facilitate buckling. Common activities that may produce buckling include catching a falling or suddenly displaced weight; missing a stair with a sudden mechanical jolt; rapid lifting; fatigued muscle control during repetitive or sudden activity; and driving for longer distances with road vibration.

The basic understanding of mechanical stability for the spine was pioneered by Bergmark (1989). He posed that multimuscle, multijoint equilibrium required two sets of motor control systems: the large torso muscles that attach between body regions, e.g., thorax to pelvis, as global drivers of posture and motion; and the small intrinsic spinal muscles that pass between the individual spinal segments responsible for coordinating local joint action consistent with global motion. Failure of these two systems to effectively coordinate joint activity and maintain stable equilibrium permits the joint to undergo buckling action. The consequence is an increased local tissue strain/stress which presents as a set of complaints determined by the identity of the tissue itself. Another way to think about these effects clinically is to consider that the same cause of pain in an individual may result in different symptoms in a comparable person doing a similar task. The basic mechanical phenomenon ('buckling') is the same, but the structure that was 'hurt' will differ based on local factors, including its direction and severity.

Much remains to be learned about the biomechanical buckling model and how the local forces are distributed and undergo mechanotransduction at the cellular level. Animal (Solomonow et al. 2008, Youssef et al. 2008), ex-vivo (Ogon et al. 1997, Wilder et al. 1989), computer modeling (Howarth et al. 2004), and a single observation of in-vivo (McGill 2007) evidence in support of the epiphenomenon are now available at the level of the organism and the organ.

Therapeutic factors

The mechanical principles that underlie factors of tissue loading during activity (see Table 6.3) are in force during the application of physical treatment, whether they be manually applied or directed as in exercise therapy. The difference is not in the underlying principles, but in the controlled focus of the load application directed to alter the underlying tissue strains associated with harmful effects from injury. Factors of therapeutic loading may be divided into two strategic categories (Table 6.4) for all mechanical therapies, regardless of the method.

In the case of exercise as the vehicle to apply loads, the usual intention is to increase the compliance of some tissue components (fascia, ligament, tendon, muscle) to promote an increased range of functional motion. For others, exercise will promote an increase in muscular strength and tone to stabilize and protect the tissues. Manual therapies take a number of forms, based on different theoretical constructs, all designed to alter local tissue strains, promote normal function, and permit symptom resolution and healing. Figure 6.4 organizes examples of prominent

Table 6.4 Categories of strategic control factors that apply when administering clinical treatment loads, whether by manual method or through direction as in exercise therapy, that focus the efforts to a targeted area for therapeutic benefit

Provider-based factors	Patient-based factors
Provider body mass and strength	Patient body mass
	Reactive muscle tone
Choice of procedure (e.g., orientation and direction of loads applied)	Initial posture positioning
	Initial motion state – static or dynamic
Preload amplitude	
Speed of application	Site of application
Duration of procedure	
Repetition of procedure	

mechanotherapy intervention systems by modes of mechanical stimulation in common with the tissues.

Gravitational loading uses guided postural training, body segment position and movement training, or self-stretching techniques to provide a coordinated structural rearrangement of tissues. Intended effects range from modification of muscle tone and reducing local tissue strains to encouraging postural positions that empower overall relaxation and enhancing respiratory function. Relative joint positions are held for specific intervals to promote the desired change, or involve slow movements, also termed quasi-static, as in self-stretching methods.

The mechanisms and benefits of exercise have long been studied. Relative isolation of muscle groups is sought through selection of joint position and directions of movement or resistance. Rate and range of motion, frequency and intensity of effort, and duration of performance may all be varied to achieve different local and physiological effects.

When loads are applied by an operator, controlled effects are achieved by combining provider- and patient-based factors (Table 6.4). Therapeutic loads are directed more focally and can systematically accentuate the timing, speed, deformation, total forces, and moments that are applied (Triano & Schultz 1997). Transcutaneous procedures allow a restricted region of mechanical stimulation to the fascia and muscle for immediate local effects (Langevin et al. 2005).

The amplitude of forces being applied or transmitted through the target body segments during manual procedures has been a topic of research in the past three decades for both high-velocity, low-amplitude (HVLA) and mobilization procedures. Mobilization forces are applied over a series of cycles. Peak amplitudes were reported over a broad range from 20 N at preload to 550 N at peak loading. Segmental, absolute (1 cm), and relative displacements (0.1 cm) were measured (Lee & Svensson 1993). Intersegmental rotations of vertebral segments were estimated

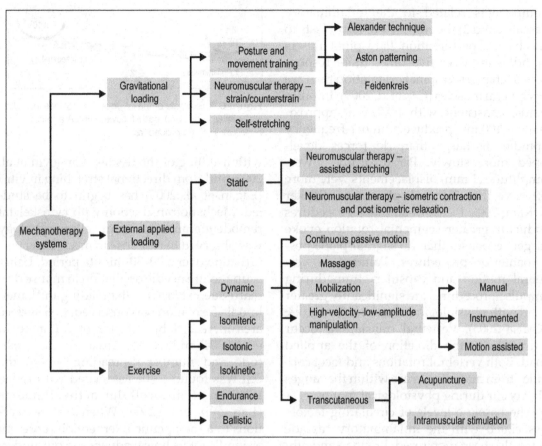

Figure 6.4 Mechanotherapy systems of intervention organized by common mechanical characteristics, consistent with the physiological factors of Table 6.3 and control strategies identified in Table 6.4.

at 0.1°–1.8°. For HVLA procedures, forces are delivered with both compression and biaxial shear components (Triano & Schultz 1997; van Zoest & Gosselin 2003). Treatment mean force to the thoracic spine has ranged from 399 N (Gal et al. 1997) to 1213 N (Kirstukas & Backman 1999). Peak transmitted loads for three separate procedures targeting the low back ranged from 385 N to 515 N (Triano & Schultz 1997). The mean time to peak force has been given from 96 to 183 ms (Herzog 2000; Kirstukas & Backman 1999, van Zoest & Gosselin 2003). Peak rates of force development of 7101 N/s to the thoracic region have been reported (Gal et al. 1997), and three different procedures in the lumbar spine ranged from 1807 N/s to 2483 N/s (Triano & Schultz 1997).

The benefits of varying the control factors are based on the experience of skilled operators. Despite the large variation of force amplitudes and speeds reported across operators and procedures, recent evidence suggests that individual trained operators can systematically vary the forces they apply (Triano et al. 2006). The differences in clinical application seem to be related to the stature of the patient (Triano, unpublished data).

Studies of physiologic biomarker responses to HVLA procedures suggest that different outcomes can be determined by varying the parameters of control. Only a few biomarkers associated with manual therapy have been studied. They include three types of measure: 1) responses associated with joint motion; 2) circulating components related to the inflammatory cascade; and 3) the response of fibroblasts to mechanical perturbation. Paraspinal muscle spindles are over five times more responsive to changes in spinal orientation than are peripheral muscles (Cao et al. 2009). Impulse loads, consistent with HVLA at approximately 100 ms, produce a higher-frequency spindle discharge than do forces developed more slowly. Paradoxically, lower-amplitude (1 mm) displacements were more effective than 2 mm displacements (Pickar & Kang 2006; Pickar et al. 2007). Procedures inducing greater segmental rotation evoke larger responses than do sagittal-plane posteroanterior procedures. Patterns of vertebral motion and capsular strain during impulse procedures are significantly greater than with physiological rotations (Ianuzzi & Khalsa 2005). Vertebral translations occur primarily in the direction of the applied load. Both vertebral rotations and facet capsule strain magnitudes are within the ranges that occur during physiological motion.

The baseline levels of circulating factors associated with the inflammatory cascade have also been monitored. Brennan and others (Brennan et al. 1991, Triano et al. 1976) demonstrated an increase in white blood cell chemiluminescence in response to particulate challenge lasting up to 45 minutes after manipulation applied to the thoracic and lumbar spine regions. A threshold effect was observed, a 400 N force being required to trigger a response. Similar effects were not observed when the same level of force was applied to the gluteal muscle (Triano, unpublished data). Other mediators showing effects from HVLA included an increase in TNF-α and substance P. Altered balance of the cytokines from the inflammatory cascade (Fig. 6.5) has been observed for up to 2 hours in comparison to sham maneuvers (Teodorczyk-Injeyan et al. 2006). In contrast to the early work by Brennan et al. (1991), TNF-α did not show a response to HVLA.

Fibroblast behavior as a biomarker in response to mechanical perturbation associated

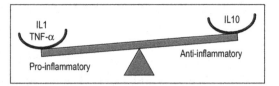

Figure 6.5 Example of the balance of cytokines involved in the inflammatory cascade following HVLA and not observed in sham procedures.

with needling of the tissues (Langevin et al. 2005) and from directional stretching in vitro (Eagan et al. 2007) has begun to be studied. Mechanotransduction with cytoskeletal remodeling and change in cell morphology was observed in response to mechanical perturbation over a 20–30-minute period. Using acupuncture needle oscillation in mouse dermal tissue, extensive cell spreading and lamellipodia formation was observed. Cell surface area increased by a factor of 2 (Langevin et al. 2004) and was sensitive to cycle amplitude and number. Spreading within the cell was found to be associated with redistribution of intracellular actin filaments (Langevin et al. 2006). Whereas these reactions to a therapeutic intervention represent a significant technical advance in our understanding of potential effects, a more startling observation made by this group was that the local mechanical stimulus cascaded from one cell to another. That is, lamellipodia formation and spreading occurring in one cell close to the stimulus was seen to influence the next more distant cell to do the same over a range of approximately 4 cm (Langevin, personal communication). This has led to speculation about the presence of a body-wide cellular signaling system (Langevin et al. 2004).

Working in vitro, fibroblasts were exposed to symmetrical and asymmetrical planar strain. Symmetrical strain exhibited a significant decrease in proliferation, production of inflammatory interleukin (IL)-6 secretion and macrophage-derived chemoattractant/chemokine secretion (Eagan et al. 2007). These changes suggest load directional preferences, at least from prolonged strain conditions. Studies on more transient loads as seen with therapeutic efforts remain to be carried out.

Conclusions

Strong biological evidence shows that all tissues and cells are able to sense their mechanical environment and to respond to it. Physical stimulus is interpreted directly by the cell in addition to triggering neurosensory efferents that inform the system as a whole of the local conditions. Stretch-sensitive membrane channels alter the ionic balance across the membrane and interact directly with the cytoskeletal infrastructure. Transmembrane integrins connect the extracellular matrix directly to the CSK. Tissue layers are organized cross-sectionally with a collagen-reinforced matrix that aggregrates superficially into fascial sheets and planes. Loads are carried through the layers by the connective tissue surrounding neurovascular tracts that supply the tissues, and by interconnections of fascia. Epimuscular force transmission is the best-studied cross-sectional force transfer mechanism. Beginning with shear loading in the endomysium, force is collected and shared with surrounding structures. The result is, as yet, an incompletely understood pattern of force distribution that results in local concentrations or dissipation of strain that cannot be directly predicted from empirical observation of the anatomy. The final response of the cell is influenced by the geometry and properties of the tissues in which it resides and contributes to the more centrally driven neurological and endocrine coordination.

Manual therapies rely on body tissues to absorb, dissipate, and respond to interventional procedures. Recent work has begun to characterize the biomechanical factors associated with manual treatments. There is a wide disparity between the reported forces applied during manual procedures and those necessary at the microstrain level to affect a triggering of the mechanosensitive ligand receptors in cell membranes. The difference itself implies that there is significant dissipation of loads within the tissues during therapy. Tissues appear to be load direction, intensity and speed dependent in their responses. Skilled operators are able to systematically modify the various parameters of therapeutic loading to accentuate or minimize the active parameter.

A gaping hole in our knowledge needs to be filled before the information that has been developed on the biomechanics of manual treatment and cellular mechanotransduction can meaningfully inform clinical practice. That gap is in the area of mechanobiology of load transfer from the site of application to the targeted tissues. How much effective loading reaches the tissue of interest? What part do higher centers play in coordinating response to various loading forces and vectors of forces? Which type of load is important? What are the effective joint angles necessary to optimally load target tissues? What are the effective parameters of dosage necessary to trigger desirable physiological responses? What are the mechanisms for remote effects from mechanical treatment? What modifications will be needed to the delivery of manual care to optimize outcomes?

These questions have been daunting for physicians and therapists who use manual loading of the body to effect change. The new technological approaches to interrogating the body and its responses to treatment must be coupled with clinical trials to determine the clinically relevant factors. Armed with the combined mechanistic and practical clinical information, providers in the next 20 years should be more able to determine which patients will respond well to manual therapy and select therapies with more reliable and predictable outcomes than is possible today.

References

Bakris, G., Dickholtz Sr., M., Meyer, P.M., et al., 2007. Atlas vertebra realignment and achievement of arterial pressure goal in hypertensive patients: a pilot study. J. Hum. Hypertens. 21 (5), 347–352.

Bergmark, A., 1989. Stability of the lumbar spine. A study in mechanical engineering. Acta Orthop. Scand. Suppl. 230, 1–54.

Brennan, P.C., Kokjohn, K., Kaltinger, C.J., et al., 1991. Enhanced phagocytic cell respiratory burst induced by spinal manipulation: potential role of substance P. J. Manipulative Physiol. Ther. 14 (7), 399–408.

Burkholder, T.J., 2007. Mechanotransduction in skeletal muscle. Front. Biosci. 174–191.

Cao, D.Y., Khalsa, P.S., Pickar, J.G., 2009. Dynamic responsiveness of lumbar paraspinal muscle spindles during vertebral movement in the cat. Exp. Brain Res.

Chaffin, D.B., Andersson, G., 1984. Occupational Biomechanics. John Wiley & Sons.

Degenhardt, B.F., Kuchera, M.L., 2006. Osteopathic evaluation and manipulative treatment in reducing the morbidity of otitis media: a pilot study. J. Am. Osteopath. Assoc. 106 (6), 327–334.

Eagan, T.S., Meltzer, K.R., Standley, P.R., 2007. Importance of strain direction in regulating human fibroblast proliferation and cytokine secretion: a useful in vitro model for soft tissue injury and manual medicine treatments. J. Manipulative Physiol. Ther. 30 (8), 584–592.

Gal, J., Herzog, W., Kawchuk, G., Conway, P.J., Zhang, Y.T., 1997. Movements of vertebrae during manipulative thrusts to unembalmed human cadavers. J. Manipulative Physiol. Ther. 20 (1), 30–40.

Hamill, O.P., Martinac, B., 2001. Molecular basis of mechanotransduction in living cells. Physiol. Rev. 81 (2), 68–740.

Hawk, C., Khorsan, R., Lisi, A.J., Ferrance, R.J., Evans, M.W., 2007. Chiropractic care for nonmusculoskeletal conditions: a systematic review with implications for whole systems research. J. Altern. Complement. Med. 13 (5), 491–512.

Henderson, C.N., Cramer, G.D., Zhang, Q., DeVocht, J.W., Fournier, J.T., 2007. Introducing the external link model for studying spine fixation and misalignment: part 1 - Need, rationale, and applications. J. Manipulative Physiol. Ther. 30 (3), 239–245.

Henderson, C.N., Cramer, G.D., Zhang, Q., DeVocht, J.W., Fournier, J.T., 2007. Introducing the external link model for studying spine fixation and misalignment: part 2, Biomechanical features. J. Manipulative Physiol. Ther. 30 (4), 279–294.

Herzog, W., 1998. Movements of vertebrae during manipulative thrusts to unembalmed human cadavers. J. Manipulative Physiol. Ther. 21 (5), 373–374.

Herzog, W., 2000. The mechanical, neuromuscular, and physiologic effects produced by spinal manipulation. In: Herzog, W. (Ed.), Clinical Biomechanics of Spinal Manipulation. Churchill Livingstone, Philadelphia, pp. 191–207.

Howarth, S.J., Allison, A.E., Grenier, S.G., Cholewicki, J., McGill, S.M., 2004. On the implications of interpreting the stability index: a spine example. J. Biomech. 37 (8), 1147–1154.

Huang, H., Kamm, R.D., Lee, R.T., 2004. Cell mechanics and mechanotransduction: pathways, probes, and physiology. Am. J. Physiol. Cell Physiol. 287 (1), C1–C11.

Huang, S., Ingber, D.E., 2005. Cell tension, matrix mechanics, and cancer development. Cancer Cell 8 (3), 175–176.

Huijing, P.A., 2007. Epimuscular myofascial force transmission between antagonistic and synergistic muscles can explain movement limitation in spastic paresis. J. Electromyogr. Kinesiol. 17 (6), 708–724.

Huijing, P.A., van de Langenberg, R.W., Meesters, J.J., Baan, G.C., 2007. Extramuscular myofascial force transmission also occurs between synergistic muscles and antagonistic muscles. J. Electromyogr. Kinesiol. 17 (6), 680–689.

Ianuzzi, A., Khalsa, P.S., 2005. High loading rate during spinal manipulation produces unique facet joint capsule strain patterns compared with axial rotations. J. Manipulative Physiol. Ther. 28 (9), 673–687.

Ingber, D.E., 1997. Tensegrity: the architectural basis of cellular mechanotransduction. Annu. Rev. Physiol. 59, 575–599.

Ingber, D.E., 2003. Mechanobiology and diseases of mechanotransduction. Ann. Med. 35 (8), 564–577.

Jaalouk, D.E., Lammerding, J., 2009. Mechanotransduction gone awry. National Review of Molecular and Cellular Biology 10 (1), 63–73.

Jalali, S., del Pozo, M.A., Chen, K., Miao, H., Li, Y., Schwartz, M.A., et al., 2001. Integrin-mediated mechanotransduction requires its dynamic interaction with specific extracellular matrix (ECM) ligands. Proc. Natl. Acad. Sci. USA 98 (3), 1042–1046.

Kamm, R.D., Kaazempur-Mofrad, M.R., 2004. On the molecular basis for mechanotransduction. Mech. Chem. Biosyst. 1 (3), 201–209.

Katsumi, A., Orr, A.W., Tzima, E., Schwartz, M.A., 2004. Integrins in mechanotransduction. J. Biol. Chem. 279 (13), 12001–12004.

Kimberly, P.E., 2006. Outline of Osteopathic Manipulative Procedures. Walsworth Publishing, Mareline.

Kirstukas, S.J., Backman, J., 1999. Physician-applied contact pressure and table force response during unilateral thoracic manipulation. J. Manipulative Physiol. Ther. 22 (5), 269–279.

Langevin, H.M., Cornbrooks, C.J., Taatjes, D.J., 2004. Fibroblasts form a body-wide cellular network. Histochem. Cell Biol. 122 (1), 7–15.

Langevin, H.M., Bouffard, N.A., Badger, G.J., Iatridis, J.C., Howe, A.K., 2005. Dynamic fibroblast cytoskeletal response to subcutaneous tissue stretch ex vivo and in vivo. Am. J. Physiol. Cell Physiol. 288 (3), C747–C756.

Langevin, H.M., Storch, K.N., Cipolla, M.J., White, S.L., Buttolph, T.R., Taatjes, D.J., 2006. Fibroblast spreading induced by connective tissue stretch involves intracellular redistribution of alpha- and beta-actin. Histochem. Cell. Biol. 125 (5), 487–495.

Lee, M., Svensson, N.L., 1993. Effect of loading frequency on response of the spine to lumbar posteroanterior forces. J. Manipulative Physiol. Ther. 16 (7), 439–446.

Lotz, J.C., Staples, A., Walsh, A., Hsieh, A.H., 2004. In: Mechanobiology in intervertebral disc degeneration and regeneration. Conference Proceedings, Institute of Electrical and Electronics Engineers English Medical and Biological Society 7. pp. 5459.

Maniotis, A.J., Chen, C.S., Ingber, D.E., 1997. Demonstration of mechanical connections between integrins, cytoskeletal filaments, and nucleoplasm that stabilize nuclear structure. Proc. Natl. Acad. Sci. 94 (3), 849–854.

Mayers, T.W., 2009. Anatomy Trains, Myofascial Meridians for Manual and Movement Therapists. second ed. Elsevier, New York.

McGill, S.M., 2007. Evidence Based Prevention and Rehabilitation. Low Back Disorders. Kinetics Publishers, Champaign.

Noll, D.R., Degenhardt, B.F., Johnson, J.C., Burt, S.A., 2008. Immediate effects of osteopathic manipulative treatment in elderly patients with chronic obstructive pulmonary disease. J. Am. Osteopath. Assoc. 108 (5), 251–259.

Ogon, M., Bender, B.R., Hooper, D.M., et al., 1997. A dynamic approach to spinal instability. Part II: Hesitation and giving-way during interspinal motion. Spine 22 (24), 2859–2866.

Pickar, J.G., Kang, Y.M., 2006. Paraspinal muscle spindle responses to the duration of a spinal manipulation under force control. J. Manipulative Physiol. Ther. 29 (1), 22–31.

Pickar, J.G., Sung, P.S., Kang, Y.M., Ge, W., 2007. Response of lumbar paraspinal muscles spindles is greater to spinal manipulative loading compared with slower loading under length control. Spine J. 7 (5), 583–595.

Preuss, R., Fung, J., 2005. Can acute low back pain result from segmental spinal buckling during sub-maximal activities? A review of the current literature. Man. Ther. 10 (1), 14–20.

Rijkelijkhuizen, J.M., Meijer, H.J., Baan, G.C., Huijing, P.A., 2007. Myofascial force transmission also occurs between antagonistic muscles located within opposite compartments of the rat lower hind limb. J. Electromyogr. Kinesiol. 17 (6), 690–697.

Shaw, W.S., van der Windt, D.A., Main, C.J., Loisel, P., Linton, S.J., 2009. Early patient screening and intervention to address individual-level occupational factors ('blue flags') in back disability. J. Occup. Rehabil. 19 (1), 64–80.

Solomonow, D., Davidson, B., Zhou, B.H., Lu, Y., Patel, V., Solomonow, M., 2008. Neuromuscular neutral zones response to cyclic lumbar flexion. J. Biomech. 41 (13), 2821–2828.

Sovak, G., Triano, J.J., 2009. Non-uniform psoas deformation under tensile load corresponds to superficial dense connective tissue morphology. Proceedings ACC-RAC Conference, Las Vegas, Mar 14.

Suki, B., Ito, S., Stamenovic, D., Lutchen, K.R., Ingenito, E.P., 2005. Biomechanics of the lung parenchyma: critical roles of collagen and mechanical forces. J. Appl. Physiol. 98 (5), 1892–1899.

Tavi, P., Laine, M., Weckstrom, M., Ruskoaho, H., 2001. Cardiac mechanotransduction: from sensing to disease and treatment. Trends Pharmacol. Sci. 22 (5), 254–260.

Teodorczyk-Injeyan, J.A., Injeyan, H.S., Ruegg, R., 2006. Spinal manipulative therapy reduces inflammatory cytokines but not substance P production in normal subjects. J. Manipulative Physiol. Ther. 29 (1), 14–21.

Triano, J.J., 2001. Biomechanics of spinal manipulative therapy. Spine J. 1 (2), 121–130.

Triano, J.J., 2005a. The theorectical basis for spinal manipulation. In: Principles and Practice of Chiropractic. McGraw-Hill, Philadelphia.

Triano, J.J., 2005b. Buckling, A Biomechanical Model of Subluxation. In: Gatterman, M.I. (Ed.), Foundations of Chiropractic: Subluxation. Mosby.

Triano, J.J., 2008. What constitutes evidence for best practice? J. Manipulative Physiol. Ther. 31 (9), 637–643.

Triano, J.J., Schultz, A.B., 1997. Loads transmitted during lumbosacral spinal manipulative therapy. Spine 22 (17), 1955–1964.

Triano, J.J., McGregor, M., Hondras, M.A., Brennan, P.C., 1976. Manipulative therapy versus education programs in chronic low back pain. Spine 20 (8), 948–955.

Triano, J.J., Scaringe, J., Bougie, J., Rogers, C., 2006. Effects of visual feedback on manipulation performance and patient ratings. J. Manipulative Physiol. Ther. 29 (5), 378–385.

Triano, J.J., Sovak, G., Cambridge, E., 2009a. Fascia dependent tri-axial deformation and strain of psoas under manipulation preload conditions. Proceedings ACC-RAC Conference, Las Vegas, Mar 14.

Triano, J.J., Cambridge, E., LeBlanc, F., Tran, S., Sovak, G., 2009b. Psoas non-uniform tri-axial deformation and strain under tensile preload conditions corresponds to superficial dense connective tissue morphology. Fascia Research Congress, Virie University, Amsterdam, Oct 27.

Turner, C.H., Pavalko, F.M., 1998. Mechanotransduction and functional response of the skeleton to physical stress: the mechanisms and mechanics of bone adaptation. J. Orthop. Sci. 3 (6), 346–355.

Van Zoest, G.G., Gosselin, G., 2003. Three-dimensionality of direct contact forces in chiropractic spinal manipulative therapy. J. Manipulative Physiol. Ther. 26 (9), 549–556.

Wilder, D.G., Pope, M.H., Seroussi, R.E., Dimnet, J., Krag, M.H., 1989. The balance point of the intervertebral motion segment: an experimental study. Bulletin Hospital of Joint Disease Orthopedic Institute 49 (2), 155–169.

Wilder, D.G., 1993. The biomechanics of vibration and low back pain. Am. J. Ind. Med. 23 (4), 577–588.

Yang, J.H., Briggs, W.H., Libby, P., Lee, R.T., 1998. Small mechanical strains selectively suppress matrix metalloproteinase-1 expression by human vascular smooth muscle cells. J. Biol. Chem. 273 (11), 6550–6555.

Youssef, J., Davidson, B., Zhou, B.H., Lu, Y., Patel, V., Solomonow, M., 2008. Neuromuscular neutral zones response to static lumbar flexion: muscular stability compensator. Clin. Biomech. (Bristol, Avon) 23 (7), 870–880.

Yucesoy, C.A., Baan, G., Huijing, P.A., 2008. Epimuscular myofascial force transmission occurs in the rat between the deep flexor muscles and their antagonistic muscles. Dec 3 J. Electromyogr. Kinesiol. [Epub ahead of print].

Section Two
Segmental and suprasegmental mediation of somatovisceral interactions

Spinothalamic system and viscerosomatic motor reflexes: functional organization of cardiac and somatic input

Robert D Foreman • Chao Qin • Chuanchau Jerry Jou

Introduction

Osteopathic manual manipulation is built upon the concept of reflex phenomena that involve the nervous system, viscera, and somatic tissues. Clinical studies and research reports have provided support for the existence of viscerosomatic and somatovisceral reflexes. These reflexes provide a two-way communication between the musculoskeletal system and the visceral organs as well as other systems. Moreover, manual manipulation is dependent not only on somatoautonomic processing and control via the nervous system, but also on the multiple and varied chemical routes of communication as well as the mechanical effects of musculoskeletal activity on viscera and on the movement of lymph and blood (Korr 1991). Although all these lines of communication are available, this chapter will address the mechanisms that are dependent on neural control related to the heart.

Normally cardiac function does not appear to be involved with the performance of the myotomes and dermatomes that are innervated by nerves from the upper thoracic spinal segments. In a similar manner, under normal circumstances the activities of the paraspinal musculature located on the upper thoracic segments do not appear to contribute to cardiac function. However, in pathological conditions such as ischemic heart disease, myocardial ischemia appears to link the heart with the upper thoracic somatic structures in a 'self-sustaining circuit of autogenic impulses' (Korr 1991). The result of this linkage is that pain is not felt as originating from the heart but is referred most commonly to the overlying somatic structures of the upper thoracic segments.

Patients with ischemic heart disease usually seek medical care when they experience the symptom of cardiac pain know as angina pectoris. The most typical manifestation is retrosternal pain described as crushing, burning, and/or squeezing (Bonica 1990, Harrison & Reeves 1968, Procacci & Zoppi 1989, Sampson & Cheitlin 1971) (Fig. 7.1A). Pain may also radiate to the throat, neck, or ulnar aspect of the left arm, sometimes reaching to the little finger. Less often, it radiates to the neck and jaw, or either the right or both arms. Angina pectoris may also be associated with the subjective sensation of anguish and fear of impending death. However, there is a great variability in the location of cardiac pain between patients and with the associated subjective sensations (Maseri et al. 1992). In addition to referred pain, functional changes can occur in muscle, skin, and bone.

Angina pectoris can also generate changes in the paraspinal muscles of the upper thoracic segments. Muscular changes resulting from the viscerosomatic reflex are characterized as a condition of exaggerated tone of the paraspinal muscles (Burns 1907). Furthermore, there appear to be at least two adjacent segments with confluent deep muscle splinting (Beal 1983). Theories in manual medicine have proposed that visceral spinal afferent pathways play a role in modifying the muscle tone of the upper thoracic paraspinal groups in response to changes in cardiac function (Beal 1989, Beal & Kleiber 1985, Cox et al. 1983, Larson 1976, Nicholas et al. 1985, 1991). Patients with cardiovascular disease have revealed a common spinal reflex 'somatic dysfunction' pattern involving spinal segments T1–T5, with the greatest incidence between T2 and T4 on the left side (Beal 1983, 1985, Beal & Kleiber 1985, Cox et al. 1983, Larson 1976) (Fig. 7.1B).

The purpose of this chapter is to describe the mechanisms that underlie the characteristics of referred pain of angina pectoris; and discuss the behavior and neural pathways of cardiosomatic motor reflexes associated with angina pectoris resulting from ischemic heart disease.

Spinal processing of cardiac nociceptive information

The section will address the neural mechanisms underlying angina pectoris by focusing on spinal processing of cardiac nociceptive impulses. Studies have shown that the C1–C2, C5–C6, and T2–T4 segments of the spinal cord are necessary for processing information in the neural hierarchy that regulates cardiac control (Foreman 1999).

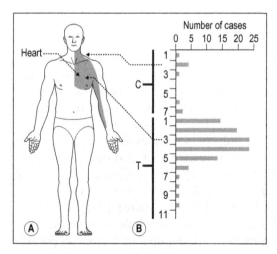

Figure 7.1 Diagrams of the general area of referred pain (A) and change in the tonicity of paraspinal muscles (B) resulting from patients experiencing angina pectoris. In (B) palpatory techniques were used in patients with ischemic heart disease to determine changes in paraspinal muscles. The abscissa is the number of cases and the ordinate is the spinal segment level from cervical segment 1 (C1) to thoracic segment 12 (T11). The arrows from the graph to the human figure indicate the location of the equivalent segments. (B) is adapted from Beal (1985).

Spinothalamic tract cells and spinal neurons have been examined to study the effects evoked by electrical stimulation of the visceral spinal or vagal afferent fibers, the application of bradykinin or other algesic chemicals into the heart or into the pericardial sac, occlusion of the coronary arteries, and stimulation of the skin and muscle in various animal models.

Activation of cardiac nociceptors

Angina pectoris often results from ischemic episodes that excite chemosensitive and mechanoreceptive receptors in the heart (see Coleridge & Coleridge 1980, Foreman 1999, Longhurst et al. 2001 for review). Ischemic episodes release a barrage of chemicals, including adenosine and bradykinin, which excite receptors of the visceral spinal afferent and vagal afferent pathways. The discovery of the chemicals that are released during periods of myocardial ischemia and activating spinal afferent fibers innervating the heart may be important for treating angina pectoris; however, there is very little information about the receptors involved. Recently, it has been proposed that the onset of angina pectoris associated with myocardial ischemia may depend on the activation of the transient receptor potential vanilloid-1 (TRPV1). This receptor is a molecular integrator of noxious stimuli that is specifically expressed in the plasma membrane of nociceptive afferent fibers and opens an important nonspecific cation channel that is activated by capsaicin (CAP), heat stimuli, and protons (Caterina et al. 1997, Pan & Chen 2004). It has been shown that TRPV1-expressing afferent nerves are distributed extensively on the epicardial surface of the rat ventricle (Zahner et al. 2003). Epicardial application of CAP excites visceral spinal afferent fibers and produces sympathoexcitatory reflexes (Pan & Chen 2004, Schultz & Ustinova 1998, Zahner et al. 2003); TRPV1 antagonists can eliminate these effects. Injections of CAP into the left atrium or pericardial sac also

activate spinal and spinoreticular neurons in cats (Bolser et al. 1989) and rats (Qin et al. 2006). These results suggest that excitation of TRPV1-containing visceral spinal afferent fibers might excite spinal neurons that receive convergent input from the heart and overlying somatic structures. To support this suggestion, we have shown that the majority of upper thoracic spinal neurons with cardiac input responded to intrapericardial administration of BK or CAP and received somatic input from structures overlying the heart (Qin et al. 2006). To determine whether TRPV1-containing fibers were responsible for transmitting this cardiac nociceptive information, resinferatoxin (RTX), an ultrapotent analog of CAP, was used to desensitize the fibers (Karai et al. 2004, Pan et al. 2003, Raisingani et al. 2005, Szallasi and Blumberg 1989, Wu et al. 2006, 2007). RTX causes TRPV1 to become permeable to cations, specifically Ca^{2+} ions, and evokes a powerful sensitization that is followed within 20 minutes by desensitization and analgesia.

Desensitization of cardiac visceral spinal afferent fibers containing TRPV1 with intrapericardial RTX eliminated excitatory neuronal responses to BK, CAP, and also to a cocktail of algesic chemicals (BK, serotonin, PGE2, histamine, and adenosine) released during myocardial ischemia (Foreman 1999, Meller & Gebhart 1992, Qin et al. 2006) (Fig. 7.2). However, selective blockade of TRPV1-containing afferent fibers with intrapericardial capsazepine significantly attenuated the activation of spinal neurons by CAP but did not affect neuronal responses to BK or to somatic manipulation. These results provided evidence that CAP-sensitive visceral spinal afferent fibers play an important role in the activation of upper thoracic spinal neurons by cardiac noxious stimuli. However, the BK-elicited spinal neuronal responses are not dependent upon TRPV1 receptors at the nerve endings of cardiac afferents. It has been proposed that visceral spinal afferent fibers containing TRPV1

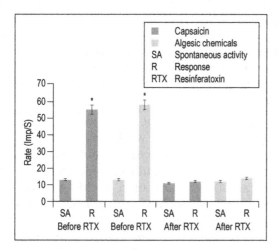

Figure 7.2 Effects of pretreatment of the heart with resinferatoxin (RTX) on excitatory responses of T3–T4 spinal neurons to intrapericardial injections of capsaicin, or a mixture of algogenic chemicals. SA, Spontaneous Activity. R, Response representing maximal activity during administration of intrapericardial chemicals that activated cardiac spinal visceral afferent fibers. Values are presented as means ± SEM. *P ≤ 0.01 compared to corresponding spontaneous activity (SA). Adapted from Qin et al. (2006).

may operate as molecular sensors, because this receptor and receptor channel complex can activate cardiac nociceptors by detecting the release of BK, ATP, serotonin, and lipid metabolites as well as changes in pH that commonly occur with tissue ischemia (Julius & Basbaum 2001, Pan & Chen 2004). In summary, these new findings are important to advance our understanding about the afferent mechanisms that may contribute to angina pectoris and the phenotypes of visceral spinal afferent neurons that are involved in the activation of sympathetic reflexes to myocardial ischemia.

Neural mechanisms of referred pain in upper thoracic spinal cord

Visceral spinal afferent fibers from the heart enter the upper thoracic spinal cord and synapse on cells of origin of ascending pathways. This review focuses on the spinothalamic tract (STT), but other pathways are excited as well (Foreman 1999). The

responses of individual STT cells, which have their origin in the gray matter of the thoracic spinal cord, to nociceptive input from the heart have been assessed by transient coronary artery occlusion or injection of algesic chemicals into the heart, followed by examination of somatic fields (Fig. 7.3) (see Foreman 1999). The STT projects to the medial and lateral thalamus and, based on positron emission tomography studies,

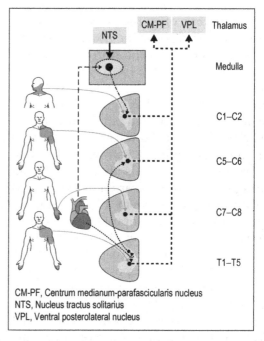

Figure 7.3 Schematic diagram of the neural mechanisms to explain the referral of pain of angina pectoris in the chest and arm (C5–C6, T1–T5) and the neck and jaw (C1–C2). The *heavy dashed line* originating from the small circle in the spinal gray matter and ascending to the thalamus represents spinothalamic tract cells arising from different spinal segments. The shaded gray area on each figurine represents somatic receptive fields and the *solid gray lines* represent somatic afferent fibers. The dotted lines represent the cardiac spinal visceral afferent fibers that enter the T1–T5 segments and the ascending pathway bypassing the C7–C8 segments and entering the upper cervical segments. The *long-dashed lines* represent the vagal afferent fibers that synapse on neurons in the nucleus tractus solitarius (NTS) and the NTS neurons descend to synapse on neurons in the C1–C2 segments (dash-dot-dash line). CM-PF, centrum medianum–parafascicular nucleus of the medial thalamus; VPL, ventral posterolateral nucleus of the lateral thalamus. Adapted from Foreman (1999).

activates several cortical areas, including the anterior cingulate gyrus, the insula, the lateral basal frontal cortex, and the mesiofrontal cortex (see Foreman 1999, Jänig 2006, Chapter 2).

In general, three main characteristics can be used to describe angina pectoris:

1. Nociceptive information originating from the heart is commonly expressed as pain in overlying somatic structures.
2. The pain is referred to proximal and axial somatic structures.
3. The pain is described as deep and aching.

The following sections will discuss the possible neurophysiological mechanisms that can be used to explain the characteristics of angina pectoris.

Convergence of somatic and visceral input

Chemical or electrical activation of cardiac visceral spinal afferent fibers excites approximately 80% of the STT cells located in the lamina I and laminae V–VII of the T1–T6 spinal segments (Ammons et al. 1985, Blair et al. 1982, Hobbs et al. 1992) (Fig. 7.4A, B).

It should be noted that these afferent fibers are most likely polymodal, and when excited they activate protective reflexes, regulate cardiac function, and elicit pain (see Jänig 2006). These STT cells also receive somatic input from the chest and upper arm (Fig. 7.4C). In addition, approximately 60% of the STT neurons in the C5–C6 segments also receive afferent input from the heart (Hobbs et al. 1992). It is important to note that STT cells in the cervical enlargement (C7, C8) are activated by somatic input from the distal forelimb and hand but receive very little input from activation of the cardiopulmonary fibers (Hobbs et al. 1992). These results might explain the clinical observations that angina pectoris generally is not referred to the distal forearm and hand (Harrison & Reeves 1968, Procacci & Zoppi 1989, Sampson & Cheitlin 1971).

Anatomical studies have shown that cardiac visceral spinal afferent fibers generally enter the T1–T5 segments but not the C5–C6 segments (Hopkins & Armour 1989, Kuo et al. 1984, Vance & Bowker 1983). Thus, information transmitted in the upper thoracic spinal visceral afferent fibers may activate a propriospinal pathway that makes synaptic connections with the C5–C6 STT cells (Nowicki & Szulczyk 1980) and/or branches of the T2 and T3 afferent fibers may travel for several segments in the zone of Lissauer and then terminate on C5–C6 STT neurons (Sugiura et al. 1989). This last possibility is less likely because the branches

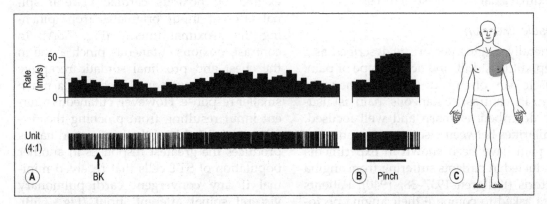

Figure 7.4 Responses of T3 spinothalamic tract cell to intracardiac injections of bradykinin that activated cardiac spinal visceral afferent fibers **(A)** and to pinching **(B)** the skin and muscle of a typical somatic receptive field **(C)**. The upper tracings in **(A)** and **(B)** are the rate of discharge (Imp/s) of extracellular action potentials of the spinothalamic tract cell and the bottom tracings represent the individual action potentials (4:1, each line represents four action potentials. The shaded area in **(C)** is the somatic receptive field. Adapted from Blair et al. (1982).

would need to bypass the cervical enlargement in order to reach the upper cervical segments. However, it is possible that during fetal development neurochemical messages from cells in the cervical enlargement (C7–C8) may prevent branches from forming synapses in these segments, but at present this is speculative. In summary, visceral and somatic input converges onto a common pool of STT cells; this provides a substrate to explain pain referred to overlying somatic structures.

Referral to proximal and axial somatic structures

Human studies have shown that the pain of angina pectoris generally radiates to the chest more than 95% of the time and to the left proximal shoulder 30–60% of the time. Pain is felt much less frequently further down the arm (Bennet & Atkinson 1966, Sampson & Cheitlin 1971, Sylvén 1989). It has been shown that stimulation of the cardiopulmonary visceral spinal afferent fibers strongly activated approximately 80% of the C5–C6 and T1–T5 STT cells receiving input from proximal somatic receptive fields, but only 35% of cells with distal somatic input were weakly excited (Hobbs et al. 1992). These results support the clinical observations that angina pectoris most commonly radiates to proximal axial somatic structures.

Muscle-like pain

Generally, angina pectoris is described as a deep, diffuse, dull, and aching type of pain. Muscle pain often is described in the same way. In contrast, cutaneous pain is usually described as sharp and well focused. Similarities between visceral pain and muscle pain have been shown in experiments conducted in patients suffering from angina pectoris (Kellgren 1937–38, 1940). Patients were asked to compare their angina pectoris pain with pain generated by injecting a hypertonic saline solution into the muscles surrounding the interspinous ligament of the left eighth cervical or first thoracic

segment. These patients noted that the onset, continuation, character, and segmental localization of the muscle pain were similar to the pain they experienced with angina pectoris (Kellgren 1937–38). Clinical and experimental studies have shown that diseases of visceral organs result in hyperalgesia of the overlying muscle. In patients calculosis of the upper urinary tract leads to the development of muscle hyperalgesia, but with less cutaneous involvement (Giamberardino et al. 1994, Vecchiet et al. 1989). Experimental studies have also shown that noxious stimulation of the ureter results in central sensitization of spinal neurons and muscle hyperalgesia (Giamberardino et al. 1996, 1997, Laird et al. 1996). The development of muscle hyperalgesia described in these studies may depend on viscerosomatic motor reflexes in a manner similar to the changes in the tonicity of thoracic paraspinal muscles resulting from activation of cardiosomatic reflexes, as described in the introduction and in a subsequent section.

Studies conducted to examine segments processing noxious cardiac input in the STT cells of the upper thoracic spinal cord supported the findings that pinching the proximal muscles can generate a strong noxious input (Hobbs et al. 1992). The predominant somatic afferent input to STT cells that are excited by noxious cardiac visceral spinal afferent input originates from pinching the proximal muscle (Fig. 7.5A). In contrast, noxious cutaneous pinch alone in the chest and proximal somatic receptive fields of the upper arm generated a much smaller response. However, cutaneous afferent input resulting from pinching the distal receptive fields of the fingers and hands produces the greatest responses in another population of STT cells that received minimal if any convergent cardiopulmonary visceral spinal afferent input (Fig. 7.5B). In summary, visceral spinal afferent input from cardiopulmonary fibers converged onto STT cells with proximal muscle input, whereas visceral afferent input has minimal

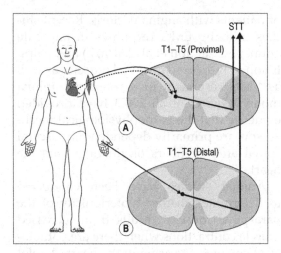

Figure 7.5 Activation of spinothalamic (STT) neurons with proximal receptive fields (solid line) **(A)** or distal receptive fields **(B)** to electrical stimulation of cardiopulmonary afferents (long dashed line). **(A)** Noxious muscle stimulation and to a much less extent cutaneous stimulation of the upper arm activated STT neurons that received convergent input from the cardiopulmonary afferent fibers. **(B)** In contrast, cutaneous, but not noxious, muscle stimulation of the hand (distal) activated STT cells; these cells did not receive cardiopulmonary input.

effect on STT cells receiving primarily distal cutaneous inputs (Fig. 7.5). As a result of this arrangement, nociceptive input generated during myocardial ischemia and infarction most likely mimics muscle pain. Thus, angina pectoris is most commonly felt as a deep, diffuse, aching pain that is generally referred to proximal and axial structures such as muscle, ligaments, and tendons.

Neural mechanisms of referred pain in the upper cervical spinal cord

Osteopathic literature, dental case studies, and interruption of cardiac spinal visceral afferent fibers to treat angina pectoris led us to examine an explanation for pain referral to the neck and jaw region during myocardial ischemic episodes. Manual medicine physicians have shown in a population of patients with cardiovascular disease that the segmental distribution of increased paraspinal tone in the majority of them was from segments T1 to T5, however, a few of the

patients had paraspinal tonicity changes in the C1–C3 segments (Beal 1985, Fig. 7.1B). Articles in the dental literature also report that myocardial ischemia elicits craniofacial pain as the only complaint in approximately 6% of dental patients (Kreiner & Okeson 1999, Kreiner et al. 2007, Tzukert et al. 1981). A recent case report has suggested that the vagal afferents may mediate angina pectoris expressed as jaw and tooth pain (Myers 2008). Early clinical observations of neck pain being unmasked after sympathectomy (to interrupt spinal visceral afferents from the heart) to reduce angina pectoris led to the hypothesis that STT cells in the C1–C2 region receive cardiac input (Lindgren & Olivecrona 1947, White et al. 1933, White & Bland 1948). Thus, these observations served as a basis for exploring neural mechanisms of referred pain in the cervical spinal cord. To address this hypothesis recordings of extracellular potentials were made from STT cells located in the C1–C2 spinal segments (Chandler et al. 1999, 2000). Coronary occlusion, injection of algesic chemicals into the heart before and after bilateral vagotomy, or electrical stimulation of cardiopulmonary visceral spinal afferent fibers and thoracic vagal afferents were used to activate the neurons.

Electrical stimulation of vagal and cardiac sympathetic nerves showed that STT and non-STT spinal neurons in C1–C2 were more responsive to stimulation of vagal afferents than of spinal cardiac afferents, and that the somatic fields for these cells were located primarily in the jaw and neck regions (Chandler et al. 1996, Qin et al. 2001). In addition, vagotomy markedly reduced the nociceptive input produced by algesic chemicals injected into the heart, as evidenced by reduced activity of STT and non-STT spinal neurons in the cervical region (Chandler et al. 2000, Qin et al. 2001) (Fig. 7.6).

Because only 6% of the vagal afferents project directly to the C1–C2 spinal neurons, the rest most likely ascend into the nucleus

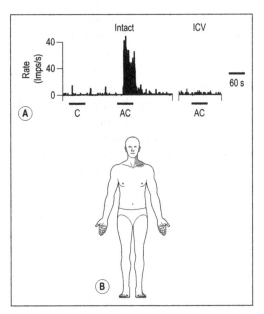

Figure 7.6 Effects of cervical vagotomy on evoked responses of a C2 spinal neuron to intrapericardial injections of algesic chemicals that activated cardiac visceral spinal afferent fibers. **(A)** Saline injection into the pericardial sac (C = Control) did not change cell activity. Intrapericardial injection of algesic chemicals (Intact, AC) evoked a strong response of the C2 neuron; this response was eliminated after ipsilateral cervical vagotomy (ipsilateral cervical vagotomy (ICV). The tracing represents the rate of discharge (Rate; imp/s) of the neuron. The shaded area in **(B)** represents a typical location of somatic receptive fields that activate C1–C2 neurons. Adapted from Qin et al. (2001).

tractus solitarius and then synapse on cells with axons projecting to the C1–C2 segments (McNeill et al. 1991) (Fig. 7.3). This finding suggests that the vagus plays an important role in relaying this information from the heart to the C1–C2 region. These results also support clinical observations that information transmitted in the vagus contributes to the referral of pain to the neck and jaw in some patients suffering from angina pectoris.

Cardiosomatic motor reflexes

This section focuses on cardiosomatic reflexes that may underlie tonicity changes observed in the thoracic paraspinal muscles of patients with angina pectoris. Recent studies utilizing EMG responses in an acute animal model (Jou et al. 2001a, b) and palpitation of thoracic paraspinal muscles as well as EMG responses in a conscious animal model (Gwirtz et al. 2007) have provided evidence that the pathophysiological mechanisms are primarily dependent on visceral spinal afferent fibers originating from the heart.

Animal studies have been conducted to determine whether hypertonicity of the paraspinal muscles results from increased muscle contractions when there are pathological changes occurring in the heart. A pilot study has shown that myocardial ischemia resulting from occlusion of the left coronary artery evoked EMG activity in the thoracic paraspinal muscles (Schoen & Finn 1978). In a more detailed study, infusion of algogenic chemicals (which are normally released during myocardial ischemia) into the pericardial sac evoked EMG activity in several paraspinal muscles of a rat, including the acromiotrapezius, splenius, rhomboideus thoracis, spinotrapezius, rhomboideus capitis, and thoracic latissimus dorsi (Jou et al. 2001a). Of these paraspinal muscles, the spinotrapezius at the T2–T4 vertebral level showed the highest percentage of positive EMG responses to the noxious cardiac stimulus.

Intrapericardial injections of noxious algogenic chemicals produced EMG responses that consisted of single-motor unit potentials and compound motor potentials (Jou et al. 2001a) (Fig. 7.7A).

A single-motor unit potential is the discharge of a single motor unit, whereas a compound motor potential is the summation of several single-motor units discharging at the same time. Generally speaking, the single-unit pattern of EMG activities consists of a low-amplitude and a prolonged discharge (>75 s). The prolonged discharge of the single-unit pattern of the EMGs may contribute to the development of chronic referred pain (Graven-Nielsen et al. 1997, Hoheisel et al. 1993, Marchettini et al. 1996).

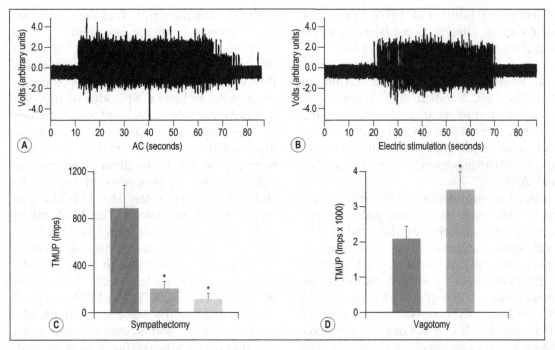

Figure 7.7 Effects of stimulation and nerve transections to determine neural pathways of the cardiosomatic motor reflexes. Noxious chemical stimulation of cardiac afferents with algesic chemicals (AC) **(A)** and electrical stimulation (Elec. Stim.) of the left sympathetic chain **(B)** evoked EMG activities in the paraspinal muscle **(A)** (spinotrapezius in rat). **(C)** Total motor unit potential EMG responses (TMUP) to intrapericardial injections of algesic chemicals in intact animals (dark gray bar) and 60 minutes (middle bar) and 120 minutes (third bar) after transections of cardiac spinal visceral afferent fibers (sympathectomy). **(D)** TMUP evoked by algesic chemicals in intact nerves (first bar) and 60 min after bilateral vagotomy (second bar). For C and D the data were analyzed by repeated ANOVA followed by Tukey's comparison: *P≤ 0.01, **P≤ 0.05. Adapted from Jou et al. (2001b).

This sustained pattern of EMG activity may also produce the characteristics of non-painful hypertonic muscle that can be palpated in patients with chronic heart disease (Beal 1985, Larson 1976). In contrast, the high-amplitude and complex characteristic of compound motor potentials, as well as their relatively brief discharge interval, is most commonly observed in the EMG responses of fatigued, ischemic, and painful muscles (Hudson et al. 1978, Zimmermann 1991). Thus, the complex component of the EMG response may contribute to the muscle pain that patients experience during the early phase of angina pectoris. In summary, the spasm-like characteristics and the sustained EMG activity suggest that noxious cardiac stimuli evoke reflex contractions of the spinotrapezius (paraspinal) muscles, resulting in the generation of muscle hypertonicity and hyperalgesia.

Neural pathways

Clinical practitioners of manual medicine have proposed but have not proved the neural pathways that are used to produce hypertonic paraspinal muscles in patients with chronic heart disease. Thus, transections and electrical stimulation have been performed in animal studies to determine the afferent neural pathways and their role in the generation of cardiosomatic motor reflexes. Convergence of muscle and cardiac visceral spinal afferents onto spinothalamic tract neurons may play an important role in referred muscle pain (Hobbs et al. 1992). In contrast, vagal cardiac afferents have been shown to inhibit the transmission of nociceptive information from spinal cardiac afferent fibers onto spinothalamic tract cells (Ammons et al. 1983a,b; Randich & Gebhart 1992). Thus, the studies were conducted to determine whether cardiac visceral spinal afferent fibers and vagal cardiac afferents had similar roles in cardiosomatic motor reflexes (Jou et al. 2001b).

Electrical stimulation of the left sympathetic chain near the stellate ganglion that contains the majority of the cardiac visceral spinal afferent fibers (Lindgren & Olivecrona, 1947, White et al. 1933, White & Bland 1948) evoked contractions in the spinotrapezius muscles (Fig. 7.7B). To support this finding, cardiosomatic motor reflexes to intrapericardial injections of algogenic chemicals were markedly suppressed after transection of spinal cardiac visceral afferent fibers (Fig. 7.7C).

In contrast to activation of the cardiosomatic motor reflexes via the cardiac visceral spinal afferent fibers, vagal afferent stimulation did not elicit the paraspinal EMG activity or change the ongoing EMG activity. However, vagal afferent stimulation suppressed evoked EMG activity resulting from activation of the spinal cardiac afferent fibers. In addition, vagal transection increased EMG responses to cardiac spinal nociceptive stimuli compared to the EMG responses with the intact vagal pathways (Fig. 7.7D). These results provide evidence that ongoing activity transmitted in vagal afferent fibers produces tonic suppression of the muscle contractions. This effect was unveiled when a major EMG response was evoked with noxious cardiac stimulation.

A chronic conscious animal model of myocardial ischemia supports and expands the finding that spinal visceral cardiac afferent fibers produces cardiosomatic motor reflexes of the paraspinal muscles (Gwirtz et al. 2007). Chronically instrumented canines with an intact peripheral nervous system or with selective interruption of the spinal cardiac afferents from the left ventricle were examined for changes in EMG activity and blinded manual palpatory assessments (MPA) before, during, and after episodes of myocardial ischemia. Episodes of myocardial ischemia were associated with increases in heart rate and reductions in regional myocardial contractile function. The MPA were performed on the tissue overlying the transverse spinal processes of the T2–T5 and T11–T12 segments. The T11–T12 segments served as controls. The MPA rating system was developed from standard manual medicine techniques (Ettlinger & Gintis 1991) and in agreement with manual medicine specialists (Gwirtz et al. 2007). As stated by Gwirtz et al. (2007), 'An MPA rating of '1' indicated that the tissue was soft, pliable, plastic, mobile, and symmetric (uniform) and that no somatic dysfunction is evident. A MPA rating of '5' indicated that the tissue was hard, irregular, not pliable, resistant to induced movement, bilateral, and marked somatic dysfunction is evident.' In the control state of neurally intact animals, muscle tension and texture at the T2–T5 and T11–T12 segments were soft and compliant as estimated by MPA (Fig. 7.8).

However, during the episodes of myocardial ischemia the physician conducting the MPA stated that the muscle texture was less compliant, firmer, and the muscle tension felt moderate to heavy in the T2–T5 segments (Fig. 7.8A). These changes were much less apparent in the T11–T12 segments (Fig. 7.8A). In addition, EMG recordings correlated with the MPA observations as demonstrated by an increase in amplitude for the measurements made in the T2–T5 segments compared to the amplitude for the T11–T12 segments (Fig. 7.8B). In contrast to the neurally intact animals, the animals with interruption of cardiac visceral spinal afferents innervating the left ventricle did not present with any palpatory or EMG changes during episodes of myocardial ischemia. The muscle texture and tension were soft

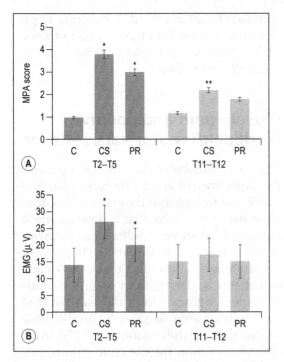

Figure 7.8 Manual palpatory assessments (MPA) **(A)** and EMG recordings **(B)** obtained during stenosis of the left circumflex coronary artery. The measurements were made at the T2–T5 segments (dark shaded bars) and the T11–T12 segments (light shaded bars). The T11–T12 segments served as controls. C, control; CS, coronary stenosis; PR, 15 minutes post release. Values are means ±SE. *$P \leq 0.05$ stenosis vs. control; **$P \leq 0.05$ coronary stenosis vs. 15 post release. Adapted from Gwirtz et al. (2007).

and compliant at the T2–T5 as well as the T11–T12 segments (not shown in Fig. 7.8).

Proposed pathways for cardiosomatic motor reflexes

The results of the studies described in the previous paragraphs are illustrated in Figure 7.9 to propose how cardiosomatic reflexes may function. These reflexes most likely activate motor neurons that innervate the paraspinal muscles, including the T2–T5 segments in humans (Beal 1985) and primarily the spinotrapezius muscle in rats. Most likely episodes of myocardial ischemia excite spinal cardiac nociceptive afferent neurons that enter the upper thoracic dorsal horn (Fig. 7.9, 1). These fibers synapse

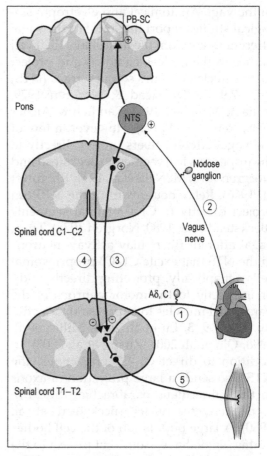

Figure 7.9 Summary diagram of functional spinal visceral and vagal afferent pathways of the cardiosomatic motor reflexes. The cardiac spinal afferent pathway (1) excites paraspinal muscle (5). Vagal afferent fibers (2) activate the nucleus tractus solitarii (NTS)→C1–C2 descending pathway (3) and the NTS→ parabrachial–subceruleus nucleus (PB-SC) descending inhibitory pathway (4); both descending systems inhibit motor activity (5). T1–T5, thoracic paraspinal muscles.

on interneurons in the spinal cord, mediating excitatory reflexes in motor neurons that contract paraspinal muscles of the upper thoracic segments (Fig. 7.9, 5).

As described in the previous section, our studies also show that activation of the vagal afferent fibers can modulate the motor activity of paraspinal muscles. Figure 7.9 shows the possible pathways involved in processing this information transmitted in the vagi. Anatomical and electrophysiological studies report that most of the vagal afferent fibers from the heart have their cell bodies in the nodose ganglion and project to the nucleus of the solitary tract (NTS) (Fig. 7.9, 2; Beckstead & Norgren 1979, Kalia & Mesulam 1980, Randich & Aicher 1988, Ren et al. 1990a). However, a few of the vagal afferent fibers project directly to the upper cervical segments (Beckstead and Norgren 1979, McNeill et al. 1991, Rhoton et al. 1966). Relay neurons from the NTS can project directly to C1–C3 spinal segments (Beckstead et al. 1980, Norgren 1978). Thus, vagal afferent fibers may activate neurons in the NTS that excite C1–C3 propriospinal cells synaptically, projecting directly and/or indirectly to the motor neurons of the paraspinal muscles to suppress their activity (Fig. 7.9, 3, Lu et al. 2004, Miller et al. 1998, Qin et al. 2004, Zhang et al. 2003). In addition to direct C1–C3 projections, the NTS also sends a large projection of axons to the subceruleus parabrachial (SC-PB)/locus ceruleus nuclei (Beckstead et al. 1980). A large population of the cell bodies in this region have axons that project to the spinal cord (Hancock & Fougerousse 1976, Takeuchi et al. 1980, Westlund & Coulter 1980, Westlund et al. 1984). Thus, activation of vagal afferent fibers can excite neurons of the SC-PB, which in turn suppress spinal neuronal processing (Fig. 7.9, 4, Ren et al. 1990b) and reduce muscle activity (Fig. 7.9, 5).

In summary, spinal cardiac fibers form the afferent limb of the reflexes to skeletal muscle that evoke EMG activity, whereas vagal cardiac afferent fibers form the afferent limb to inhibit the motor neurons innervating the paraspinal skeletal muscle. This inhibition is mediated via the NTS and cervical segments C1 and C2 and/or the parabrachial/subceruleus nucleus. Thus, increased levels of EMG activity evoked reflexly by noxious cardiac stimulation could be attributed to excitation of cardiac spinal afferents or suppressed vagal afferent activity, or both. It can also be speculated that myocardial ischemia might disturb the balance in transmission of information between the spinal cardiac and the vagal afferent pathways.

Muscle pain and positive feedback/feedforward reflexes

The contributions of muscle nociception to the experience of angina pectoris have been addressed throughout the previous sections. Here we hypothesize that a possible mechanism of positive feedback/feedforward spinal reflexes might explain the hypertonicity of paraspinal muscles that are palpated in patients suffering from angina pectoris. This idea originates from the positive feedback reflexes associated with chronic work-related myalgia (Johansson et al. 2003). In this clinical condition muscle contractions, possibly accompanied by the release of inflammatory chemicals, lead to sensitization of muscle nociceptors. In addition, 'shear' forces between non-synchronized contractions of motor units may excite nociceptors and contribute to the muscle pain and change in muscle tonicity. Long-term non-synchronized contractions of motor units may sensitize the muscle nociceptors (Johannson et al. 2003). These positive somatomotor reflex loops (Fig. 7.10, 2) critically involve the nociceptors in the muscles. Continuous feedback occurring in these loops may lead to the development of vicious cycles. The cycles may be enhanced by long-term changes in muscle morphology and sensitization of the nociceptors (Johansson et al. 2003). Based on this information and the processing of cardiac information described in the previous paragraphs, we have proposed the following positive feedback/feedforward hypothesis to explain the increased tonicity and muscle pain that is associated with ischemic heart disease (Fig. 7.10).

Ischemic episodes increase the activity of the spinal cardiac nociceptive afferent fibers. The bombardment of this noxious cardiac

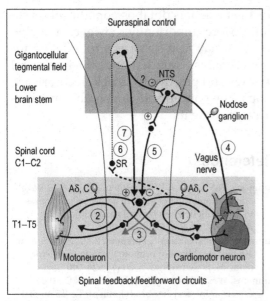

Figure 7.10 A hypothesis about possible cardiosomatic pathways providing positive feedforward reflexes during ischemic heart disease. Under normal conditions spinal cardiocardiac (1) and somatosomatic (2) feedback circuits participate in the regulation of the heart and muscle. During ischemic episodes a key point in the hypothesis is that spinal interneurons (3) provide a feedforward cardiosomatic reflex. Myocardial ischemia excites nociceptive cardiac Aδ and C afferent fibers that activate the cardiocardiac feedback loop (2). This afferent information can also sensitize interneurons (3; light arrows) setting in motion the feedforward reflex by exciting motor neurons that cause contractions of the paraspinal muscles. These contractions activate the muscle Aδ and C afferent fibers that lead to activation of the somatosomatic circuit (2). Thus, the important point is that both circuits are enhanced via the feedforward pathway involving spinal interneurons (3; light arrows) when myocardial ischemia activates cardiac afferent fibers. The circuits are modulated by supraspinal control. Under normal conditions the vagal (4) →NTS→C1–C2 propriospinal pathway (5) may suppress the feedback and feedforward circuits. However, myocardial ischemia excites the spinoreticular (SR) (6)→supraspinal→descending pathway (7) and suppresses the vagal→NTS→C1–C2 pathway via a collateral (?) that inhibits neuronal activity in the NTS. The result is an enhancement of the positive feedback (1,2) and feedforward circuits (3) that contribute to the sustained tonicity of paraspinal muscles in patients suffering from ischemic heart disease.

information could generate positive cardiomotor feedback reflexes (Fig. 7.10, 1) and sensitization of wide dynamic range interneurons (Fig. 7.10, 3) in the spinal cord that also receive convergent input from muscle nociceptors.

The sensitization of the interneurons could activate the somatic motor neurons that increase the contractions of the muscle. The prolonged excitement of the muscle might activate and sensitize small-diameter muscle afferent fibers. These afferent fibers transmit the information to the same wide dynamic range spinal neurons that further enhances the feedback to the muscle as well as to the heart (Fig. 7.10, 2). This cycle of nociceptive information from the heart and from the muscle afferents establishes a vicious cycle that produces muscle pain and tonicity, and at the same time intensifies the pain of angina pectoris.

Supraspinal pathways might also contribute to the enhancement of positive feedback reflexes (Fig. 7.10). As discussed in a previous section, activation of cardiac vagal afferents suppresses the spinal neuronal processing of cardiac nociceptive information (Fig. 7.10, 4, 5). However, if the balance between vagal cardiac afferent activity and spinal cardiac afferent activity is compromised, the spinal responses to nociceptive cardiac input are enhanced. This change might contribute to the enhancement of positive feedback/feedforward reflexes involving paraspinal skeletal muscles and their innervation by motor neurons (Fig. 7.10, 2), and the heart and its innervation by sympathetic cardiomotor neurons (Fig. 7.10, 1). Furthermore, activation of nociceptive cardiac afferents increases the activity of the spinoreticular pathway (Foreman et al. 1984) (Fig. 7.10, 6), which in turn activates reticulospinal neurons originating in the gigantocellular tegmental field (Blair 1987) (Fig. 7.10, 7). These neurons project to the spinal cord and possibly to the NTS, and may enhance both positive reflex circuits (pathway 7 in Fig. 7.10, Blair 1987); they may furthermore inhibit the NTS–spinal cord pathway (pathways 4 and 5 in Fig. 7.10), leading in this way to a disinhibition of the positive feedback reflex circuits (Foreman et al. 1984). It is proposed that the reticulospinal pathway may be an important contributor to the enhancement of the positive feedback reflexes because it is a major descending pathway that is important for motor control (Peterson 1979, 1984). Thus, this supraspinal loop may contribute to the positive feedback/feedforward reflexes resulting in increased muscle tonicity and muscle pain. Future studies will be necessary to test this hypothesis.

Summary

Convergence of visceral TRPV1-containing fibers and somatic afferent fibers onto spinothalamic tract cells supports the convergence projection theory to explain referred pain associated with angina pectoris. During pain referred to the chest and upper arm, cardiac nociceptive information is transmitted via visceral spinal afferent fibers onto the upper thoracic spinothalamic tract cells that receive primarily deep (muscle) input from proximal somatic receptive fields. With pain referred to the jaw and neck, cardiac nociceptive information is transmitted primarily via vagal afferent fibers onto upper cervical spinothalamic tract cells receiving somatic input from the neck and jaw region. Increased excitation of cardiac visceral spinal afferent fibers can generate spasm-like muscle contractions, and decreased activation of vagal cardiac afferent fibers can augment muscle contractions. The evoked muscle contractions might provide additional nociceptive input from muscle afferents to induce angina-like referred pain by activating the contraction-sensitive afferent fibers that excite spinothalamic tract cells. Therefore, strong excitation of cardiac visceral spinal afferent fibers and/or decreased input of vagal cardiac afferent fibers, in addition to the convergence-projection theory, could potentially explain cardiac referred pain. Furthermore, this mechanism might also be responsible for the increased paraspinal muscle tone found in patients with chronic cardiac disease. The neural mechanism that underlies cardiac referred pain serves as an explanation for the once anecdotal osteopathic observations. More importantly, however, the new insights may also serve as a foundation for the mechanisms underlying somatovisceral reflexes and positive feedback/feedforward loops, key concepts of osteopathic manipulative treatments.

References

Ammons, W.S., Blair, R.W., Foreman, R.D., 1983a. Vagal afferent inhibition of spinothalamic cell responses to sympathetic afferents and bradykinin in the monkey. Circ. Res. 53 (5), 603–612.

Ammons, W.S., Blair, R.W., Foreman, R.D., 1983b. Vagal afferent inhibition of primate thoracic spinothalamic neurons. J. Neurophysiol. 50 (4), 926–940.

Ammons, W.S., Girardot, M.N., Foreman, R.D., 1985. Effects of intracardiac bradykinin on T2–T5 medial spinothalamic cells. Am. J. Physiol. 249 (2), Pt 2: R147–R152.

Beal, M.C., 1983. Palpatory testing for somatic dysfunction in patients with cardiovascular disease. J. Am. Osteopath. Assoc. 82 (11), 822–831.

Beal, M.C., 1985. Viscerosomatic reflexes: A review. J. Am. Osteopath. Assoc. 85 (12), 786–801.

Beal, M.C., 1989. Incidence of spinal palpatory findings: A review. J. Am. Osteopath. Assoc. 89 (8), 1027–1030 1033–5.

Beal, M.C., Kleiber, G.E., 1985. Somatic dysfunction as a predictor of coronary artery disease. J. Am. Osteopath. Assoc. 85 (5), 302–307.

Beckstead, R.M., Norgren, R., 1979. An autoradiographic examination of the central distribution of the trigeminal, facial, glossopharyngeal, and vagal nerves in the monkey. J. Comp. Neurol. 184, 455–472.

Beckstead, R.M., Morse, J.R., Norgren, R., 1980. The nucleus of the solitary tract in the monkey: Projections to the thalamus and brainstem nuclei. J. Comp. Neurol. 190, 259–282.

Bennett, J.R., Atkinson, M., 1966. The differentiation between oesophageal and cardiac pain. Lancet 2 (7), 473, 1123–1127.

Blair, R.W., 1987. Responses of feline medial medullary reticulospinal neurons to cardiac input. J. Neurophysiol. 58, 1149–1167.

Blair, R.W., Weber, R.N., Foreman, R.D., 1982. Responses of thoracic spinothalamic neurons to intracardiac injection of bradykinin in the monkey. Circ. Res. 51 (1), 83–94.

Bolser, D.C., Chandler, M.J., Garrison, D.W., Foreman, R.D., 1989. Effects of intracardiac bradykinin and capsaicin on spinal and spinoreticular neurons. Am. J. Physiol. Heart Circ. Physiol. 257, H1543–H1550.

Bonica, J.J., 1990. In: Management of Pain. Lea & Febiger, London, pp. 133–179.

Burns, L., 1907. Viscerosomatic and somatovisceral spinal reflexes. J. Am. Osteopath. Assoc. 7, 51–60.

Caterina, M.J., Schumacher, M.A., Tominaga, M., Rosen, T.A., Levine, J.D., Julius, D., 1997. The capsaicin receptor: a heat-activated ion channel in the pain pathway. Nature 389, 816–824.

Chandler, M.J., Zhang, J., Foreman, R.D., 1999. Vagal, sympathetic and somatic sensory inputs to upper cervical (C1–C3) spinothalamic tract neurons in monkeys. J. Neurophysiol. 76, 2555–2567.

Chandler, M.J., Zhang, J., Qin, C., Yuan, Y., Foreman, R.D., 2000. Intrapericardiac injections of algogenic chemicals excite primate C1–C2 spinothalamic tract neurons. Am. J. Physiol. Regul. Integr. Comp. Physiol. 279 (2), R560–R568.

Coleridge, H.M., Coleridge, J.C.G., 1980. Cardiovascular afferents involved in regulation of peripheral vessels. Annu. Rev. Physiol. 42, 413–427.

Cox, J.M., Gorbis, S., Dick, L.M., Rogers, J.C., Rogers, F.J., 1983. Palpable musculoskeletal findings in coronary artery disease: results of a double-blind study. J. Am. Osteopath. Assoc. 82, 832–836.

Ettlinger, H., Gintis, B., 1991. Osteopathic Approaches to Diagnosis and Treatment. Lippincott, Philadelphia, PA.

Foreman, R.D., 1999. Mechanisms of cardiac pain. Annu. Rev. Physiol. 61, 143–167.

Foreman, R.D., Blair, R.W., Weber, R.N., 1984. Viscerosomatic convergence onto T2–T4 spinoreticular, spinoreticular-spinothalamic, and spinothalamic tract neurons in the cat. Exp. Neurol. 85, 597–619.

Giamberardino, M.A., de Bigontina, P., Martegian, I.C., Vecchiet, L., 1994. Effects of extracorporeal shock-wave lithotripsy on referred hyperalgesia from renal/ureteral calculosis. Pain 56, 77–83.

Giamberardino, M.A., Dalal, A., Valente, R., Vecchiet, L., 1996. Changes in activity of spinal cells with muscular input in rats with referred muscular hyperalgesia from ureteral calculosis. Neurosci. Lett. 203 (2), 89–92.

Giamberardino, M.A., Valente, R., Affaitati, G., Vecchiet, L., 1997. Central neuronal changes in recurrent visceral pain. Int. J. Clin. Pharmacol. Res. 17 (2–3), 63–66.

Graven-Nielsen, T., Arendt-Nielsen, L., Svensson, P., Jensen, T.S., 1997. Quantification of local and referred muscle pain in humans after sequential i.m. injections of hypertonic saline. Pain 69 (1–2), 111–117.

Gwirtz, P.A., Dickey, J., Vick, D., Williams, M.A., Foresman, B., 2007. Viscerosomatic interaction induced by myocardial ischemia in conscious dogs. J. Appl. Physiol. 103 (2), 511–517.

Hancock, M.B., Fougerousse, C.L., 1976. Spinal projections from the nucleus locus coeruleus and nucleus subcoeruleus in the cat and monkey as demonstrated by the retrograde transport of horseradish peroxidase. Brain Res. Bull 1, 229–234.

Harrison, T.R., Reeves, T.J., 1968. Patterns and causes of chest pain. In: Principles and Problems of Ischemic Heart Disease. YearBook Medical, Chicago, pp. 197–204.

Hobbs, S.F., Chandler, M.J., Bolser, D.C., Foreman, R.D., 1992. Segmental organization of visceral and somatic input onto C3–T6 spinothalamic tract cells of the monkey. J. Neurophysiol. 68 (5), 1575–1588.

Hoheisel, U., Mense, S., Simons, D.G., Yu, X.M., 1993. Appearance of new receptive fields in rat dorsal horn neurons following noxious stimulation of skeletal muscle: a model for referral of muscle pain? Neurosci. Lett. 153 (1), 9–12.

Hopkins, D.A., Armour, J.A., 1989. Ganglionic distribution of afferent neurons innervating the canine heart and cardiopulmonary nerves. J. Auton. Nerv. Syst. 26 (3), 213–222.

Hudson, A.J., Brown, W.F., Gilbert, J.J., 1978. The muscular pain-fasciculation syndrome. Neurology 28 (11), 1105–1109.

Janig, W., 2006. The Integrative Action of the Autonomic Nervous System: Neurobiology of Homeostasis. Cambridge University Press, Cambridge, pp. 65–85.

Johansson, H., Arendt-Nilsson, L., Bergenheim, M., et al., 2003. Epilogue: An integrated model for chronic work-related myalgia: 'Brussels Model'. In: Johansson, H., Windhorst, U., Djupsjöbacka, M., Passatore, M. (Eds.), Chronic Work-Related Myalgia: Neuromuscular Mechanisms behind Work-Related Chronic Pain Syndromes. Gävle University Press, Gävle, pp. 291–300.

Jou, C.J., Farber, J.P., Qin, C., Foreman, R.D., 2001a. Intrapericardial algogenic chemicals evoke cardiac-somatic motor reflexes in rat. Auton. Neurosci. 94 (1–2), 52–61.

Jou, C.J., Farber, J.P., Qin, C., Foreman, R.D., 2001b. Afferent pathways for cardiac-somatic motor reflexes in rats. Am. J. Physiol. Regul. Integr. Comp. Physiol. 281 (6), R2096–R2102.

Julius, D., Basbaum, A.I., 2001. Molecular mechanisms of nociception. Nature 413, 203–210.

Kalia, M., Mesulam, M.M., 1980. Brain stem project, ions of sensory and motor components of the vagus complex in the cat: II. Laryngeal, tracheobronchial, pulmonary, cardiac, and gastrointestinal branches. J. Comp. Neurol. 193 (2), 467–508.

Karai, L., Brown, D.C., Mannes, A.J., et al., 2004. Deletion of vanilloid receptor 1-expressing primary afferent neurons for pain control. J. Clin. Invest. 113, 1344–1352.

Kellgren, J.H., 1937–38. Observations on referred pain arising from muscle. Clin. Sci. 3, 175–190.

Kellgren, J.H., 1940. Somatic simulating visceral pain. Clin. Sci. 4, 303–309.

Korr, I.M., 1991. Osteopathic research: The needed paradigm shift. J. Am. Osteopath. Assoc. 91 (2), 156 161–8, 170–1.

Kreiner, M., Okeson, J.P., 1999. Toothache of cardiac origin. J. Orofac. Pain 13, 201–207.

Kreiner, M., Okeson, J.P., Michelis, V., Lujambio, M., Isberg, A., 2007. Craniofacial pain as the sole symptom of cardiac ischemia: a prospective multicenter study. J. Am. Dent.Assoc. 138, 174–179.

Kuo, D.C., Oravitz, J.J., DeGroat, W.C., 1984. Tracing of afferent and efferent pathways in the left inferior cardiac nerve of the cat using retrograde and transganglionic transport of horseradish peroxidase. Brain Res. 321 (1), 111–118.

Laird, J.M., Roza, C., Cervero, F., 1996. Spinal dorsal horn neurons responding to noxious distension of the ureter in anesthetized rats. J. Neurophysiol. 76 (5), 3239–3248.

Larson, N.J., 1976. Summary of site and occurrence of paraspinal soft tissue changes of patients in the intensive care unit. J. Am. Osteopath. Assoc. 75 (9), 840–842.

Lindgren, I., Olivecrona, H., 1947. Surgical treatment of angina pectoris. J. Neurosurg. 4, 19–39.

Longhurst, J.C., Tjen-A-Looi, S.C., Fu, L.W., 2001. Cardiac sympathetic afferent activation provoked by myocardial ischemia and reperfusion. Mechanisms and reflexes. Ann. N.Y. Acad. Sci. 940, 74–95.

Lu, F., Qin, C., Foreman, R.D., Farber, J.P., 2004. Chemical activation of C1–C2 spinal neurons modulates intercostal and phrenic nerve activity in rats. Am. J. Physiol. Regul. Integr. Comp. Physiol. 286 (6), R1069–R1076.

Marchettini, P., Simone, D.A., Caputi, G., Ochoa, J.L., 1996. Pain from excitation of identified muscle nociceptors in humans. Brain Res. 740 (1–2), 109–116.

Maseri, A., Crea, F., Kaski, J.C., Davies, G., 1992. Mechanisms and significance of cardiac ischemic pain. Prog. Cardiovasc. Dis. 35 (1), 1–18.

McNeill, D.L., Chandler, M.J., Fu, Q.G., Foreman, R.D., 1991. Projection of nodose ganglion cells to the upper cervical spinal cord in the rat. Brain Res. Bull 27, 151–155.

Meller, S.T., Gebhart, G.F., 1992. A critical review of the afferent pathways and the potential chemical mediators involved in cardiac pain. Neuroscience 48, 501–524.

Miller, K.E., Douglas, V.D., Richards, A.B., Chandler, M.J., Foreman, R.D., 1998. Propriospinal neurons in the C1–C2 spinal segments project to the L5–S1 segments of the rat spinal cord. Brain Res. Bull 47 (1), 43–47.

Myers, D.E., 2008. Vagus nerve pain referred to the craniofacial region. A case report and literature review with implications for referred cardiac pain. Br. Dent. J. 204 (4), 187–189.

Nicholas, A.S., DeBias, D.A., Ehrenfeuchter, W., et al., 1985. A somatic component to myocardial infarction. BMJ (Clinical research ed.) 291, 13–17.

Nicholas, A.S., DeBias, D.A., Greene, C.H., 1991. Somatic component to myocardial infarction: three year follow up. Br. Med. J. 302, 1581.

Norgren, R., 1978. Projections from the nucleus of the solitary tract in the rat. Neuroscience 3, 207–218.

Nowicki, D., Szulczyk, P., 1986. Longitudinal distribution of negative cord dorsum potentials following stimulation of afferent fibres in the left inferior cardiac nerve. J. Auton. Nerv. Syst. 17 (3), 185–197.

Pan, H.L., Chen, S.R., 2004. Sensing tissue ischemia: another new function for capsaicin receptors? Circulation 110 (13), 1826–1831.

Pan, H.L., Khan, G.M., Alloway, K.D., Chen, S.R., 2003. Resiniferatoxin induces paradoxical changes in thermal and mechanical sensitivities in rats: mechanism of action. J. Neurosci. 23, 2911–2919.

Peterson, B.W., 1979. Reticulospinal projections to spinal motor nuclei. Annu. Rev. Physiol. 41, 127–140.

Peterson, B.W., 1984. The reticulospinal system and its role in the control of movement. In: Barnes, C.D. (Ed.), Brainstem Control of Spinal Cord Function. Academic Press, New York, pp. 27–86.

Procacci, P., Zoppi, M., 1989. Heart pain. In: Textbook of Pain. Churchill Livingstone, Edinburgh, pp. 410–419.

Qin, C., Chandler, M.J., Miller, K.E., Foreman, R.D., 2001. Responses and afferent pathways of superficial and deeper c(1)-c(2) spinal cells to intrapericardial algogenic chemicals in rats. J. Neurophysiol. 84 (4), 1522–1532.

Qin, C., Kranenburg, A., Foreman, R.D., 2004. Descending modulation of thoracic visceroreceptive transmission by C1–C2 spinal neurons. Auton. Neurosci. 114 (1–2), 11–16.

Qin, C., Farber, J.P., Miller, K.E., Foreman, R.D., 2006. Responses of thoracic spinal neurons to activation and desensitization of cardiac TRPV1-containing afferents in rats. Am. J. Physiol. Regul. Integr. Comp. Physiol. 291 (6), R1700–R1707.

Raisinghani, M., Pabbidi, R.M., Premkumar, L.S., 2005. Activation of transient receptor potential vanilloid 1 (TRPV1) by resiniferatoxin. J. Physiol. 567, 771–786.

Randich, A., Aicher, S.A., 1988. Medullary substrates mediating antinociception produced by electrical stimulation of the vagus. Brain Res 445, 68–76.

Randich, A., Gebhart, G.F., 1992. Vagal afferent modulation of nociception. Brain Res. Rev. 17 (2), 77–99.

Ren, K., Randich, A., Gebhart, G.F., 1990a. Modulation of spinal nociceptive transmission from nuclei tractus solitarii: a relay for effects of vagal afferent stimulation. J. Neurophysiol. 63 (5), 971–986.

Ren, K., Randich, A., Gebhart, G.F., 1990b. Electrical stimulation of cervical vagal afferents. I. Central relays for modulation of spinal nociceptive transmission. J. Neurophysiol. 64, 1095–1114.

Rhoton Jr., A.L., O'Leary, J.L., Ferguson, J.P., 1966. The trigeminal, facial, vagal, and glossopharyngeal nerves in the monkey. Arch. Neurol. 14, 530–540.

Sampson, J.J., Cheitlin, M.D., 1971. Pathophysiology and differential diagnosis of cardiac pain. Prog. Cardiovasc. Dis. 13 (6), 507–531.

Schoen, R.E., Finn, W.E., 1978. A model for studying a viscerosomatic reflex induced by myocardial infarction in the cat. J. Am. Osteopath. Assoc. 78, 122–123.

Schultz, H.D., Ustinova, E.E., 1998. Capsaicin receptors mediate free radical induced activation of cardiac afferent endings. Cardiovasc. Res. 38, 348–355.

Sugiura, Y., Terui, N., Hosoya, Y., 1989. Difference in distribution of central terminals between visceral and somatic unmyelinated (C) primary afferent fibers. J. Neurophysiol. 62 (4), 834–840.

Sylvén, C., 1989. Angina pectoris. Clinical characteristics, neurophysiological and molecular mechanisms. Pain 36 (2), 145–167.

Szallasi, A., Blumberg, P.M., 1989. Resiniferatoxin, a phorbol-related diterpene, acts as an ultrapotent analog of capsaicin, the irritant constituent in red pepper. Neuroscience 30, 515–520.

Takeuchi, Y., Uemura, M., Matsuda, K., Matsushima, R., Mizuno, N., 1980. Parabrachial nucleus neurons projecting to the lower brain stem and the spinal cord. A study in the cat by the Fink-Heimer and the horseradish peroxidase methods. Exp. Neurol. 70 (2), 403–413.

Tzukert, A., Hasin, Y., Sharav, Y., 1981. Orofacial pain of cardiac origin. Oral Surg. Oral Med. Oral Pathol. 51, 484–486.

Vance, W.H., Bowker, R.C., 1983. Spinal origins of cardiac afferents from the region of the left anterior descending artery. Brain Res. 258, 96–100.

Vecchiet, L., Giamberardino, M.A., Dragani, L., Albe-Fessard, D., 1989. Pain from renal/ureteral calculosis: evaluation of sensory thresholds in the lumbar area. Pain 36 (3), 289–295.

Westlund, K.N., Coulter, J.D., 1980. Descending projections of the locus coeruleus and subcoeruleus/medial parabrachial nuclei in monkey: axonal transport studies and dopamine-B-hydroxylase immunocytochemistry. Brain Res. Rev. 203, 235–265.

Westlund, K.N., Bowker, R.M., Ziegler, M.G., Coulter, J.D., 1984. Origins and terminations of descending noradrenergic projections to the spinal cord of monkey. Brain Res. 292 (1), 1–16.

White, J.C., Bland, E.F., 1948. The surgical relief of severe angina pectoris. Medicine (Baltimore) 27, 1–42.

White, J.C., Garrey, W.E., Atkins, J.A., 1933. Cardiac innervation: experimental and clinical studies. Arch. Surg. 26, 765–786.

Wu, M., Komori, N., Qin, C., Farber, J.P., Linderoth, B., Foreman, R.D., 2006. Sensory fibers containing vanilloid receptor-1 (VR-1) mediate spinal cord stimulation-induced vasodilation. Brain Res. 1107, 177–184.

Wu, M., Qin, C., Foreman, R.D., Farber, J.P., 2007. Transient receptor potential vanilloid receptor-1 does not contribute to slowly adapting airway receptor activation by inhaled ammonia. Auton. Neurosci. 133, 121–127.

Zahner, M.R., Li, D.P., Chen, S.R., Pan, H.L., 2003. Cardiac vanilloid receptor 1-expressing afferent nerves and their role in the cardiogenic sympathetic reflex in rats. J. Physiol. 551, 515–523.

Zhang, J., Chandler, M.J., Foreman, R.D., 2003. Cardiopulmonary sympathetic and vagal afferents excite C1–C2 propriospinal cells in rats. Brain Res. 969 (1–2), 53–58.

Zimmermann, M., 1991. Pathophysiological mechanisms of fibromyalgia. Clin. J. Pain 7 (Suppl. 1), S8–S15.

8

Central convergence of viscerosomatic inputs from spinal and vagal sources

Charles H Hubscher

Introduction

The traditional view of the nervous system treats cutaneous structures and the internal visceral organs as separate entities. The skin forms a barrier with the external environment and provides precise information (e.g., mechanical intensity, temperature, spatial dimensions) that is conveyed to higher centers in the brain for processing via a number of well-defined pathways. Sensory afferent information conveyed centrally from the urogenital tract, upper and lower gastrointestinal tracts, and other viscera is involved in the regulation of internal organs and organ reflexes via sympathetic and parasympathetic efferent outputs. Specific sensations, such as pleasure, hunger/satiety, urges related to the need to urinate/defecate, and visceral pain, also involve higher-order processing. It is well known, however, that cutaneous and visceral systems do not function independently. For example, different types of somatic manipulation (such as different forms of manual therapy, acupuncture) produce precise changes in a variety of visceral systems (Berkley 1993). Integration in the CNS therefore includes not only the processing of information for the coordination of multiple organ systems (viscerovisceral interactions), for example, but also for the processing of inputs from both somatic territories and internal organs (viscerosomatic interactions).

Central convergence of viscerosomatic inputs is found beginning at all three main ports of entry into the CNS: spinal gray matter, dorsal column nuclei, and solitary nucleus. These regions can influence each other through direct interconnections as well as indirectly via overlapping target regions across the entire neuraxis (Fig. 8.1). The interactions and contributions of these various ports of entry for affective/motivational systems and sensation, from pleasure to pain, are not well understood. One functional role associated with viscerosomatic convergence, for example, is referred pain of visceral origin, whereby convergence may be an efficient means through which visceral nociceptive information utilizes ascending somatic nociceptive systems. In this chapter, central convergence of viscerosomatic inputs will be reviewed at these three main ports of entry into the CNS, as well as within three of the major central relay areas (medullary reticular formation, thalamus, hypothalamus). The contribution of spinal versus vagal sources of input to the CNS for pelvic visceral sensations/functions is discussed within the context of our ongoing studies on spinal cord injury.

Viscerosomatic inputs to the CNS: three ports of entry

Spinal processing

The lumbosacral segments (L5–S1 in the rat) of the spinal cord in males contain a center for erection and the expulsive part of ejaculation. Numerous studies have been carried out to study the various elements of the spinal neural circuitry mediating these functions. For example, erection and ejaculation have been shown to be mediated by preganglionic parasympathetic motor axons in the pelvic nerve and somatic motor axons in the pudendal nerve supplying the striated perineal muscles of the pelvic floor (Coolen et al. 2004, de Groat & Booth 1993, Giuliano & Rampin 2004, McKenna 1998, Steers 2000). Animal experiments in which electrical stimulation is applied to the nerve that supplies

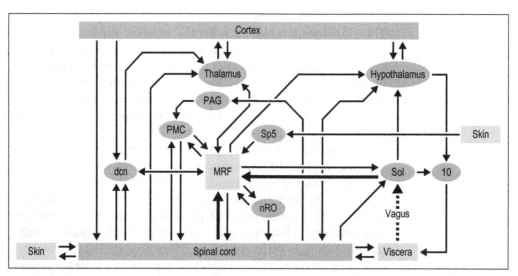

Figure 8.1 Summary of pathways that convey visceral and somatic information within the CNS. Note that all three ports of entry in the CNS (spinal cord, dcn, sol) have reciprocal interconnections with the brain stem MRF region, which contains many neurons with a high degree of somatovisceral convergence. Also note that the diagram is simplified for illustrative purposes and that not all CNS regions/pathways are represented. dcn, dorsal column nuclei; MRF, medullary reticular formation; nRO, nucleus raphe obscurus; PAG, periaqueductal gray; PMC, pontine micturition center; sol, solitary nucleus; Sp5, spinal trigeminal nucleus; 10, dorsal motor nucleus of the vagus.

the penis, the dorsal nerve of the penis (DNP), reveals expression of a neural activity marker (Fos protein) in the dorsal horn, dorsal gray commissure and sacral parasympathetic nucleus (Rampin et al. 1997). Individual spinal cord interneurons in the dorsal horn and intermediate zone of primarily L6–S1 that receive input from DNP afferents have been studied in vivo with electrophysiological recordings (Johnson 1989). All penile interneurons exhibit receptive fields on the penis that are significantly larger than the receptive fields for single primary afferent neurons, thereby demonstrating a central convergence of penile sensory input. In addition, most penile interneurons have receptive fields on both sides of the body, and their electrical characteristics strongly suggest a monosynaptic input from both ipsilateral and contralateral DNP fibers (Johnson 1989). There is also an extensive representation from the distal glans ('cup') region in these spinal cord interneurons. DNP afferents produce bilateral (crossed and uncrossed) reflex facilitation of pudendal motoneurons located in L5–L6.

In addition to the lumbosacral region of the spinal cord in male rats, a lumbar (L3–L4) reflex region for ejaculation has been identified that depends on input from afferent systems releasing substance P (Truitt & Coolen 2002). These lumbar neurons are located lateral to the central canal in lamina X and in the medial portion of lamina VII, and have projections to neurons involved in the emission as well as the expulsion phase of ejaculation.

In females, organ-specific and organ-characteristic information is conveyed in a rostrocaudal topographic array to the caudal spinal cord (Berkley & Hubscher 1995b, Berkley et al. 1993c). In vivo electrophysiological recordings as well as neuroanatomical tracing studies indicate that there is an extensive system of neurons in thoracolumbar and lumbosacral spinal cord that receive female reproductive organ inputs (Berkley et al. 1993b, Lee & Erskine 1996, 2000). The

cervix, for example, which is innervated by both the hypogastric and the pelvic nerves, has inputs to dorsal horn neurons at both levels, although the neurons are concentrated ventrally in the dorsal horn at T13–L1 and throughout the dorsal horn at L4–L5 and L6–S1 segments (Berkley et al. 1993b). Cervix-responsive dorsal horn neurons in both regions receive convergent inputs from other pelvic organs such as the colon (51%) as well as cutaneous regions, although the receptive fields tend to be larger at T13–L1 and more confined to the perineum for the neurons at L6–S2 located in the dorsal part of the dorsal horn (Berkley et al. 1993b). Many cervix-responsive neurons at L6–S2, for example, respond to uterine distension by being inhibited. This uterine input originates from distant roots (uterus innervated by the hypogastric nerve), as shown in experiments where T13–L2 roots were sectioned bilaterally (Wall et al. 1993). How these interactions sculpt the actions of these neurons for various aspects of reproduction is unclear.

A somatic region that is consistently seen to converge with neurons having inputs originating from the female reproductive tract, particularly at the T13–L1 region but also in the deep dorsal horn at the L6–S2 region, is the hind paws (Berkley et al. 1993b). This is true throughout the neuraxis (see summary of studies on Relay Nuclei section below) as well as for penile-responsive neurons in male rats. The stimulus is deep pressure (squeezing) of the toes with a moderate (presumably noxious) force. Thus, the neural circuitry is such that stimuli or pathology affecting the pelvic organs can modulate the processing of inputs from the feet, and vice versa.

The dorsal column nuclei

The dorsal column nuclei (gracile – lower body; cuneate – upper body) is a region traditionally designated as receiving somatotopically organized input related to active touch and kinesthesia. Neurons in the gracile nucleus (Gr), however, have also been shown to receive afferent input from the external genitalia, internal reproductive organs, colon, pancreas, and kidney (Al-Chaer et al. 1996a, Berkley & Hubscher 1995a, Bradshaw & Berkley 2000, Cothron et al. 2008, Rong et al. 2004, Simon & Schramm 1984, Wang & Westlund 2001). Thus, in addition to the spinal cord, the dorsal column nuclei in the caudal brain stem are another port of entry into the CNS where somatic and visceral interactions and modulation of inputs can occur.

Evidence for such convergence and thus the potential for interactions once again comes from experimental studies in animal models. In male rats, several neuroanatomic tracing studies have shown that injection of a tracer such as fluorogold or horseradish peroxidase (HRP) into the pelvic or pudendal nerve labels axons within Gr medially near the level of obex (Ding et al. 1999, Ueyama et al. 1985, 1987). More Gr labeling was found in response to the application of HRP to the cut end of the perineal nerve branch than to the DNP sensory branch (Ueyama et al. 1985, 1987). An extensive search of the Gr using extracellular recordings in urethane-anesthetized animals (Cothron et al. 2008) revealed only a small proportion of electrode tracks (41 of 319 in 12 rats) in the medial third of the nucleus around obex containing neurons responsive to penile stimulation. These neurons did, however, also respond to stimulation of a variety of somatic territories, but not the distal colon (Fig. 8.2). The lack of responses to colon is probably related to the medial location of the penile-responsive neurons in Gr. In another electrophysiologic recording study of somatovisceral interactions in the Gr of male rats (Rong et al. 2004), none of the 43 neurons (out of 212 tested) that were excited or inhibited by colorectal distension responded to stimulation of the scrotum (i.e., the most common somatic convergent territory for penile-responsive neurons). The somatic receptive fields for the Gr neurons responding to colorectal distension were

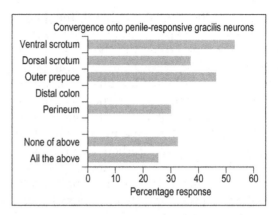

Figure 8.2 The histogram shows the proportion of convergent overlap of various body regions for neurons in the gracile nucleus that respond to stimulation of the penis. The percent response represents the proportion of the number of penile-responsive single neurons tested in the gracile nucleus that fired to at least twice the background level of neural activity upon stimulation (only a few were inhibited). For example, of all the gracile neurons that were found to respond to stimulation of the penis, 37% also responded to stimulation of the dorsal scrotum. Note that although there are some neurons that only respond to penile stimulation, others respond to multiple somatic territories of the hindquarters (bar marked 'all of above'). Adapted from Cothron et al. (2008).

centered on the outer leg from the hip to the foot, and tended to be located lateral and caudal relative to obex. Of particular note is the finding, using both electrophysiological and neuroanatomical tracing techniques, that penile inputs to Gr are both ipsi- and contralateral, whereas cutaneous inputs are only ipsilateral (Cothron et al. 2008).

Interestingly, although a study in cats also found penile projections to Gr, the inputs from the clitoris in females were not in an analogous position (Kawatani et al. 1994). Many neurons in the rodent Gr have been shown to receive input from the female internal reproductive organs and colon (Berkley & Hubscher 1995a, Bradshaw & Berkley 2000, Hubscher 1994). In addition, the responses to reproductive organ stimulation (cervix pressure, vaginal and uterine distension) vary across the estrous cycle (latencies and proportion of excitatory/ inhibitory responses), suggesting a possible role in mating (Bradshaw & Berkley 2000).

The hormonal influences are probably due to fluctuations in levels of 17β-estradiol (Bradshaw & Berkley 2003). The most common somatic receptive fields for Gr neurons responding to stimulation of the female internal reproductive organs are the ipsilateral foot/toes, followed by the leg (including ankle), tail, and perineum. A typical example showing a somatovisceral convergent neuronal response in Gr is provided in Figure 8.3. Note that the foot/toes were also a common convergent territory for female

reproductive organ responsive neurons at the thoracolumbar and lumbosacral levels of the spinal cord, albeit bilateral.

The solitary nucleus

The solitary nucleus (NTS) is another region within the caudal medulla (just below Gr) that receives primary afferent inputs. However, unlike Gr, which receives primary inputs from small cutaneous receptive fields, the NTS receives visceral and pelvic organ inputs. The NTS is known as

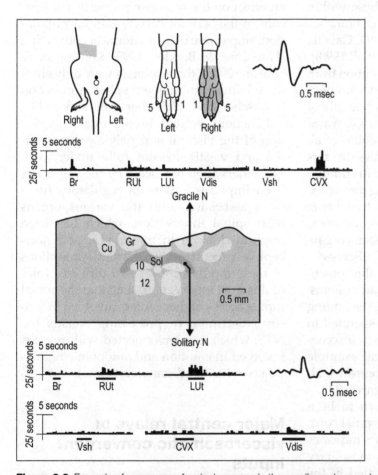

Figure 8.3 Example of responses of a single neuron in the gracile nucleus and a single neuron in the solitary nucleus. For each neuron recorded, responses to stimulation (touch, pressure) over the entire surface of the body were tested, as well as responses to probing and/or balloon distension of various pelvic visceral territories. Note the contrast in the responses of the two neurons in these adjacent brainstem regions, i.e., a lack of responses to somatic stimulation (touch) in the solitary nucleus. Br, brush; Cu, cuneate nucleus; CVX, cervix pressure; Gr, gracile nucleus; LUt, left uterine horn distension; Rut, right uterine horn distension; Vdis, vaginal distension; Vsh, vaginal shear; 10, dorsal motor nucleus of the vagus; 12, hypoglossal nucleus. Adapted from Hubscher and Berkley (1994) and Berkley and Hubscher (1995).

a region that processes gustatory, cardio-vascular, and respiratory information as well as information from the esophagus, stomach, cecum, small intestine, colon, cervix, uterus, and vaginal canal, with a general viscerotopic organization from rostral (gustatory) to caudal (pelvic organs) (Altschuler et al. 1989, 1991, 1993, Cechetto 1987, Collins et al. 1999, Hubscher & Berkley 1994, Jean 1991, Lu & Bieger 1998, Norgren & Leonard 1973, Novin et al. 1981, Zhang et al. 1992).

The NTS receives primary afferent input via the nodose ganglion from viscera innervated by the vagus, including those within the pelvic region (via the abdominal branches of the vagus (Altschuler et al. 1993, Gabella & Pease 1973, Ortega-Villalobos et al. 1990)). For example, a vagal–solitary projection from the uterus has been demonstrated with neuroanatomic tracing and other types of animal experiments (Collins et al. 1999, Guevara-Guzman et al. 2001, Ortega-Villalobos et al. 1990). Electrophysiological studies in rats indicate NTS neurons responsive to stimulation of the pelvic viscera, including the cervix, vaginal canal, uterus, and colon (Hubscher & Berkley 1994). Of the responsive neurons, 29% respond to more than one visceral organ, demonstrating the existence of viscerovisceral convergence and hence the potential for interactions between organ systems. Consistent with the literature was the finding that none of the NTS neurons responded to stimulation of somatic territories (no somatovisceral convergence). A typical example illustrating this point (and the contrast with the nearby Gr) is presented in Figure 8.3.

The NTS has also been shown to be a relay of inputs coming from the spinal cord. Retrograde tracing from the NTS indicates that neurons comprising the spinosolitary pathway include cell bodies located in the superficial dorsal horn, laminae IV–VII, the dorsal commissural nucleus of lamina X (thoracolumbar levels), and within the vicinity of the sacral parasympathetic nuclear region (Esteves et al. 1993, Menetrey & Basbaum 1987, Menetrey & de Pommery 1991). Lesion studies indicate that different pathways probably exist for different portions of the reproductive tract. Electrophysiological recording of responses to pelvic organ stimulation in the NTS pre and post combinations of acute complete spinal transection and bilateral vagotomy were made (Hubscher & Berkley 1995). The lack of responses to uterine distension post vagotomy is consistent with anatomic tracing and other studies (Collins et al. 1999, Guevara-Guzman et al. 2001, Ortega-Villalobos et al. 1990). In addition, although bilateral vagotomy had an effect on the response properties of neurons in the NTS for cervix/vaginal stimulation, suggestive of an anatomical connection (Hubscher & Berkley 1995, Komisaruk & Sansone 2003), the responses were only eliminated after a subsequent spinal transection (Hubscher 1994, Hubscher & Berkley 1995).

Functions related to the dual innervation of the visceral and pelvic organs (spinal and vagal) are not fully understood. The innervation of viscera by the vagus has been implicated more in regulatory functions associated with the various organs than spinal innervation, which has been implicated more in mechanical and nociceptive processing. The rostral projections of these inputs support two different roles of this dual innervation, such that the spinal inputs access higher centers involved in sensory/discriminitve processing, versus the NTS, which is interconnected with regions involved in emotion and autonomic regulation (see further discussion below).

Major central relays of viscerosomatic convergent inputs

Medullary reticular formation

The medullary reticular formation (MRF) is a region in the rostral medulla of the brain stem that is known to contribute to numerous body functions. These functions include ascending control of cortical arousal, descending control of motor activity, and the control of autonomic activity (Jones 1995). The MRF in the rat has been shown to have direct reciprocal interconnections with all three ports of entry described in the previous section (spinal cord, Gr, NTS) (Aicher et al. 1995, Antal et al. 1996, Basbaum & Fields 1979, Casey 1969, Chaouch et al. 1983, Gallager & Pert 1978, Hermann et al. 2003, Jean 1991, Mtui et al. 1995, Odutola 1977, Tomasulo & Emmers 1972). Thus, MRF neurons receive convergent inputs from multiple somatic and visceral territories, which include regions innervated by spinal as well as cranial nerves. The MRF is known to process and relay a vast array of viscerosomatic sensory inputs involved in nociception (Bowsher 1976, Chan 1985, Hubscher & Johnson 1996, Peschanski & Besson 1984, Zhuo & Gebhart 1990). Many MRF neurons in both male and female rats, for example, respond to distension of the distal colon (Hubscher 2006b, Kaddumi & Hubscher 2006). All of the colon-responsive single MRF neurons receive bilateral nociceptive-specific somatic inputs from widespread regions of the body.

The MRF has been implicated to be involved in the neural circuitries mediating eliminative functions, including urination, defecation, and ejaculation. For urogenital processing in male rats, electrical stimulation of the MRF has been shown to produce field potentials in the lumbosacral spinal cord near pudendal motor nuclei (Tanaka & Arnold 1993), reduce pudendal motor neuron reflex discharges (Johnson & Hubscher 1998), and activate postganglionic sympathetic fibers contained within the motor branch of the pudendal nerve (Johnson & Hubscher 2000). Large MRF lesions that include the ventral nucleus reticularis gigantocellularis, gigantocellularis pars alpha, and lateral paragigantocellular nuclei affect ejaculatory bursts in perineal muscles (Marson & McKenna 1990).

Electrophysiological data from extracellular single unit recordings in the rostral ventromedial medulla in male rats has demonstrated a significant degree of viscerosomatic and viscerovisceral convergence. Somatic convergent territories are not just confined to the hind quarters but include rostral skin areas such as the ears and forepaws (Hubscher 2006b, Hubscher & Johnson 1996, Kaddumi & Hubscher 2006). Many of these viscerosomatic MRF neurons receive input from cutaneous territories across the entire body, including the face. The majority of the viscerosomatic neuronal responses are to noxious levels of stimulation. There is also a high degree of viscerovisceral convergence in the MRF. Single unit recordings in MRF indicate that 62% of neurons responding to distension of the urinary bladder also respond to stimulation of the urethra, penis, and distal colon (Hubscher 2006b, Kaddumi & Hubscher 2006), suggesting that this CNS region is probably important for the coordination of visceral functions.

Viscerosomatic convergent neurons in the MRF in female rats respond to electrical stimulation of the dorsal nerve of the clitoris, which is the sensory pudendal branch equivalent of the DNP in males. A summary illustrating the convergence of pudendal/pelvic nerve inputs at one anteroposterior level of the MRF is presented in Figure 8.4. Note the predominance of the pelvic nerve input in females, which probably reflects the importance of the vaginocervical responses to mating. This region has been shown to be involved in female circuitry responsible for the lordosis mating posture (Daniels et al. 1999, Modianos & Pfaff 1979, Schwartz-Giblin et al. 1996). As with the reproductive organ inputs to Gr, there are estradiol-associated differences in the responses of MRF neurons to viscerosomatic stimulation (Hubscher 2006b). Most interesting was the finding that the hormonal response variations for somatic and visceral territories were in opposite directions (estradiol-associated hypersensitivity and hyposensitivity, respectively), which

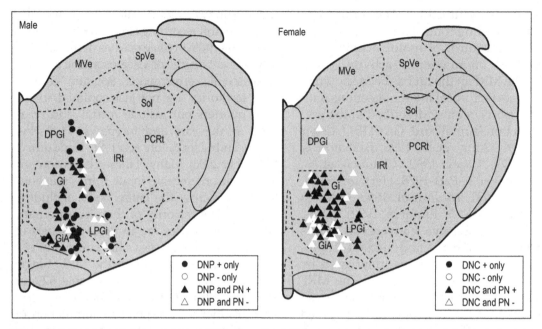

Figure 8.4 Summary of single medullary reticular formation (MRF) neurons responsive to bilateral electrical stimulation of the sensory branch of the pudendal nerve (dorsal nerve of the penis (DNP) in male rats; DNC, dorsal nerve of the clitoris in females) and the viscerocutaneous branch of the pelvic nerve (PN). Note the greater degree of convergence of pudendal and pelvic neural inputs to MRF in the female versus male rats, which could be associated with their importance in relation to the territories they innervate for mating (DNP in males but both DNC and PN in females). The section represents units located at 2.6 to 3.0 mm rostral to obex. Filled and unfilled symbols represent excitatory and inhibitory responses, respectively. DPGi, dorsal paragigantocellular nucleus; Gi, nucleus reticularis gigantocellularis; GiA, Gi pars alpha; IRt, intermediate reticular nucleus; LPGi, lateral paragigantocellular nucleus; MVe, medial vestibular nucleus; PCRt, parvocellular reticular nucleus; Sol, solitary nucleus; SpVe, spinal vestibular nucleus. Adapted from Hubscher (2006b) and Hubscher and Johnson (1996).

is consistent with what is expected during mating (for example, the reduced sensitivity of the cervix). The absence of hormonal effects for some of the viscerosomatic inputs combined with different effects depending on the source for the same individual neurons suggests that estradiol is acting elsewhere, such as within the spinal cord itself (see Hubscher 2006b).

There is also convergence from vagal inputs in the MRF. A majority of viscerosomatic convergent MRF neurons respond to stimulation of the abdominal branches of the vagus (Kaddumi & Hubscher 2006). Following a chronic complete mid-thoracic spinal transection, irritation of the urinary bladder affected the number of neurons in the MRF responding to vagal stimulation, suggesting a route that may explain

generalized sensations below the level of injury that have been documented in patients with complete spinal cord injury. Note that these changes occurred despite the lack of response to direct (mechanical and electrical nerve) pelvic visceral stimulation. An illustration of potential pathways to the MRF with transection is provided in Figure 8.5. An fMRI study of female patients with complete spinal cord injury (ASIA criteria) at or above T10 indicates activation of the NTS and many forebrain regions with vaginal–cervical self-stimulation (Komisaruk et al. 2004).

Thalamus

The thalamus is a region of well-defined nuclei that conveys a multitude of sensory information to the cerebral cortex. The

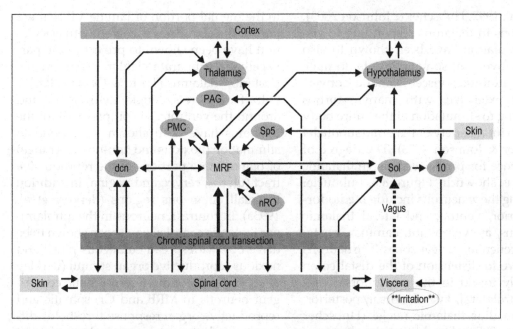

Figure 8.5 Pathway diagram illustrating the effect of chronic spinal transection at T8 on the central inputs from the pelvic viscera. Note that there are several ways (a few illustrated with open arrows) whereby a visceral stimulus (such as one resulting from chemical irritation) can access neurons in the medullary reticular formation (MRF) and other brain regions, therefore bypassing a complete spinal lesion. Abbreviations as in Figure 8.1.

thalamus consists of various groups of nuclei that have been implicated in many different processes, including somatosensory, emotion, memory, motor control, auditory, and visual functions. All three ports of entry described above have direct as well as indirect projections to a variety of thalamic subnuclei. For example, spinothalamic, spinoreticulothalamic, and dorsal column–medial lemniscal pathways provide a vast array of viscerosomatic inputs to medial and lateral thalamic nuclei (Al-Chaer et al. 1998, Apkarian & Shi 1994, Berkley 1985, Berkley et al. 1980, Berkley & Hand 1978, Cliffer et al. 1991, 1992, Craig & Burton 1981, Giesler et al. 1979, 1981, Granum 1986, Katter et al. 1996, Kevetter & Willis 1982, Peschanski & Besson 1984, Wang et al. 1999). In addition, the NTS also has projections directly to midline/intralaminar thalamic nuclei (Ruggiero et al. 1998). Neurons in medial and lateral thalamus are an integral part of information processing related to affective/motivational

and sensory discriminative aspects of pain, respectively (Apkarian et al. 1995, Vahle-Hinz et al. 1995). These functional implications for nociceptive thalamic neurons are based on sources of inputs to some of the subregions within medial and lateral thalamus (spino-reticulothalamic vs spinothalamic, respectively; Peschanski & Besson 1984), response properties for many of the neurons such as receptive field size/degree of convergence (large, bilateral, complex versus small, unilateral, respectively – references in Apkarian et al. 1995, Guilbaud et al. 1994, Willis & Coggeshall 1991) and outputs to cortex (see review by Willis 1995).

Pelvic visceral inputs to medial and lateral thalamus in rats and other species include the penis, bladder, kidney, colon, esophagus, intestines, and cardiovascular structures (Al-Chaer et al. 1996b, Berkley et al. 1993a, 1995, Bruggemann et al. 1993, 1994, 1998, Chandler et al. 1992, Chernigovskiy & Onischenko 1967, Horie & Yokota 1990,

Horn et al. 1997, Hubscher & Johnson 2003). All neurons in thalamus responding to visceral stimulation have been shown to also receive convergent somatic inputs. In male rats, for example, viscerosomatic convergence is extensive, with many neurons responding to stimulation of the entire body (bilateral) for a variety of thalamic subnuclei (Hubscher & Johnson 2003). The degree of convergence for penile-responsive thalamic neurons is shown in Figure 8.6. Subnuclei containing these neurons include mediodorsal, anterior, ventral, and lateral thalamic subregions, as well as intralaminar, posterior and reticular nuclear zones. The neurons responsive to distension of the distal colon were only found in the mediodorsal central, ventrolateral, lateral–dorsal/posterior, and submedius thalamic nuclei (Hubscher & Johnson 2003). In addition, lumbar neurons at L3 and L4 segmental levels located lateral to the central canal in lamina X and

in the medial portion of lamina VII that are part of the circuitries involved with ejaculation have been shown to project to the parvocellular subparafascicular region in the posterior thalamus (Truitt & Coolen 2002).

In female rats, single neurons in and around the ventrobasal complex (VB) of the thalamus have been shown to respond to stimulation (noxious and non-noxious range) of one or more portions of the reproductive tract (uterus, cervix, and vagina) in addition to small cutaneous regions (Berkley et al. 1993a). In contrast, neurons in the intralaminar thalamic complex have been shown to be driven by widespread cutaneous pinch and noxious reproductive organ stimuli (Berkley et al. 1995). As with viscerosomatic convergent neurons in MRF and Gr, somatic and reproductive organ response thresholds differed with the presence versus absence of 17β estradiol (Reed et al. 2009). These differences are illustrated graphically in Figure 8.7. Note that, as with the MRF, the somatic and visceral hormonal effects on response thresholds were in opposite directions.

Hypothalamus

The hypothalamus is associated with many visceral and pelvic functions, including sexual behaviors and functions, gastric modulation, cardiovascular function, taste, and pain, just to name a few (Ackerman et al. 1998, Barone et al. 1995, Blaustein et al. 1994, Bullitt 1990, Cechetto 1987, Dafny et al. 1996, van der Plas et al. 1995). The hypothalamus in the rat receives direct projections from two of the three main ports of entry to the CNS. Spinohypothalamic axons ascend via a medial and lateral route, with the majority projecting via the latter contralaterally (Burstein et al. 1996, Katter et al. 1996, Zhang et al. 1995). Visceral information from the NTS also projects directly to the hypothalamus (Norgren 1978, Nosaka 1984, Ricardo & Koh 1978, Ter Horst et al. 1989). The hypothalamus can also receive input indirectly from the NTS and spinal cord via

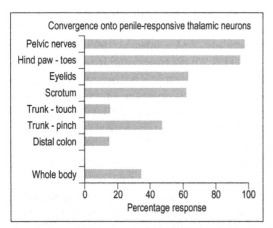

Figure 8.6 Summary showing some of the regions in the male rat that provide convergent input to penile-responsive neurons in the thalamus. As in the gracile nucleus (Fig. 8.2), many neurons in the thalamus responding to penile stimulation respond to stimulation of a variety of body regions. However, in contrast to the gracile neurons recorded in males, the convergent territories extend beyond the pelvic/pudendal innervated territories of the body. Note that many thalamic neurons respond to multiple somatic territories (bilateral), some of which encompass skin over the entire length of the rat's body (bar marked 'whole body'). Adapted from Hubscher and Johnson (2003).

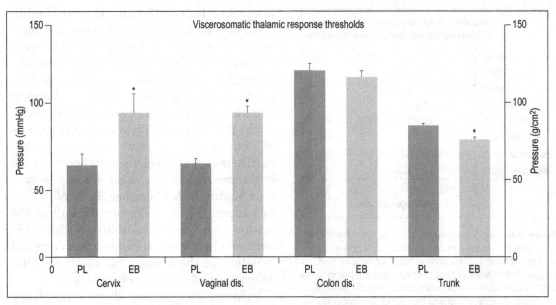

Figure 8.7 Summary showing the response thresholds to pelvic visceral organ stimulation (distension [dis.] pressures and cervix probe pressure in mmHg) and somatic trunk stimulation (Electro-vonFrey with rigid tip, from IITC Inc., Woodland Hills, CA). Asterisk (*) indicates significant differences between 17β estradiol-treated female ovariectomized rats and placebo (PL)-treated ovariectomized rats, evidence that hormonal status can alter neuronal response properties. These observed effects may be contributing to some of the neural mechanisms that underlie sex differences in pain, which has been observed both in numerous experimental animal studies as well as in clinical settings. Note that estradiol-treated rats had lower response thresholds (indicating more sensitivity) to trunk stimulation and higher response thresholds (indicating less sensitivity) for reproductive organ stimulation. Testing was done during terminal electrophysiological recordings in the thalamus under urethane anesthesia. Terminal experiments were done 6 weeks after ovariectomy/implantation of 60-day time-release pellets obtained from Innovative Research of America (Sarasota, FL). Adapted from Reed et al. (2009).

the parabrachial nucleus (Bester et al. 1995, Saper & Loewy 1980) and periaqueductal gray (Cameron et al. 1995). The hypothalamus has outputs projecting to a vast array of CNS areas, including the NTS, parabrachial nucleus, MRF, and spinal cord (Basbaum & Fields 1979, Saggu & Lundy 2008, van der Kooy et al. 1984, Vertes & Crane 1996).

All of the above interconnections give the hypothalamus access to a wide array of viscerosomatic inputs. Neurons in the preoptic area of the hypothalamus, for example, contribute to mating behavior, the neuroendocrine control of the reproductive cycle, and antinociception (Docke et al. 1984, Moss & Foreman 1976, Murphy et al. 1999). In vivo electrophysiological recordings demonstrate that neurons in the preoptic area responding to the search stimuli, bilateral electrical stimulation of the viscerocutaneous branch of

the pelvic nerve, and/or sensory branch of the pudendal nerve (i.e., dorsal nerve of the clitoris), receive a high degree of viscerosomatic convergence, including inputs from the abdominal branches of the vagus, cervix, vagina, distal colon, and skin territories on the perineum and trunk (Fig. 8.8). In addition, as with other CNS regions in female rats, the mean neuronal response thresholds for vaginal and cervical stimulation, but not colon distension, were significantly higher for animals tested during proestrus, the estrous stage when estradiol levels are elevated (Chadha & Hubscher 2008).

Ascending visceral pathways

Limited information is available on the location of ascending spinal pathways that convey information originating from the viscera,

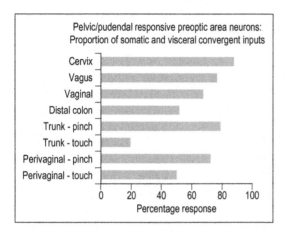

Figure 8.8 Histogram showing some of the somatic and visceral regions in the female rat that provide convergent input to hypothalamic neurons in the preoptic area that respond to bilateral electrical stimulation of the pelvic nerve and/or pudendal nerve (sensory branch, dorsal nerve of the clitoris). Note that many of these neurons respond to multiple somatic (bilateral) and visceral territories and how extensive the overlap is at this level of the neuraxis. The percent response represents the proportion of convergence from a given territory with neurons that are responsive to electrical stimulation of both the pelvic and pudendal nerves. Adapted from Chadha and Hubscher (2008).

including those within the pelvic region. The results of several studies, taken together, indicate that there are likely many spinal pathways that convey these inputs to the brain, and these projections are probably all bilateral. Pathways include most, if not all, of the following: dorsal column, postsynaptic dorsal column, spinoreticular, spinothalamic, spinosolitary, spinoparabrachial, spinohypothalamic, spinoamygdalar, spinomesencephalic, and spinocerebellar projections (Berkley & Hubscher 1995b, Hubscher 2006a, Menetrey & de Pommery 1991). Viscerosomatic convergent inputs to the cortex include primary somatosensory and insular cortex (Bruggemann et al. 1997, Ito 1998).

In addition to spinal pathways, visceral information enters the brain via the vagus nerve through an additional port of entry, the NTS within the caudal medulla. The normal functional significance of this dual projection may relate to sensory/autonomic

integration for coordinating multiple bodily functions, including reproductive and eliminative events. In a chronic spinal transection model, responses in the rostral medulla to mechanical stimulation of below-lesion-level territories are lost. However, chemical irritation of a visceral organ below the level of the spinal lesion can still alter responses of neurons in the brain stem, suggesting that below-lesion regions have access to the brain, probably via a vagal–solitary projection (Kaddumi & Hubscher 2007). Note that this access did not occur as a result of the noxious mechanical stimulus (bladder distension) but can be attributed to the chemical irritation of the urinary bladder following infusion of 2% solution of acetic acid.

Evidence suggesting that spinosolitary and vagal–solitary pathways subserve different functions comes from studies on a variety of different visceral organs. For example, it has been shown that gastric vagal afferent fibers do not have response thresholds in the noxious range (Ozaki et al. 1999), and that the mechanosensitive vagal afferents increase their excitability with gastric inflammation (Kang et al. 2004). Thus, the vagal input may normally be relaying non-nociceptive regulatory information from the various pelvic/visceral organs, versus the nociceptive/mechanical properties of the stimulus which are being conveyed via ascending spinal pathways (Hubscher et al. 2004, Ness & Gebhart 1987). Interestingly, low-intensity electrical stimulation of vagal afferent fibers (abdominal branches) reduces visceromotor responses to colorectal distension (Chen et al. 2008). The finding that the vagus may exert an antinociceptive effect on viscera is consistent with a study of intestinal pressure thresholds in patients who had undergone vagotomy versus healthy controls (Holtmann et al. 1998).

Concluding remarks

The central relay and processing of viscerosomatic inputs is complex and involves multiple sites along the neuraxis, including regions involved in hormonal regulation. Central convergence of viscerosomatic inputs is found beginning at all three main ports of entry into the CNS: the spinal gray matter, dorsal column nuclei, and solitary nucleus (Fig. 8.1). These regions can influence each other through direct interconnections as well as indirectly via overlapping target regions across the entire neuraxis. Thus, at any given moment a dynamic system is in place whereby pathology associated with one organ or somatic territory can affect the physiology and functioning of another (Berkley 2005, Malykhina 2007, Pezzone et al. 2005, Qin et al. 2003, 2007, 2005, Ustinova et al. 2007, Winnard et al. 2006). Likewise, as a result of somatovisceral convergence at all levels of the neuraxis, any manipulation of any somatic region or any rehabilitation strategy will probably affect the central neural circuitries associated with the processing or information originating from a variety of visceral organs, including inputs involved in cardiovascular, respiratory, urinary, and sexual function. Also, a therapeutic intervention affecting one system may modify the physiology and functioning of another. These system interactions must be kept in mind for example during the design of combination therapies for the treatment of pain patients, which may include a mix of drug therapies, somatic manipulations (such as massage, physical therapy, regional nerve blocks), and situational adjustments (such as diet, behavioral therapy, self-education) (Berkley & Holdcroft 1999). A better understanding of the mechanisms underlying the system crosstalk between multiple somatic and visceral territories will affect the treatment of many conditions that often present concomitantly.

References

Ackerman, A.E., Lange, G.M., Clemens, L.G., 1998. Effects of paraventricular lesions on sex behavior and seminal emission in male rats. Physiology and Behavior 63, 49–53.

Aicher, S.A., Reis, D.J., Nicolae, R., Milner, T.A., 1995. Monosynaptic projections from the medullary gigantocellular reticular formation to sympathetic preganglionic neurons in the thoracic spinal cord. J. Comp. Neurol. 363 (4), 563–580.

Al-Chaer, E.D., Lawand, N.B., Westlund, K.N., Willis, W.D., 1996a. Pelvic visceral input into the nucleus gracilis is largely mediated by the postsynaptic dorsal column pathway. J. Neurophysiol. 76 (4), 2675–2690.

Al-Chaer, E.D., Lawand, N.B., Westlund, K.N., Willis, W.D., 1996b. Visceral nociceptive input into the ventral posterolateral nucleus of the thalamus: a new function for the dorsal column pathway. J. Neurophysiol. 76 (4), 2661–2674.

Al-Chaer, E.D., Feng, Y., Willis, W.D., 1998. A role for the dorsal column in nociceptive visceral input into the thalamus of primates. J. Neurophysiol. 79 (6), 3143–3150.

Altschuler, S.M., Bao, X.M., Bieger, D., Hopkins, D.A., Miselis, R.R., 1989. Viscerotopic representation of the upper alimentary tract in the rat: sensory ganglia and nuclei of the solitary and spinal trigeminal tracts. J. Comp. Neurol. 283 (2), 248–268.

Altschuler, S.M., Ferenci, D.A., Lynn, R.B., Miselis, R.R., 1991. Representation of the cecum in the lateral dorsal motor nucleus of the vagus nerve and commissural subnucleus of the nucleus tractus solitarii in rat. J. Comp. Neurol. 304 (2), 261–274.

Altschuler, S.M., Escardo, J., Lynn, R.B., Miselis, R.R., 1993. The central organization of the vagus nerve innervating the colon of the rat. Gastroenterology 104 (2), 502–509.

Antal, M., Petko, M., Polgar, E., Heizmann, C.W., Storm-Mathisen, J., 1996. Direct evidence of an extensive GABAergic innervation of the spinal dorsal horn by fibres descending from the rostral ventromedial medulla. Neuroscience 73 (2), 509–518.

Apkarian, A.V., Shi, T., 1994. Squirrel monkey lateral thalamus. I. Somatic nociresponsive neurons and their relation to spinothalamic terminals. J. Neurosci. 14 (11 Pt 2), 6779–6795.

Apkarian, A.V., Bruggemann, J., Shi, T., Airapetian, L.R., 1995. A thalamic model for true and referred pain sensation. In: Gebhart, G.F. (Ed.), Visceral Pain, Progress in Pain Research and Management. IASP Press, Seattle, pp. 217–259.

Barone, F.C., Zarco de Coronado, I., Wayner, M.J., 1995. Gastric distension modulates hypothalamic neurons via a sympathetic afferent path through the mesencephalic periaqueductal gray. Brain Res. Bull 38 (3), 239–251.

Basbaum, A.I., Fields, H.L., 1979. The origin of descending pathways in the dorsolateral funiculus of the spinal cord of the cat and rat: further studies on the anatomy of pain modulation. J. Comp. Neurol. 187 (3), 513–531.

Berkley, K.J., 1985. Multiple systems diverging from the dorsal column nuclei in the cat. Development, Organization, and Processing in Somatosensory Pathways. Alan R. Liss, Inc, pp. 191–202.

Berkley, K.J., 1993. On the significance for viscerosomatic convergence. APS. J. 2, 239–247.

Berkley, K.J., 2005. A life of pelvic pain. Physiology and Behavior 86 (3), 272–280.

Berkley, K.J., Hand, P.J., 1978. Efferent projections of the gracile nucleus in the cat. Brain Res. 153 (2), 263–283.

Berkley, K.J., Holdcroft, A., 1999. Sex and gender differences in pain. In: Wall, P.D., Melzack, R. (Eds.), Textbook of Pain, fourth ed. Churchill Livingstone, London, pp. 951–965.

Berkley, K.J., Hubscher, C.H., 1995a. Are there separate central nervous system pathways for touch and pain? Nat. Med. 1 (8), 766–773.

Berkley, K.J., Hubscher, C.H., 1995b. Visceral and somatic sensory tracks through the neuraxis and their relation to pain: lessons from the rat female reproductive system. In: Gebhart, G.F. (Ed.), Visceral Pain. IASP Press, Seattle, pp. 195–216.

Berkley, K.J., Blomqvist, A., Pelt, A., Flink, R., 1980. Differences in the collateralization of neuronal projections from the dorsal column nuclei and lateral cervical nucleus to the thalamus and tectum in the cat: an anatomical study using two different double-labeling techniques. Brain Res. 202 (2), 273–290.

Berkley, K.J., Guilbaud, G., Benoist, J.M., Gautron, M., 1993a. Responses of neurons in and near the thalamic ventrobasal complex of the rat to stimulation of uterus, cervix, vagina, colon, and skin. J. Neurophysiol. 69 (2), 557–568.

Berkley, K.J., Hubscher, C.H., Wall, P.D., 1993b. Neuronal responses to stimulation of the cervix, uterus, colon, and skin in the rat spinal cord. J. Neurophysiol. 69 (2), 545–556.

Berkley, K.J., Robbins, A., Sato, Y., 1993c. Functional differences between afferent fibers in the hypogastric and pelvic nerves innervating female reproductive organs in the rat. J. Neurophysiol. 69 (2), 533–544.

Berkley, K.J., Benoist, J.M., Gautron, M., Guilbaud, G., 1995. Responses of neurons in the caudal intralaminar thalamic complex of the rat to stimulation of the uterus, vagina, cervix, colon and skin. Brain Res. 695 (1), 92–95.

Bester, H., Menendez, L., Besson, J.M., Bernard, J.F., 1995. Spino (trigemino) parabrachiohypothalamic pathway: electrophysiological evidence for an involvement in pain processes. J. Neurophysiol. 73 (2), 568–585.

Blaustein, J.D., Tetel, M.J., Ricciardi, K.H., Delville, Y., Turcotte, J.C., 1994. Hypothalamic ovarian steroid hormone-sensitive neurons involved in female sexual behavior. Psychoneuroendocrinology 19 (5–7), 505–516.

Bowsher, D., 1976. Role of the reticular formation in responses to noxious stimulation. Pain 2 (4), 361–378.

Bradshaw, H.B., Berkley, K.J., 2000. Estrous changes in responses of rat gracile nucleus neurons to stimulation of skin and pelvic viscera. J. Neurosci. 20 (20), 7722–7727.

Bradshaw, H.B., Berkley, K.J., 2003. The influence of ovariectomy with or without estrogen replacement on responses of rat gracile nucleus neurons to stimulation of hindquarter skin and pelvic viscera. Brain Res. 986 (1–2), 82–90.

Bruggemann, J., Vahle-Hinz, C., Kniffki, K.D., 1993. Representation of the urinary bladder in the lateral thalamus of the cat. J. Neurophysiol. 70 (2), 482–491.

Bruggemann, J., Vahle-Hinz, C., Kniffki, K.D., 1994. Projections from the pelvic nerve to the periphery of the cat's thalamic ventral posterolateral nucleus and adjacent regions of the posterior complex. J. Neurophysiol. 72 (5), 2237–2245.

Bruggemann, J., Shi, T., Apkarian, A.V., 1997. Viscero-somatic neurons in the primary somatosensory cortex (SI) of the squirrel monkey. Brain Res. 756 (1–2), 297–300.

Bruggemann, J., Shi, T., Apkarian, A.V., 1998. Viscerosomatic interactions in the thalamic ventral posterolateral nucleus (VPL) of the squirrel monkey. Brain Res. 787 (2), 269–276.

Bullitt, E., 1990. Expression of c-fos-like protein as a marker for neuronal activity following noxious stimulation in the rat. J. Comp. Neurol. 296 (4), 517–530.

Burstein, R., Falkowsky, O., Borsook, D., Strassman, A., 1996. Distinct lateral and medial projections of the spinohypothalamic tract of the rat. J. Comp. Neurol. 373 (4), 549–574.

Cameron, A.A., Khan, I.A., Westlund, K.N., Cliffer, K.D., Willis, W.D., 1995. The efferent projections of the periaqueductal gray in the rat: a phaseolus vulgaris-leucoagglutinin study. I. Ascending projections. J. Comp. Neurol. 351 (4), 568–584.

Casey, K.L., 1969. Somatic stimuli, spinal pathways, and size of cutaneous fibers influencing unit activity in the medial medullary reticular formation. Exp. Neurol. 25 (1), 35–56.

Cechetto, D.F., 1987. Central representation of visceral function. Federal Proceedings 46 (1), 17–23.

Chadha, H.K., Hubscher, C.H., 2008. Convergence of nociceptive information in the forebrain of female rats: reproductive organ response variations with stage of estrus. Exp. Neurol. 210 (2), 375–387.

Chan, S.H., 1985. Arterial pressure- and cardiac rhythm-related single-neuron activities in the nucleus reticularis gigantocellularis of the rat. J. Auton. Nerv. Syst. 13 (2), 99–100.

Chandler, M.J., Hobbs, S.F., Fu, Q.G., Kenshalo, D.R., Blair, R.W., Foreman, R.D., 1992. Responses of neurons in ventroposterolateral nucleus of primate thalamus to urinary bladder distension. Brain Res. 571 (1), 26–34.

Chaouch, A., Menetrey, D., Binder, D., Besson, J.M., 1983. Neurons at the origin of the medial component of the bulbopontine spinoreticular tract in the rat: an anatomical study using horseradish peroxidase retrograde transport. J. Comp. Neurol. 214 (3), 309–320.

Chen, S.L., Wu, X.Y., Cao, Z.J., Fan, J., Wang, M., Owyang, C., Li, Y., 2008. Subdiaphragmatic vagal afferent nerves modulate visceral pain. Am. J. Physiol. Gastrointest. Liver Physiol. 294 (6), G1441–G1449.

Chernigovskiy, V.N., Onischenko, G., (trans), 1967. Interoceptors. American Psychological Association, Washington, DC.

Cliffer, K.D., Burstein, R., Giesler, G.J., 1991. Distributions of spinothalamic, spinohypothalamic, and spinotelencephalic fibers revealed by anterograde transport of PHA-L in rats. J. Neurosci. 11 (3), 852–868.

Cliffer, K.D., Hasegawa, T., Willis, W.D., 1992. Responses of neurons in the gracile nucleus of cats to innocuous and noxious stimuli: basic characterization and antidromic activation from the thalamus. J. Neurophysiol. 68 (3), 818–832.

Collins, J.J., Lin, C.E., Berthoud, H.R., Papka, R.E., 1999. Vagal afferents from the uterus and cervix provide direct connections to the brainstem. Cell Tissue Res. 295 (1), 43–54.

Coolen, L.M., Allard, J., Truitt, W.A., McKenna, K.E., 2004. Central regulation of ejaculation. Physiology and Behavior 83 (2), 203–215.

Cothron, K.J., Massey, J.M., Onifer, S.M., Hubscher, C.H., 2008. Identification of penile inputs to the rat gracile nucleus. Am. J. Physiol. Regul. Integr. Comp. Physiol. 294 (3), R1015–R1023.

Craig, A.D., Burton, H., 1981. Spinal and medullary lamina I projection to nucleus submedius in medial thalamus: a possible pain center. J. Neurophysiol. 45 (3), 443–466.

Dafny, N., Dong, W.Q., Prieto-Gomez, C., Reyes-Vazquez, C., Stanford, J., Qiao, J.T., 1996. Lateral hypothalamus: Site involved in pain modulation. Neuroscience 70 (2), 449–460.

Daniels, D., Miselis, R.R., Flanagan-Cato, L.M., 1999. Central neuronal circuit innervating the lordosis-producing muscles defined by transneuronal transport of pseudorabies virus. J. Neurosci. 19 (7), 2823–2833.

De Groat, W.C., Booth, A.M., 1993. Neural control of penile erection. In: Maggi, C.A. (Ed.), The Autonomic Nervous System. Harwood Academic, London, pp. 465–516.

Ding, Y.Q., Shi, J., Wang, D.S., Xu, J.Q., Li, J.L., Ju, G., 1999. Primary afferent fibers of the pelvic nerve terminate in the gracile nucleus of the rat. Neurosci. Lett. 272 (3), 211–214.

Docke, F., Rohde, W., Gerber, P., Chaoui, R., Dorner, G., 1984. Varying sensitivity to the negative oestrogen feedback during the ovarian cycle of female rats: evidence for the involvement of oestrogen and the medial preoptic area. J. Endocrinol. 102 (3), 287–294.

Esteves, F., Lima, D., Coimbra, A., 1993. Structural types of spinal cord marginal (lamina I) neurons projecting to the nucleus of the tractus solitarius in the rat. Somatosens. Mot. Res. 10 (2), 203–216.

Gabella, G., Pease, H.L., 1973. Number of axons in the abdominal vagus of the rat. Brain Res. 58 (2), 465–469.

Gallager, D.W., Pert, A., 1978. Afferents to brain stem nuclei (brain stem raphe, nucleus reticularis pontis caudalis and nucleus gigantocellularis) in the rat as demonstrated by microiontophoretically applied horseradish peroxidase. Brain Res. 144 (2), 257–275.

Giesler, G.J., Menetrey, D., Basbaum, A.I., 1979. Differential origins of spinothalamic tract projections to medial and lateral thalamus in the rat. J. Comp. Neurol. 184 (1), 107–126.

Giesler, G.J., Spiel, H.R., Willis, W.D., 1981. Organization of spinothalamic tract axons within the rat spinal cord. J. Comp. Neurol. 195 (2), 243–252.

Giuliano, F., Rampin, O., 2004. Neural control of erection. Physiology and Behavior 83 (2), 189–201.

Granum, S.L., 1986. The spinothalamic system of the rat. I. Locations of cells of origin. J. Comp. Neurol. 247 (2), 159–180.

Guevara-Guzman, R., Buzo, E., Larrazolo, A., de la Riva, C., Da Costa, A.P., Kendrick, K.M., 2001. Vaginocervical stimulation-induced release of classical neurotransmitters and nitric oxide in the nucleus of the solitary tract varies as a function of the oestrus cycle. Brain Res. 898 (2), 303–313.

Guilbaud, G., Bernard, J.F., Besson, J.M., 1994. Brain areas involved in nociception and pain. In: Wall, P.D., Melzack, R. (Eds.), Textbook of Pain, third ed. Churchill Livingstone, Edinburgh, pp. 113–128.

Hermann, G.E., Holmes, G.M., Rogers, R.C., Beattie, M.S., Bresnahan, J.C., 2003. Descending spinal projections from the rostral gigantocellular reticular nuclei complex. J. Comp. Neurol. 455 (2), 210–221.

Holtmann, G., Goebell, H., Jockenhoevel, F., Talley, N.J., 1998. Altered vagal and intestinal mechanosensory function in chronic unexplained dyspepsia. Gut 42 (4), 501–506.

Horie, H., Yokota, T., 1990. Responses of nociceptive VPL neurons to intracardiac injection of bradykinin in the cat. Brain Res. 516 (1), 161–164.

Horn, A.C., Vahle-Hinz, C., Petersen, M., Bruggemann, J., Kniffki, K.D., 1997. Projections from the renal nerve to the cat's lateral somatosensory thalamus. Brain Res. 763 (1), 47–55.

Hubscher, C.H., 1994. Sensory input from pelvic reproductive organs to the gracile and solitary nuclei in the female rat (Dissertation). Florida State University, Tallahassee, p. 80.

Hubscher, C.H., 2006a. Ascending spinal pathways from sexual organs: effects of chronic spinal lesions. In: Weaver, L.C. (Ed.), Autonomic Dysfunction After Spinal Cord Injury: The Problems and Underlying Mechanisms. Elsevier, Oxford, UK, pp. 405–418.

Hubscher, C.H., 2006b. Estradiol-associated variation in responses of rostral medullary neurons to somatovisceral stimulation. Exp. Neurol. 200 (1), 227–239.

Hubscher, C.H., Berkley, K.J., 1994. Responses of neurons in caudal solitary nucleus of female rats to stimulation of vagina, cervix, uterine horn and colon. Brain Res. 664 (1–2), 1–8.

Hubscher, C.H., Berkley, K.J., 1995. Spinal and vagal influences on the responses of rat solitary nucleus neurons to stimulation of uterus, cervix and vagina. Brain Res. 702 (1–2), 251–254.

Hubscher, C.H., Johnson, R.D., 1996. Responses of medullary reticular formation neurons to input from the male genitalia. J. Neurophysiol. 76 (4), 2474–2482.

Hubscher, C.H., Johnson, R.D., 2003. Responses of thalamic neurons to input from the male genitalia. J. Neurophysiol. 89 (1), 2–11.

Hubscher, C.H., Kaddumi, E.G., Johnson, R.D., 2004. Brain stem convergence of pelvic viscerosomatic inputs via spinal and vagal afferents. NeuroReport 15 (8), 1299–1302.

Ito, S.I., 1998. Possible representation of somatic pain in the rat insular visceral sensory cortex: a field potential study. Neurosci. Lett. 241 (2–3), 171–174.

Jean, A., 1991. The nucleus tractus solitarius: neuroanatomic, neurochemical and functional aspects. Archives International Physiology Biochemistry Biophysics 99 (5), A3–A52.

Johnson, R.D., 1989. Physiology of single spinal cord sensory neurons responding to penile stimulation in the rat. Society for Neuroscience Abstracts 15, 756.

Johnson, R.D., Hubscher, C.H., 1998. Brainstem microstimulation differentially inhibits pudendal motoneuron reflex inputs. NeuroReport 9 (2), 341–345.

Johnson, R.D., Hubscher, C.H., 2000. Brainstem microstimulation activates sympathetic fibers in pudendal nerve motor branch. NeuroReport 11 (2), 379–382.

Jones, B.E., 1995. Reticular formation: cytoarchitecture, transmitters, and projections. In: Paxinos, G. (Ed.), The Rat Nervous System, second ed. Academic Press, New York, pp. 155–171.

Kaddumi, E.G., Hubscher, C.H., 2006. Convergence of multiple pelvic organ inputs in the rat rostral medulla. J. Physiol. 572 (Pt 2), 393–405.

Kaddumi, E.G., Hubscher, C.H., 2007. Urinary bladder irritation alters efficacy of vagal stimulation on rostral medullary neurons in chronic T8 spinalized rats. J. Neurotrauma 24 (7), 1219–1228.

Kang, Y.M., Bielefeldt, K., Gebhart, G.F., 2004. Sensitization of mechanosensitive gastric vagal afferent fibers in the rat by thermal and chemical stimuli and gastric ulcers. J. Neurophysiol. 91 (5), 1981–1989.

Katter, J.T., Dado, R.J., Kostarczyk, E., Giesler, G.J., 1996. Spinothalamic and spinohypothalamic tract neurons in the sacral spinal cord of rats. I. Locations of antidromically identified axons in the cervical cord and diencephalon. J. Neurophysiol. 75 (6), 2581–2605.

Kawatani, M., Tanowitz, M., de Groat, W.C., 1994. Morphological and electrophysiological analysis of the peripheral and central afferent pathways from the clitoris of the cat. Brain Res. 646, 26–36.

Kevetter, G.A., Willis, W.D., 1982. Spinothalamic cells in the rat lumbar cord with collaterals to the medullary reticular formation. Brain Res. 238 (1), 181–185.

Komisaruk, B.R., Sansone, G., 2003. Neural pathways mediating vaginal function: the vagus nerves and spinal cord oxytocin. Scand. J. Psychol. 44 (3), 241–250.

Komisaruk, B.R., Whipple, B., Crawford, A., Liu, W.C., Kalnin, A., Mosier, K., 2004. Brain activation during vaginocervical self-stimulation and orgasm in women with complete spinal cord injury: fMRI evidence of mediation by the vagus nerves. Brain Res. 1024 (1–2), 77–88.

Lee, J.W., Erskine, M.S., 1996. Vaginocervical stimulation suppresses the expression of c-fos induced by mating in thoracic, lumbar and sacral segments of the female rat. Neuroscience 74 (1), 237–249.

Lee, J.W., Erskine, M.S., 2000. Pseudorabies virus tracing of neural pathways between the uterine cervix and CNS: effects of survival time, estrogen treatment, rhizotomy, and pelvic nerve transection. J. Comp. Neurol. 418 (4), 484–503.

Lu, W.Y., Bieger, D., 1998. Vagal afferent transmission in the NTS mediating reflex responses of the rat esophagus. Am. J. Physiol. 274 (5 Pt 2), R1436–R1445.

Malykhina, A.P., 2007. Neural mechanisms of pelvic organ cross-sensitization. Neuroscience 149 (3), 660–672.

Marson, L., McKenna, K.E., 1990. The identification of a brainstem site controlling spinal sexual reflexes in male rats. Brain Res. 515 (1–2), 303–308.

McKenna, K.E., 1998. Central control of penile erection. Int. J. Impot. Res. 10 (Suppl. 1), S25–S34.

Menetrey, D., Basbaum, A.I., 1987. Spinal and trigeminal projections to the nucleus of the solitary tract: a possible substrate for somatovisceral and viscerovisceral reflex activation. J. Comp. Neurol. 255 (3), 439–450.

Menetrey, D., de Pommery, J., 1991. Origins of spinal ascending pathways that reach central areas involved in visceroception and visceronociception in the rat. Eur. J. NeuroSci. 3, 249–259.

Modianos, D., Pfaff, D., 1979. Medullary reticular formation lesions and lordosis reflex in female rats. Brain Res. 171 (2), 334–338.

Moss, R.L., Foreman, M.M., 1976. Potentiation of lordosis behavior by intrahypothalamic infusion of synthetic luteinizing hormone-releasing hormone. Neuroendocrinology (2), 176–181.

Mtui, E.P., Anwar, M., Reis, D.J., Ruggiero, D.A., 1995. Medullary visceral reflex circuits: local afferents to nucleus tractus solitarii synthesize catecholamines and project to thoracic spinal cord. J. Comp. Neurol. 351 (1), 5–26.

Murphy, A.Z., Rizvi, T.A., Ennis, M., Shipley, M.T., 1999. The organization of preoptic-medullary circuits in the male rat: evidence for interconnectivity of neural structures involved in reproductive behavior, antinociception and cardiovascular regulation. Neuroscience 91 (3), 1103–1116.

Ness, T.J., Gebhart, G.F., 1987. Characterization of neuronal responses to noxious visceral and somatic stimuli in the medial lumbosacral spinal cord of the rat. J. Neurophysiol. 57 (6), 1867–1892.

Norgren, R., 1978. Projections from the nucleus of the solitary tract in the rat. Neuroscience 3 (2), 207–218.

Norgren, R., Leonard, C.M., 1973. Ascending central gustatory pathways. J. Comp. Neurol. 150 (2), 217–237.

Nosaka, S., 1984. Solitary nucleus neurons transmitting vagal visceral input to the forebrain via a direct pathway in rats. Exp. Neurol. 85 (3), 493–505.

Novin, D., Rogers, R.C., Hermann, G., 1981. Visceral afferent and efferent connections in the brain. Diabetologia 20, 331–336.

Odutola, A.B., 1977. On the location of reticular neurons projecting to the cuneo-gracile nuclei in the rat. Exp. Neurol. 54 (1), 54–59.

Ortega-Villalobos, M., Garcia-Bazan, M., Solano-FloRes, L.P., Ninomiya-Alarcon, J.G., Guevara-Guzman, R., Wayner, M.J., 1990. Vagus nerve afferent and efferent innervation of the rat uterus: an electrophysiological and HRP study. Brain Res. Bull. 25 (3), 365–371.

Ozaki, N., Sengupta, J.N., Gebhart, G.F., 1999. Mechanosensitive properties of gastric vagal afferent fibers in the rat. J. Neurophysiol. 82 (5), 2210–2220.

Peschanski, M., Besson, J.M., 1984. A spino-reticulo-thalamic pathway in the rat: an anatomical study with reference to pain transmission. Neuroscience 12 (1), 165–178.

Pezzone, M.A., Liang, R., Fraser, M.O., 2005. A model of neural cross-talk and irritation in the pelvis: implications for the overlap of chronic pelvic pain disorders. Gastroenterology 128 (7), 1953–1964.

Qin, C., Chandler, M.J., Foreman, R.D., 2003. Effects of urinary bladder distension on activity of T3-T4 spinal neurons receiving cardiac and somatic noxious inputs in rats. Brain Res. 971 (2), 210–220.

Qin, C., Malykhina, A.P., Akbarali, H.I., Foreman, R.D., 2005. Cross-organ sensitization of lumbosacral spinal neurons receiving urinary bladder input in rats with inflamed colon. Gastroenterology 129 (6), 1967–1978.

Qin, C., Foreman, R.D., Farber, J.P., 2007. Inhalation of a pulmonary irritant modulates activity of lumbosacral spinal neurons receiving colonic input in rats. Am. J. Physiol. Regul. Integr. Comp. Physiol. 293 (5), R2052–R2058.

Rampin, O., Gougis, S., Giuliano, F., Rousseau, J.P., 1997. Spinal Fos labeling and penile erection elicited by stimulation of dorsal nerve of the rat penis. Am. J. Physiol. 272 (5 Pt 2), R1425–R1431.

Reed, W.R., Chadha, H.K., Hubscher, C.H., 2009. Effects of 17β estradiol on responses of viscerosomatic convergent thalamic neurons in the ovariectomized female rat. J. Neurophysiol. in press.

Ricardo, J.A., Koh, E.T., 1978. Anatomical evidence of direct projections from the nucleus of the solitary tract to the hypothalamus, amygdala, and other forebrain structures in the rat. Brain Res. 153 (1), 1–26.

Rong, P.J., Zhang, J.L., Zhang, H.Q., 2004. Interactions between tactile and noxious visceral inputs in rat nucleus gracilis. Neurosci. Lett. 362 (2), 162–165.

Ruggiero, D.A., Anwar, S., Kim, J., Glickstein, S.B., 1998. Visceral afferent pathways to the thalamus and olfactory tubercle: behavioral implications. Brain Res. 799 (1), 159–171.

Saggu, S., Lundy, R.F., 2008. Forebrain neurons that project to the gustatory parabrachial nucleus in rat lack glutamic acid decarboxylase. Am. J. Physiol. Regul. Integr. Comp. Physiol. 294 (1), R52–R57.

Saper, C.B., Loewy, A.D., 1980. Efferent connections of the parabrachial nucleus in the rat. Brain Res. 197 (2), 291–317.

Schwartz-Giblin, S., McCarthy, M.M., Robbins, A., 1996. The medullary reticular formation is a site of muscle relaxant action of diazepam on deep back and neck muscles in the female rat. Brain Res. 710 (1–2), 178–188.

Simon, O.R., Schramm, L.P., 1984. The spinal course and medullary termination of myelinated renal afferents in the rat. Brain Res. 290 (2), 239–247.

Steers, W.D., 2000. Neural pathways and central sites involved in penile erection: neuroanatomy and clinical implications. Neuroscience Biobehavioral Reviews 24 (5), 507–516.

Tanaka, J., Arnold, A.P., 1993. An electrophysiological study of descending projections to the lumbar spinal cord in adult male rats. Exp. Brain Res. 96 (1), 117–124.

Ter Horst, G.J., de Boer, P., Luiten, P.G., van Willigen, J.D., 1989. Ascending projections from the solitary tract nucleus to the hypothalamus. A phaseolus vulgaris lectin tracing study in the rat. Neuroscience 31 (3), 785–797.

Tomasulo, K.C., Emmers, R., 1972. Activation of neurons in the gracile nucleus by two afferent pathways in the rat. Exp. Neurol. 36 (1), 197–206.

Truitt, W.A., Coolen, L.M., 2002. Identification of a potential ejaculation generator in the spinal cord. Science 297 (5586), 1566–1569.

Ueyama, T., Arakawa, H., Mizuno, N., 1985. Contralateral termination of pudendal nerve fibers in the gracile nucleus of the rat. Neurosci. Lett. 62 (1), 113–117.

Ueyama, T., Arakawa, H., Mizuno, N., 1987. Central distribution of efferent and afferent components of the pudendal nerve in rat. Anatomical Embryology (Berlin) 177 (1), 37–49.

Ustinova, E.E., Gutkin, D.W., Pezzone, M.A., 2007. Sensitization of pelvic nerve afferents and mast cell infiltration in the urinary bladder following chronic colonic irritation is mediated by neuropeptides. Am. J. Physiol. Renal Physiology 292 (1), F123–F130.

Vahle-Hinz, C., Bruggemann, J., Kniffki, K.D., 1995. Thalamic processing of visceral pain. In: Bromm, B., Desmedt, J.E. (Eds.), Pain and the Brain. From Nociception to Cognition. Raven Press, Ltd., New York, pp. 125–141.

Van der Kooy, D., Koda, L.Y., McGinty, J.F., Gerfen, C.R., Bloom, F.E., 1984. The organization of projections from the cortex, amygdala, and hypothalamus to the nucleus of the solitary tract in rat. J. Comp. Neurol. 224 (1), 1–24.

Van der Plas, J., Wiersinga-Post, J.E., Maes, F.W., Bohus, B., 1995. Cardiovascular effects and changes in midbrain periaqueductal gray neuronal activity induced by electrical stimulation of the hypothalamus in the rat. Brain Res. Bull 37 (6), 645–656.

Vertes, R.P., Crane, A.M., 1996. Descending projections of the posterior nucleus of the hypothalamus: Phaseolus vulgaris leucoagglutinin analysis in the rat. J. Comp. Neurol. 374 (4), 607–631.

Wall, P.D., Hubscher, C.H., Berkley, K.J., 1993. Intraspinal modulation of neuronal responses to uterine and cervix stimulation in rat L1 and L6 dorsal horn. Brain Res. 622 (1–2), 71–78.

Wang, C.C., Westlund, K.N., 2001. Responses of rat dorsal column neurons to pancreatic nociceptive stimulation. NeuroReport 12 (11), 2527–2530.

Wang, C.C., Willis, W.D., Westlund, K.N., 1999. Ascending projections from the area around the spinal cord central canal: A phaseolus vulgaris leucoagglutinin study in rats. J. Comp. Neurol. 415 (3), 341–367.

Willis, W.D., 1995. Pain and the brain: From nociception to cognition. In: Bromm, B., Desmedt, J.E. (Eds.), Advances in Pain Research and Therapy. Raven Press, New York, pp. 1–19.

Willis, W.D., Coggeshall, R.E., 1991. Sensory Mechanisms of the Spinal Cord. Plenum Press, New York.

Winnard, K.P., Dmitrieva, N., Berkley, K.J., 2006. Cross-organ interactions between reproductive, gastrointestinal, and urinary tracts: modulation by estrous stage and involvement of the hypogastric nerve. Am. J. Physiol. Regul. Integr. Comp. Physiol. 291 (6), R1592–R1601.

Zhang, X., Fogel, R., Renehan, W.E., 1992. Physiology and morphology of neurons in the dorsal motor nucleus of the vagus and the nucleus of the solitary tract that are sensitive to distension of the small intestine. J. Comp. Neurol. 323 (3), 432–448.

Zhang, X., Kostarczyk, E., Giesler, G.J., 1995. Spinohypothalamic tract neurons in the cervical enlargement of rats: descending axons in the ipsilateral brain. J. Neurosci. 15 (12), 8393–8407.

Zhuo, M., Gebhart, G.F., 1990. Characterization of descending inhibition and facilitation from the nuclei reticularis gigantocellularis and gigantocellularis pars alpha in the rat. Pain 42 (3), 337–350.

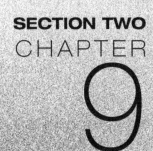

Role of oxytocin and oxytocin-related effects in manual therapies

Kerstin Uvnäs-Moberg • Maria Petersson

The relaxation and growth or the calm and connection response

All types of manual therapy involve touching the patient. In this chapter we suggest that all therapies involving gentle skin contact will lead to activation of a basic psychophysiological reaction in response to activation of cutaneous sensory nerves. This basic reaction pattern is probably from an evolutionary perspective very old, and forms an antithesis to the fight and flight response and other defensive reactions (Cannon 1929, Selye 1976). The effects include stimulation of social behavior, decreased anxiety, increased pain threshold, wellbeing, decreased activity in the hypothalamopituitary–adrenal (HPA) axis, lowered blood pressure, vasodilatation of cutaneous vessels, and increased function in the endocrine system of the gastrointestinal tract. In addition, anabolic, storage metabolism, healing of wounds and restorative processes are promoted. Learning is also stimulated.

Corticotropin-releasing factor (CRF) and vasopressin play an important integrative function in defense and stress reactions. We propose that oxytocin produced in the nucleus paraventricularis (PVN), mainly via oxytocinergic nerves projecting to many important regulatory areas in the central nervous system (CNS), plays a similar integrative function in a reaction pattern that runs opposite to and forms an antithesis to the defense reactions. The physiological aspects of this reaction pattern have been named the *relaxation and growth response* and, when behavioral expressions are included, the *calm and connection response* (Uvnäs-Moberg 1997, 2003).

Noxious versus non-noxious stimulation of sensory nerves and the experience of fear versus trust

Release of CRF and vasopressin can be induced by physical damage to the skin or other noxious stimuli by activation of cutaneous sensory nerves. In contrast, oxytocin is released in response to non-noxious sensory stimulation of the skin, e.g., by touch, stroking, and warmth. In addition, mental experiences of danger or threat can, via processing in the hippocampus and amygdala axis, induce stress responses and defense. By analogy, we suggest that the oxytocin release and oxytocin-related effect patterns can be induced by mental experiences of love, trust, and safety (Uvnäs-Moberg et al. 2005).

The role of touch and trust in manual therapies

Because physical interaction forms part of all therapeutic sessions involving manual therapies, the oxytocin-related effect pattern may be induced in all such treatments, in addition to more specific effects related to the different therapies. In addition, the therapist's behavior and contact with the patient will be of utmost importance for the outcome. When the patient feels safe and trusts the therapist, the patient's oxytocin release, and hence the psychophysiological effect pattern integrated by oxytocin, will be further promoted.

In the following we will review some animal and human data regarding the effects of gentle sensory stimulation and of administration of oxytocin in animals and humans. We will also describe how gentle touch and a friendly and trustworthy behavior may activate oxytocin release and hence induce the effect spectrum integrated by oxytocin.

Sensory nerves mediating effects of non-noxious sensory stimulation

Activation of myelinated Aβ fibers induces a sensation of touch in specific areas in the primary somatosensory cortex of the brain. Sensory fibers mediating the sensation of touch do not, however, give rise only to awareness of which part of the body has been touched, but also to sensations of a calming, pleasant, and relaxing nature. Obviously these feelings and sensations are not related to the activation of the primary somatosensory cortex but rather are mediated by activation of older parts of the brain. The sensations are not distinctly localized from an anatomical perspective, but are diffuse and appear with a certain delay, and may not even become apparent. They can be compared with the feelings of wellbeing and relaxation that follow the ingestion of a good meal.

In addition, some physiological effects related to anti-stress and growth stimulation are induced in response to touch. The physiological, behavioral, and emotional effects that follow gentle stimulation of the skin may be induced via activation of collaterals from the myelinated afferent nerves that project to more basal parts of the brain.

Recently it has been demonstrated that also a subgroup of the thinner and more slowly conducting C fibers (CT = C tactile) mediates pleasant feelings and can be activated by touch, not only in animals but also in humans. From an evolutionary perspective, CT fibers are older than the thicker and more rapidly conducting A and B fibers, and are mainly connected to older parts of the brain, where they influence emotions. The CT fibers are activated especially in response to slow and light stroking (around

40 cm/min) and have been shown to activate areas in the insular cortex, which are related to the sensations of wellbeing (Craig 2003, Olausson et al. 2002, Vallbo et al. 1999).

Effects of non-noxious sensory stimulation in animals

Noxious stimulation is well known to induce both defense reactions and physiological reactions, which are compatible with activity and stress, via an increased activity in the HPA axis, relevant aspects of the sympathoneural system and of the sympathoadrenal (SA) system. Non-noxious stimulation, however, also induces effects of physiological nature. In anesthetized rats brushing or stroking reduces activity in the SA system and in the HPA axis, as evidenced by lowered levels of adrenaline and of corticosterone in the circulation (Araki et al. 1984, Kurosawa et al. 1982, Tsuchiya et al. 1991). Blood pressure is also reduced (Kurosawa et al. 1995). In addition, efferent vagal nerve activity is increased by low-intensity electrical stimulation and by stroking, as evidenced by an influence on the levels of vagally controlled gastrointestinal hormones (Uvnäs-Moberg et al. 1992).

In conscious rats also, physiological effects are induced in response to non-noxious stimulation. Stroking of the abdomen – but not of the back – at a frequency of 40 strokes per minute for 5 minutes, reduces blood pressure and pulse rate for several hours. These results suggest that it is easier to inhibit cardiovascular activity by stroking the chest and abdomen than by stroking the back. Further basal insulin, gastrin, and somatostatin levels are lowered and energy expenditure is decreased. These findings indicate that the treatment influences certain aspects of the sympathetic and parasympathetic nervous system. In addition, nociceptive thresholds are increased.

Behavioral effects are also induced by stroking: for example it induces a sedative effect by reducing spontaneous motor activity. This effect is dependent on the amount of stroking given, as no effect was observed after 2 minutes of stroking but was seen after 5 minutes. Weight gain is observed in response to repeated treatments with stroking, and the increase in nociceptive thresholds is further enhanced (Ågren et al. 1995, Holst et al. 2002, 2005, Kurosawa et al. 1995, Lund et al. 1999, 2002, Uvnäs-Moberg et al. 1992, 1993, 1996a).

Effects of non-noxious sensory stimulation can also be observed as a consequence of maternal interaction with pups. Stress-related effects in rat pups, such as elevated levels of corticosterone and decreased levels of growth hormone as a consequence of separation from their mothers, are prevented if the pups are exposed to extra stroking (Pauk et al. 1986, van Oers et al. 1998). The mothers are also kept calm when they are in close contact with their offspring (Lonstein 2005).

Stroking of rat pups may even induce lifelong effects. When pups were exposed to daily stroking on the ventral side of the abdomen for 1 week postnatally, blood pressure was significantly reduced in adulthood (Holst et al. 2002). Further, rat pups exposed to mothers that are highly interacting during the first week of life become less anxious, more social, and more tolerant to stress than pups of mothers who interact less (Champagne & Meaney 2008).

Oxytocin

Oxytocin – a neurotransmitter and a hormone

Oxytocin is a nonapeptide produced in the PVN and the supraoptic nucleus (SON) within the hypothalamus. Magnocellular neurons within the SON and PVN project to the neurohypophysis, whence oxytocin is released into the circulation. In addition, a widespread network of parvocellular, oxytocinergic nerve fibers project from the PVN to many areas within the brain. The median eminence, the amygdala, the hippocampus, the olfactory bulb, the striatum, the nucleus accumbens (NA), the raphe nuclei, the locus ceruleus, the vagal motor and sensory nuclei, and the spinal cord are all reached by oxytocinergic fibers (Buijs et al. 1985).

Oxytocin may induce effects in many areas of the brain, as oxytocin receptors are widely distributed in the brain (Freund-Mercier et al. 1987). Recently it has been demonstrated that large quantities of oxytocin are also released from cell bodies and dendrites of oxytocin-producing cells in the SON and PVN. It has therefore been suggested that oxytocin may also reach neurons that are not adjacent to the release sites by diffusion or volume transmission (Ludwig & Leng 2006).

It is well known that the mammary glands and the uterus are richly provided with oxytocin receptors. Oxytocin receptors are, however, also found in many peripheral organs, e.g. in the kidneys, pancreas, stomach, thymus, adipocytes, heart, ventricle and blood vessels (Bonne & Cohen 1975, Elands et al. 1990, McCann et al. 2002, Stock et al. 1990, Stoeckel & Freund-Mercier 1989, Yazawa et al. 1996).

The PVN is also reached by afferent pathways from the NTS, the locus ceruleus, other parts of the hypothalamus, and even from the dorsal horn of the spinal cord, suggesting that the release of oxytocin is controlled from many different areas in the CNS (Swanson & Sawchenko 1980, 1983, Sawchenko & Swanson 1982).

The distribution of afferent and efferent projection patterns and the distribution of oxytocin receptors are similar in females and males (Sawchenko & Swanson 1982, Sofroniew 1983, Swanson & Sawchenko 1980, 1983), but the effects of oxytocin may differ between males and females owing to the effects of sex hormones. Estrogens may increase the release of oxytocin and also the responsiveness and/or number of oxytocin receptors (Schumacher et al. 1993).

Effects of oxytocin in animals

Oxytocin modulates many physiological and behavioral functions. Administration of oxytocin to animals has been demonstrated to induce a multitude of effects, which depend in part on the experimental situation and whether the effects mimic circulating actions of oxytocin or the effects of oxytocin as a neurotransmitter in the CNS.

Oxytocin administered intracerebroventricularly, or in high doses systemically to induce effects in the CNS, has been demonstrated to reduce blood pressure and activity in the HPA axis. The effect of oxytocin on the HPA axis seems to be exerted at many levels (see below and Fig. 9.1). It also influences the release of gastrointestinal hormones, increases nociceptive thresholds, and reduces inflammation and levels of anxiety, as well as inducing calm and stimulating learning.

When oxytocin is administered repeatedly long-term effects may be induced. Five daily injections of oxytocin reduce blood pressure and activity in the HPA axis and increase nociceptive thresholds for weeks after the last treatment. In response to repeated treatments oxytocin also influences the levels of gastrointestinal hormones, increases weight gain, and shortens wound healing time.

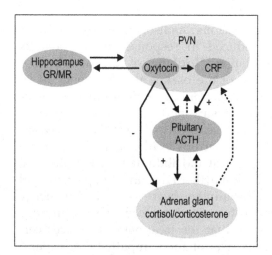

Figure 9.1 Schematic regulation of the hypothalamopituitary–adrenal (HPA) axis and the inhibition of oxytocin at several levels. ACTH, adrenocorticotropic hormone; CRF, corticotrophin-releasing factor; GR, glucocorticoid receptor; MR, mineralocorticoid receptor; PVN, paraventricular nucleus of the hypothalamus.

Further, it improves learning by conditioning (Björkstrand et al. 1996, Petersson et al. 1996a,b, 1998, 1999a,b, 2001, Szeto et al. 2008, Uvnäs-Moberg et al. 1992, 1996b, 2000).

Oxytocin knockout mice have an increased release of corticosterone in response to stress and show more anxiety-like behavior, further supporting the role of oxytocin as an anxiolytic and anti-stress agent (Amico et al. 2008). In addition, oxytocin stimulates various kinds of interactive social behavior and bonding between mother and young, and between males and females (Carter 1998).

Oxytocin mediates effects not only via the classic uterine oxytocin receptor, but probably also via oxytocin receptors with other characteristics, as not all oxytocin effects exerted in the brain are blocked by antagonists directed towards the classic oxytocin receptor. Moreover, administration of oxytocin to rats increases α_2-adrenoreceptor function in several brain regions, such as the amygdala, NTS, and locus ceruleus, as measured by autoradiography and electrophysiology. It is likely that this effect underlies some of the oxytocin-induced anti-stress effects (Petersson et al. 2005). Oxytocin also influences cholinergic, serotonergic (5HT), and opioidergic transmission. Some of the long-term effects may be induced by altering the function of these classic signaling systems. In addition, dopamine, opioids, acetylcholine, and 5HT influence the release of oxytocin, and antidepressant drugs, such as serotonin reuptake inhibitors (SSRI), have been shown to release oxytocin (Uvnäs-Moberg et al. 1999).

Taken together, these data show, first, that oxytocin induces a response pattern characterized by anti-stress effects and stimulation of growth and restorative processes (*the growth and relaxation response*) and also behavioral actions involving calm and increased social behavior (the *calm and connection response*) (Uvnäs-Moberg 1997, 2003); and second, that the function of the oxytocinergic system is strongly connected with the activity of other, more classic, signaling systems (Bagdy & Kalogeras 1993, Clarke et al.

1978, Crowley et al. 1991, Uvnäs-Moberg et al. 1999, Wright & Clarke 1984).

Effects of oxytocin in humans

Since the beginning of the 19th century oxytocin has been known to stimulate uterine contractions during labor and to induce milk letdown in breastfeeding women, being administered as an infusion to induce or augment labor and as a nasal spray to promote milk letdown. Recently the oxytocin nasal spray has also been administered to men, and several effects have been documented. The oxytocin has an anxiolytic effect and dampens activity in the amygdala. It also reduces activity in the HPA axis, as well as increasing social skills, e.g. the ability to read and evaluate the emotional valence of faces, in both healthy and autistic men. In other studies the administration of oxytocin spray has been demonstrated to increase trust and generosity in men and to reduce abdominal pain in women (Heinrichs et al. 2003, Kosfeld et al. 2005, Ohlsson et al. 2005, Rimmele et al. 2009). Oxytocin administered as an intravenous infusion also reduces anxiety and increases social skills, effects that last for weeks after administration (Hollander et al. 2007, Jonas et al. 2008a).

Thus the administration of oxytocin to humans not only stimulates uterine contractions and milk ejection via circulating effects, but also induces a behavioral and physiological effect pattern. The fact that the effect pattern induced by oxytocin in humans is identical to that induced in animals supports the assumption that oxytocin exerts important regulatory and integrative functions in the brain.

Link between oxytocin and effects induced by non-noxious sensory stimulation

Interestingly, as described above, the administration of oxytocin has been demonstrated to induce an effect spectrum similar to that induced by non-noxious sensory stimulation. As will be described below, oxytocin is also released by non-noxious sensory stimulation, and therefore some of the effects induced by non-noxious sensory stimulation may be mediated by oxytocin released in the brain.

Oxytocin release in response to non-noxious sensory stimulation in animal experiments

It is well known that oxytocin is released during parturition and in response to suckling in lactating animals, and in response to sexual interaction. Oxytocin can, however, also be released in response to other types of non-noxious and pleasant sensory stimulation. When anesthetized rats were exposed to gentle stroking on their backs or afferent electrical stimulation of the sciatic or the vagal nerves, oxytocin levels in plasma increased more than twofold (Stock & Uvnäs-Moberg 1988), and when they were exposed to electroacupuncture, thermal stimulation, or vibration, oxytocin levels increased in both plasma and cerebrospinal fluid (Uvnäs-Moberg et al. 1993).

As mentioned above, 5 minutes of stroking on the abdomen of conscious rats (40 strokes per minute) induces a multitude of behavioral and physiological effects (Box 9.1; note that weight gain is only observed in response to repeated treatments). Oxytocin is also released by this type of stimulation, and the effects of stroking may therefore involve an oxytocinergic mechanism. The elevation of pain threshold and the calming and anxiolytic-like effects caused by stroking on the abdomen are probably exerted in the

Box 9.1 Effects of stroking

Increased social interaction
Sedative and anxiolytic-like effects
Increased nociceptive thresholds
Decreased heart rate and blood pressure
Reduced corticosterone levels
Changed levels of cholecystokinin, gastrin, and insulin
Enhanced weight gain
Improved learning

periaqueductal gray (PAG), amygdala, and LC, by oxytocin released from oxytocinergic fibers originating in the PVN. The connection between oxytocin and the effects induced by stroking are supported by findings that some of the effects, e.g. the elevation of pain threshold, caused by the stroking treatment are blocked if the animals are given an oxytocin antagonist beforehand. In further support of a role for oxytocin in the increase in pain threshold caused by stroking is the fact that increased oxytocin levels in response to stroking have been demonstrated in the PAG, an area in the brain that is of central importance for nociception (Lund et al. 2002).

The effect on pulse rate and blood pressure in response to stroking may be due to an effect in the NTS mediated by oxytocin released from efferent oxytocinergic fibers originating in the paraventricular nucleus of the hypothalamus (PVN), in response to activation of the sensory afferents. The activity of the sympathetic and the parasympathetic nervous system is influenced by this effect, with consequent changes in cardiovascular function.

It is important to state that the effects induced by oxytocin on physiological and behavioral function in response to sensory stimulation are exerted in the brain. Therefore, circulating levels of oxytocin are not always a relevant marker for the release of oxytocin in the brain. Oxytocin may be released into the brain in many situations without a concomitant release into the circulation. A parallel secretion of oxytocin into both the brain and into the circulation has, however, been shown during suckling, feeding, parturition, and vaginocervical stimulation (Kendrick et al. 1986, 1988). In rats, electroacupuncture, vibration, and thermal stimuli significantly increase oxytocin levels in the cerebrospinal fluid (Uvnäs-Moberg et al. 1993).

Human models of touch and oxytocin-related effects

Touch, light pressure, and mechanical and thermal stimulation of the skin are integral parts of close human relationships irre-spective of age and gender. Data regard-ing the behavioral and physiological effects induced by closeness in the breastfeed-ing situation, during skin-to-skin contact between mothers and infants after birth, dur-ing kangaroo care, and finally in response to massage in humans are described.

Breastfeeding

Breastfeeding is associated with a pulsa-tile release of oxytocin into the circulation, aimed at stimulating milk ejection. At the same time, oxytocin is released within the brain from oxytocinergic neurons, dendrites and nerve fibers in order to induce behav-ioral and physiological adaptations in the mother (Jonas et al. 2008a, b).

During breastfeeding the mother experi-ences pleasure and a sense of wellbeing. In addition, her levels of anxiety are reduced and her social skills increased. The wellbeing may be related to a release of dopamine in the nucleus accumbens (NA) induced by oxyto-cin, and the decrease in anxiety and increase in social skills may be related to effects by oxytocin induced in the amygdala and other areas in the brain related to social behavior.

Also an anti-stress pattern is induced, as reflected by a fall in cortisol levels and blood pressure, indicating a suckling-related reduction in activity in the HPA axis and in aspects of the sympathetic nervous system involved in the regulation of blood pressure (Amico et al. 1994, Johansson et al. 2009, Jonas et al. 2008b, Nissen et al. 1996). Suckling is also accompanied by increased levels of some gastrointestinal hormones (for example insulin, CCK, and gastrin) as a consequence of activation of vagal pregan-glionic neurons (Uvnäs-Moberg 1996). All the effects mentioned above are exerted in response to oxytocin being released from nerves at different sites in the brain.

Effect of skin-to-skin contact versus suckling

During breastfeeding the mother receives sensory stimulation not only when the baby suckles, but also when the baby is lying in skin-to-skin contact with her. Interestingly, most of the adaptive effects previously observed during breastfeeding and ascribed to the suckling stimulus are indeed also trig-gered by touch and closeness. Cortisol lev-els and blood pressure fall and the mother becomes less anxious and more interac-tive (Johansson et al. 2009). Oxytocin lev-els are increased and exhibit a few pulses in response to hand massage performed by the infant (Matthiesen et al. 2001, Nissen et al. 1996). In contrast, milk ejection is not induced by skin-to-skin contact only, as it requires the more intense, pulsatile oxytocin release that occurs in response to suckling.

Dissociation between effect of suckling and skin-to-skin contact on cortisol release

When the effect of suckling and skin-to-skin contact on the HPA axis were compared, some interesting observations were made: circulating oxytocin levels were negatively correlated with ACTH levels, but not with cortisol levels; the duration of skin-to-skin contact was related to the fall in cortisol levels but not to ACTH levels; there was a strong correlation between the fall in blood pressure and the fall in cortisol levels. Together, these data suggest that suckling and skin-to-skin contact may influence the HPA axis in differ-ent ways (Johansson et al. 2009).

In an experimental cow model we have been able to show that stroking of the abdo-men results in a decreased release of cortisol without a concomitant decrease of ACTH into the circulation (Wredle et al. to be pub-lished). We therefore suggest that cortisol secretion is influenced not only by ACTH levels, but also by the sympathoadrenal system (Nussdorfer 1996) (Fig. 9.2).

HPA axis and the inhibitory role of oxytocin

During suckling large amounts of oxytocin are released. Oxytocin released by nerve fibers in the median eminence inhibits the release of CRF by neurons within the PVN

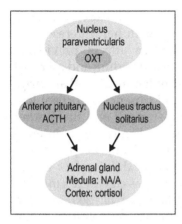

Figure 9.2 Oxytocin may reduce activity within the hypothalamopituitary–adrenal (HPA) axis both through effects directly at the HPA axis and through effects in the nucleus tractus solitarius. A, adrenaline; NA, noradrenaline.

and also the release of ACTH in the anterior pituitary gland, and thereby the release of cortisol from the adrenal cortex. During skin-to-skin contact the release of oxytocin into the circulation is much smaller than during suckling (Matthiesen et al. 2001, Nissen et al. 1996, 1998). As ACTH levels are not influenced in response to skin-to-skin contact, it is possible that only small amounts of oxytocin are released into the PVN to influence CRF secretion and into the median eminence to reduce the release of ACTH. In contrast, the oxytocinergic nerves projecting to the autonomic centers in the brainstem, e.g. the NTS, may still be activated by skin-to-skin contact to reduce blood pressure and the activity of the sympathoadrenal system. Interestingly, oxytocin fibers also reach the preganglionic sympathetic ganglia (Hosoya et al. 1995).

The suggestion that oxytocin may influence the secretion of corticosterone via an ACTH-independent mechanism is strengthened by the fact that in experiments performed in rats, repeated injections of oxytocin reduced the levels of corticosterone, whereas the levels of ACTH remained unchanged (Petersson et al. 1999b). These data demonstrated that oxytocin may reduce cortisol/corticosterone levels without influencing the secretion of ACTH. In addition, repeated

intracerebroventricular administration of oxytocin increases oxytocin levels in the adrenal glands (authors' unpublished observation) and reduces corticosterone production locally in the adrenal cortex (Stachowiak et al. 1995), suggesting that oxytocin may influence the secretion of corticosterone.

Skin-to-skin contact after birth

When infants are placed in skin-to-skin contact after birth, they express an inborn prefeeding behavior, which includes vocalizations, movements towards the mother, and massage and sucking of the breast (Widström et al. 1987). In addition, they become calmer and stop crying (Christensson et al. 1995). The mother responds to the infant's approaching behavior by increasing their circulating oxytocin levels: the more sucking and massage of the breast, the more oxytocin is released (Matthiesen et al. 2001).

Mothers in the same room as their newborn infants exhibit a fluctuating chest skin temperature, whereas mothers whose children are in the nursery have a stable skin temperature, suggesting that the presence of the infants increases maternal temperature on the chest (Bystrova et al. 2003, 2007). The infants respond to the mothers' varying skin temperature by increasing their own skin temperature, the greatest rise being observed in the infant's foot temperature. In contrast, foot temperature in infants being kept in the nursery fell. Furthermore, maternal axillary temperature correlated with foot temperature in infants having skin-to-skin contact: the higher the maternal temperature, the higher the infant's temperature. However, if the infants were wearing clothes the effect of maternal temperature was reduced, suggesting that the clothing exerted an insulating effect (Bystrova et al. 2007, Jonas et al. 2007).

These data have been interpreted as follows: skin-to-skin contact gives rise to an activation of afferent cutaneous nerves responding to touch, light pressure, and warm temperature in the infant. The fact that skin temperature was more influenced at peripheral sites such as the foot, compared to axillary skin temperature, suggests that maternal temperature must have influenced the activity of sympathetic neurons supplying the vasculature of the skin in the infant. Labor and birth are very stressful to the infant, as evidenced by high levels of circulating catecholamines and peripheral vasoconstriction. When the infant is allowed skin-to-skin contact, 'the stress of being born' is counteracted and skin temperature increased, in particular at peripheral sites such as the feet, as a consequence of cutaneous vasodilation. The infants are also less sensitive to pain during skin-to-skin contact, and the levels of gastrointestinal hormones are influenced as a consequence of vagal nerve activation (Bystrova et al. 2003, 2007, Törnhage et al. 1996).

Taken together, these data suggest that skin-to-skin contact between mother and infant leads to increased activity in the newborn's oxytocinergic system, which coordinates a pattern of behavioral and physiological effects. Oxytocin promotes the infant's social behavior, makes it calm, reduces its sensitivity to pain, reduces its stress levels, and stimulates vagal nerve activity. These changes are important adaptations for the newborn baby. A corresponding effect is observed in the mother, who becomes more interactive and calmer as a response to the skin-to-skin contact. As mentioned above, the same effects occur during breastfeeding, which, however, is a stronger stimulus than skin-to-skin contact and which also stimulates milk production and ejection.

Kangaroo treatment

Premature infants are often treated by periods of closeness (kangaroo care) with mothers and fathers as an alternative to being kept in incubators. Repeated studies demonstrate that infants so treated become less sensitive to pain, calmer, have reduced cortisol levels, increase in weight, and develop motor and cognitive skills more quickly when compared to infants being kept in incubators. They also develop a stronger attachment to

their parents. The parents also bond more rapidly with their infant, and the mother produces more milk. All these effects can be attributed to a release of oxytocin in the brain in connection with skin-to-skin contact, and a consequent integration and facilitation of an appropriate effect pattern (Hall & Kirsten 2008).

Effects of massage in humans

The effect of massage in humans has been investigated in many controlled studies. Field (2002) has demonstrated how massage causes beneficial effects in both men and women, children and adults, e.g., that massage has an anxiolytic and an antidepressant effect, and that it promotes social interaction and increases attachment between individuals. It also reduces cortisol levels. Premature infants receiving massage increase in weight and develop more quickly than control infants. In other studies massage has been shown to induce wellbeing, to reduce aggression, and to increase positive social interaction in a preschool setting, and to ameliorate the relationship between staff and patients (Field 2002, von Knorring et al. 2009). Altogether, massage seems to induce the same effects as non-noxious sensory stimulation in animals, as administration of oxytocin in animals and humans, and as breastfeeding or skin-to-skin contact and kangaroo care give rise to in parents and infants. These data strongly suggest that massage activates the oxytocinergic system in the brain.

An increase in circulating oxytocin levels is not necessary to induce effects in response to massage

During parturition and breastfeeding oxytocin is released both into the brain and into the circulation, leading to effects both in the periphery and in the brain in these situations. On the other hand, there is no real role for oxytocin in the circulation during massage, and therefore oxytocin is released mainly into the CNS. Still, a short-lasting rise in plasma oxytocin in response to massage has been found in some studies (Uvnäs-Moberg 2004).

The peak of this response occurs at variable time points, therefore it is necessary to collect and analyze repeated blood samples in order to be able to record the rise in oxytocin. On the other hand, it is possible to observe the consequences of oxytocin released into the brain, such as increased activation of social behavior, reduced levels of anxiety, decreased levels of cortisol and lowered blood pressure, and also of changed levels of gastrointestinal hormones in response to massage.

Release of oxytocin and oxytocin-linked effects in social communication: the role of attachment and mental representations

As discussed above oxytocin is released in both mothers and offspring in response to suckling and skin-to-skin contact (Lupoli et al. 2001). Oxytocin is also released in both partners during sex (Murphy et al. 1987). After a while a bond is formed between mothers and infants, and also between males and females in animal species that are capable of pair-bonding. This means that during lactation mother and infant are continuously exposed to oxytocin, and at the same time to the effects caused by oxytocin, such as wellbeing and pleasure, anti-stress effects such as decreased activity in the HPA axis, lowered blood pressure, and stimulation of growth and restorative processes, as are adults who are bonded to each other. The oxytocin-related wellbeing and reduced levels of anxiety and stress contribute to keeping the bond alive, as some of the effects are short-lasting and need reinforcement to be maintained. When the effects fade, as a consequence of separation, the bonded individuals want to reunite in order to feel well.

Oxytocin is also released in response to sensory stimulation in intimate relationships, and possibly in groups of humans (Holt-Lunstad et al. 2008). In rats, oxytocin-related effects have been demonstrated in the cage mates of an oxytocin-injected rat, suggesting that oxytocin-treated animals eject pheromones which stimulate oxytocin release and oxytocin-related effects in their companions (Ågren et al. 1997). In humans, visual cues are more likely to trigger similar oxytocin-mediated effects in groups.

When oxytocin is released in response to sensory stimulation, irrespective of the type of social relationship, it triggers and coordinates a response pattern including wellbeing, anti-stress, and growth-promoting effects (Uvnäs-Moberg 1997, 2003).

As mentioned above, the effects of oxytocin are partly mediated via activation of other signaling systems. For example, oxytocin stimulates dopaminergic, opioidergic, serotonergic, and cholinergic transmission, and inhibits (nor)adrenergic activity in certain areas of the central nervous system. The role of oxytocin is to trigger and coordinate effect patterns, e.g., in response to different types of sensory stimulation. Some of the effects of oxytocin are long-lasting and may contribute to stress buffering, and also to the stimulation of anabolic metabolism and restorative processes and growth, which have been shown to follow good relationships. In fact, the prevalence of some diseases, such as cardiovascular disease, is lower in individuals who are involved in good relationships (Holt-Lunstad et al. 2008, Knox & Uvnäs-Moberg 1998).

Most likely the effects of the partnership between mother and offspring, and also between two pair-bonded individuals, are reinforced by other sensory signals such as olfactory, auditory, and visual inputs. A kind of conditioned reflex is formed, and secondary sensory stimuli take over the role of the primary sensory stimulation in a pavlovian manner to release oxytocin and to induce the effect spectrum described above.

In humans the effects of a bond may become more or less permanent, owing to the formation of mental representations. In this case the 'bonded' individual may be able to trigger the effects, which were originally induced by sensory stimulation, via the mental representations, without the other individual's presence. These 'memories' are of course more stable and may induce more long-lasting effects. The effects on physiology and behavior will of course depend on the type of mental images that are imprinted. If 'good memories' prevail the individual may, according to the terminology of John Bowlby, be securely attached, and if the memories are less positive they may be insecurely attached.

The Doula concept – a model for supportive interaction

The duration of birth is shortened, fewer medical interventions are needed, and the mother feels better and more competent and relates better to her infant if she has been allowed to have a supporting person (a doula) accompanying her during labor (Klaus & Kennell 1997). In part, these effects are due to the fact that the doula holds the mother and touches her, which may reinforce the activity in the maternal oxytocin system via stimulation of sensory nerves.

Another aspect of the effects induced by the doula is that the mother feels safe if she has with her someone who is empathic, who supports her, holds her, and above all does not leave her. As mentioned above, oxytocin induces trust in humans as well as more social and generous behavior (Kosfeld et al. 2005). Because trust is correlated with oxytocin release, maternal oxytocin release will be reinforced and as a consequence her labor will improve. Moreover, more oxytocin will be released into the brain to induce wellbeing and relaxation, and to further improve her social skills and reduce her anxiety.

Generalization of the doula effect to other types of treatment

The oxytocin system is not unique to the mother giving birth: it is a propensity of all human beings, men and women, old and young. Therefore, we must assume that oxytocin is released in the brain not only in women giving birth or breastfeeding, but also in persons who feel safe and calm and trust their companions. It is therefore likely

that in a therapeutic setting a good therapist, whatever category she or he belongs to, may stimulate central oxytocin release, if he or she succeeds in making the patient feel calm and to trust the therapist. When, by processing environmental cues in the amygdala hippocampal system, the patient unconsciously 'decides' that he or she trusts the therapist, oxytocin release is increased, social behavior is stimulated, stress levels decrease, and restorative processes are promoted (Uvnäs-Moberg et al. 2005) (Fig. 9.3).

As described above, sensory stimulation reduces anxiety, induces wellbeing, calm, relaxation, decreased sensitivity to pain, and stimulation of restorative processes. The effects that occur during different aspects of the mother–infant interaction are similar to those occurring during massage. As the majority of the effects are induced by 'skin-to-skin' contact – that is, a very subtle kind of stimulation involving warmth, light pressure, and stroking – these types of stimulation are part of any treatment involving manual therapy. Therefore, when a therapist both touches the patient and also makes him or her calm and trusting, even stronger effects may be induced, as the oxytocinergic system will be activated in two ways: via a release of oxytocin from the PVN in response to sensory stimulation, and also via the amygdala–hippocampal pathway as described above (Fig. 9.4).

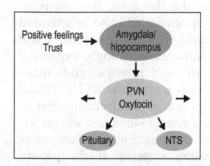

Figure 9.3 Stimulation of oxytocin release through the amygdala and hippocampal system. NTS, nucleus tractus solitarius; PVN, paraventricular nucleus of the hypothalamus.

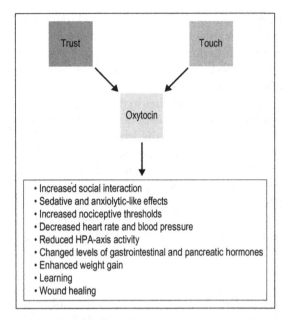

Figure 9.4 Changes triggered by trust or touch and mediated by oxytocin.

Summary and conclusion

Massage, acupuncture, chiropractic, osteopathic, and other manual therapies always include an aspect of 'hands on'. Therefore, parts of the *relaxation and growth response or the calm and connection response* will be induced as a result. This is a basic effect related to activation of the patient's own oxytocinergic system. In addition, all manual therapies also include a 'meeting' with the patient. If the therapist succeeds in making the patient feel calm and safe, i.e., if the patient trusts the therapist, the oxytocin-related effect spectrum will also be activated via 'inner touch'. This effect spectrum will of course become more strongly expressed in response to both physical and 'inner touch'. Repeated treatments will reinforce the effects, as repeated administration of oxytocin gives rise to sustained effects via facilitation of the function in other, more classic, signaling systems. If the patient forms a bond with the therapist, the effect will be further strengthened, as the positive

effects, may be linked to and activated by mental representations.

References

Agren, G., Lundeberg, T., Unväs-Moberg, K., Sato, A., 1995. The oxytocin antagonist 1-deamino-2D-Tyr-(Oet)-4-Thr-8-Orn-oxytocin reverses the increase in withdrawal response latency to thermal, but not mechanical, nociceptive stimuli following oxytocin administration or massage-like stroking in rats. Neurosci. Lett. 187, 49–52.

Agren, G., Uvnäs-Moberg, K., Lundeberg, T., 1997. Olfactory cues from an oxytocin-injected male rats can induce anti nociception in its cagemates. Neuroreport 229, 3073–3076.

Amico, J.A., Johnston, J.M., Vagnucci, A.H., 1994. Suckling-induced attenuation of plasma cortisol concentrations in postpartum lactating women. Endocr. Res. 2079–2087.

Amico, J.A., Miedlar, J.A., Hou-Ming, D., Vollmer, R.R., 2008. Oxytocin knockout mice: a model for studying stress-related and ingestive behaviours. Prog. Brain. Res. 170, 53–64.

Araki, T., Iro, M., Kurosawa, M., Sato, A., 1984. Responses of adrenal sympathetic nerve activity and catecholamine secretion to cutaneous stimulation in anesthetized rats. Neuroscience 12, 231–237.

Bagdy, G., Kalogeras, K.T., 1993. Stimulation of 5HT1A and 5HT2/5HT1c receptors induce oxytocin release in male rats. Brain Res. 611, 330–332.

Björkstrand, E., Ahlénius, S., Smedh, U., Uvnäs-Moberg, K., 1996. The oxytocin receptor antagonist 1-deamino-2-D-Tyr-(OEt)-4-Thr-8-Orn-oxytocin inhibits effects of the 5-HT1A receptor agonist 8-OH-DPAT on plasma levels of insulin, cholecystokinin and somatostatin. Regul. Pept. 63, 47–52.

Bonne, D., Cohen, P., 1975. Characterization of oxytocin receptors on isolated rat fat cells. Eur. J. Biochem. 56, 295–303.

Buijs, R.M., De Vries, G.J., Van Leeuwen, F.W., 1985. The distribution and synaptic release of oxytocin in the central nervous system. In: Amico, J.A., Robinson, A.G. (Eds.), Oxytocin: Clinical and Laboratory Studies. Elsevier, Amsterdam, pp. 77–86.

Bystrova, K., Widström, A.M., Matthiesen, A.S., et al., 2003. Skin-to-skin contact may reduce negative consequences of 'the stress of being born'; a study on temperature in newborn infants, subjected to different ward routines in St Petersburg. Acta Paediatr. 92, 320–326.

Bystrova, K., Matthiesen, A.S., Vorontsov, I., Widström, A.M., Ransjö-Arvidson, A.B., Uvnäs-Moberg, K., 2007. Maternal axillar and breast temperature after giving birth: effect of delivery ward practices and relation to infant temperature. Birth 34, 291–300.

Cannon, W.B., 1929. Bodily Changes in Pain, Hunger, Fear and Rage. Appleton, New York.

Carter, C.S., 1998. Neuroendocrine perspectives on social attachment and love. Psychoneuroendocrinology 23, 779–818.

Champagne, F.A., Meaney, M.J., 2008. Transgenerational effects of social environment on variations in maternal care and behavioural response to novelty. Behav. Neurosci. 121, 1353–1363.

Christensson, K., Cabrera, T., Christensson, E., Uvnäs-Moberg, K., Winberg, J., 1995. Separation distress call in the human neonate in the absence of maternal body contact. Acta Paediatr. 84, 468–473.

Clarke, G., Fall, C.H.D., Lincoln, D.W., Merrick, L.P., 1978. Effects of cholinoceptor antagonists on the suckling-induced and experimentally evoked release of oxytocin. Br. J. Pharmacol. 63, 519–527.

Crowley, W.R., Parker, S.L., Armstrong, W.E., Wang, W., Grosvenor, C.E., 1991. Excitatory and inhibitory dopaminergic regulation of oxytocin secretion in the lactating rat: Evidence for respective mediation by D1 and D2 dopamine receptor subtypes. Neuroendocrinology 53, 493–502.

Craig, A.D., 2003. Pain mechanisms: labeled lines versus convergence in central processing. Annu. Rev. Neurosci. 26, 1–30.

Elands, J., Resink, A., De Kloet, R., 1990. Neurohypophyseal hormone receptors in the rat thymus, spleen and lymphocytes. Endocrinology 126, 2703–2710.

Field, T., 2002. Massage therapy. Med. Clin. North Am. 86, 1034–1036.

Freund-Mercier, M.J., Stoeckel, M.E., Palacios, J.M., Pazos, A., Reichhart, J.M., Porte, A., Richard, P., 1987. Pharmacological characteristics and anatomical distribution of [3H]oxytocin-binding sites in the wistar brain studied by autoradiography. Neuroscience 20, 599–614.

Hall, D., Kirsten, G., 2008. Kangaroo mother care – a review. Transfus. Med. 18, 77–82.

Heinrichs, M., Baumgartner, T., Kirschbaum, C., Ehlert, U., 2003. Social support and oxytocin interacts to suppress cortisol and subjective responses to psychosocial stress. Biol. Psychiatry 54, 1389–1398.

Hollander, E., Bartz, J., Chaolin, W., et al., 2007. Oxytocin increases retention of social cognition in autism. Biol. Psychol. 61, 498–503.

Holst, S., Uvnäs-Moberg, K., Petersson, M., 2002. Postnatal oxytocin treatment and postnatal stroking reduce blood pressure in adulthood. Auton. Neurosci. 99, 85–90.

Holst, S., Lund, I., Petersson, M., Uvnäs-Moberg, K., 2005. Massage-like stroking influences plasma levels of gastrointestinal hormones, including insulin, and increases weight gain in male rats. Auton. Neurosci. 120 (1–2), 73–79.

Holt-Lunstad, J., Birmingham, W., Light, K., 2008. Influence of a warm touch support enhancement intervention among married couples on ambulatory blood pressure, oxytocin, alpha amylase and cortisol. Psychosom. Med. 70, 976–985.

Hosoya, Y., Matsukawa, O.N., Sugara, Y., Kohno, K., 1995. Oxytocinergic innervation to the upper thoracic sympathetic preganglionic neurons in the rat. A light and electron microscopic study using a combined retrograde transport and immunocytochemical technique. Exp. Brain Res. 107, 9–16.

Johansson, L., Jonas, W., Petersson, M., et al., 2009. Effects of sucking and skin-to-skin contact on maternal ACTH and cortisol levels during the second day post partum – influence of epidural analgesia and oxytocin in the perinatal period. Breastfeeding Medicine (in press).

Jonas, W., Wiklund, I., Nissen, E., Ransjö-Arvidson, A.B., Uvnäs-Moberg, K., 2007. Newborn skin temperature two days postpartum during breastfeeding related to different labour ward practices. Early Hum. Dev. 83, 55–62.

Jonas, W., Nissen, E., Ransjö-Arvidson, A.B., Matthiesen, A.S., Uvnäs-Moberg, K., 2008a. Influence of oxytocin or epidural analgesia on personality profile in breastfeeding women: a comparative study. Arch. Womens Ment. Health 11, 335–345.

Jonas, W., Nissen, E., Ransjö-Arvidson, A.B., Wiklund, I., Henriksson, P., Uvnäs-Moberg, K., 2008b. Short- and long-term decrease of blood pressure in women during breastfeeding. Breastfeeding Medicine 3, 103–109.

Kendrick, K.M., Keverne, E.B., Baldwin, B.A., Sharman, D.F., 1986. Cerebrospinal fluid levels of acetylcholinesterase, monoamines and oxytocin during labour, parturition, vaginocervical stimulation, lamb separation and suckling in sheep. Neuroendocrinology 44, 149–156.

Kendrick, K.M., Keverne, E.B., Chapman, C., Baldwin, B.A., 1988. Intracranial dialysis measurement of oxytocin, monoamine and uric release from the olfactory bulb and substantia nigra of sheep during parturition, suckling, separation from lambs and eating. Brain Res. 439, 1–10.

Klaus, M.H., Kennell, J.H., 1997. The doula: an essential ingredient of childbirth rediscovered. Acta Paediatr. 86, 1034–1036.

Knox, S., Uvnäs-Moberg, K., 1998. Social isolation and cardiovascular disease: an atherosclerotic pathway? Psychoneuroendocrinology 23, 877–890.

Kosfeld, M., Heinrichs, M., Zak, P.J., Fischbacher, U., Fehr, E., 2005. Oxytocin increases trust in humans. Nature 435, 673–676.

Kurosawa, M., Suzuki, K., Utsugi, T., Araki, T., 1982. Response of adrenal efferent nerve activity to non-noxious mechanical stimulation of the skin in rats. Neurosci. Lett. 34, 295–300.

Kurosawa, M., Lundeberg, T., Ågren, G., Lund, I., Unväs-Moberg, K., 1995. Massage-like stroking of the abdomen lowers blood pressure in anesthetized rats: Influence of oxytocin. J. Auton. Nerv. Syst. 56, 26–30.

Lonstein, J.S., 2005. Reduced anxiety in postpartum rats requires recent physical interactions with pups but is independent of suckling and peripheral sources of hormones. Horm. Behav. 47, 241–255.

Ludwig, M., Leng, G., 2006. Dendritic peptide release and peptide-dependent behaviours. Nat. Rev. Neurosci. 7, 126–136.

Lund, I., Lundeberg, T., Kurosawa, M., Uvnäs-Moberg, K., 1999. Sensory stimulation (massage) reduces blood pressure in unanaesthetized rats. J. Auton. Nerv. Syst. 78, 30–37.

Lund, I., Ge, Y., Yu, L.C., et al., 2002. Repeated massage-like stimulation induces long-term effects on nociception: contribution of oxytocinergic mechanism. Eur. J. Neurosci. 16, 330–338.

Lupoli, B., Johansson, B., Uvnäs-Moberg, K., Svennersten-Sjaunja, K., 2001. Effect of suckling on the release of oxytocin, prolactin, cortisol, gastrin, CCK, somatostatin and insulin in dairy cows and their calves. J. Dairy Res. 68, 175–187.

Matthiesen, A.S., Ransjö-Arvidsson, A.B., Nissen, E., Uvnäs-Moberg, K., 2001. Postpartum maternal oxytocin release by newborns: effect of infant hand massage and sucking. Birth 28, 13–19.

McCann, S.M., Antunes-Rodrigues, J., Jankowski, M., Gutkowska, J., 2002. Oxytocin, vasopressin and atrial natriuretic peptide control body fluid homeostasis by action on their receptors in brain, cardiovascular system and kidney. Prog. Brain Res. 139, 309–328.

Murphy, M.R., Seckl, J.R., Burton, S., Checkley, S.A., Lightman, S.L., 1987. Changes in oxytocin and vasopressin secretion during sexual activity in men. J. Clin. Endocrinol. Metab. 65, 738–741.

Nissen, E., Uvnäs-Moberg, K., Svensson, K., Stock, S., Widström, A.M., Winberg, J., 1996. Different patterns of oxytocin, prolactin but not cortisol release during breastfeeding in women delivered by Caesarean section or by the vaginal route. Early Hum. Dev. 45, 103–118.

Nissen, E., Gustavsson, P., Widstrom, A.M., Uvnäs-Moberg, K., 1998. Oxytocin, prolactin, milk production and their relationship with personality traits in women after vaginal delivery or Cesarean section. J. Psychosom. Obstet. Gynaecol. 19, 49–58.

Nussdorfer, G.G., 1996. Paracrine control of adrenal cortical function by medullary chromaffin cells. Pharmacol. Rev. 48, 495–530.

Ohlsson, B., Truedsson, M., Bengtsson, M., et al., 2005. Effects of long-term treatment with oxytocin in chronic constipation: a double blind, placebo-controlled pilot trial. Neurogastroenterol. Motil. 17, 697–704.

Olausson, H., Lamarre, Y., Backlund, H., et al., 2002. Unmyelinated tactile afferents signal touch and project to insular cortex. Nat. Neurosci. 5, 900–904.

Pauk, J., Kuhn, C.M., Fields, T.M., Schanberg, S.M., 1986. Positive effects of tactile versus kinesthetic or vestibular stimulation on neuroendocrine and ODC activity in maternally-deprived rat pups. Life Sci. 39, 2081–2087.

Petersson, M., Alster, P., Lundeberg, T., Uvnäs-Moberg, K., 1996a. Oxytocin increases nociceptive thresholds in a long-term perspective in female and male rats. Neurosci. Lett. 212, 87–90.

Petersson, M., Alster, P., Lundeberg, T., Uvnäs-Moberg, K., 1996b. Oxytocin causes a long-term decrease of blood pressure in female and male rats. Physiol. Behav. 60, 1311–1315.

Petersson, M., Lundeberg, T., Sohlström, A., Wiberg, U., Uvnäs-Moberg, K., 1998. Oxytocin increases the survival of musculocutaneous flaps. Naunyn Schmiedebergs Arch. Pharmacol. 357, 701–704.

Petersson, M., Hulting, A.L., Andersson, R., Uvnäs-Moberg, K., 1999a. Long-term changes in gastrin, cholecystokinin and insulin in response to oxytocin treatment. Neuroendocrinology 69, 202–208.

Petersson, M., Hulting, A.L., Uvnäs-Moberg, K., 1999b. Oxytocin causes a sustained decrease in plasma levels of corticosterone in rats. Neurosci. Lett. 264, 41–44.

Petersson, M., Wiberg, U., Lundeberg, T., Uvnäs-Moberg, K., 2001. Oxytocin decreases carrageenan induced inflammation in rats. Peptides 22 (9), 1479–1484.

Petersson, M., Diaz-Cabiale, Z., Fuxe, K., Uvnäs-Moberg, K., 2005. Oxytocin increases the density of high affinity alpha 2-adrenoreceptors within the hypothalamus, the amygdala and the nucleus of the solitary tract in female ovariectomized rats. Brain Res. 1049, 234–239.

Rimmele, U., Hediger, K., Heinrichs, M., Klaver, P., 2009. Oxytocin makes a face in memory familiar. J. Neurosci. 29, 38–42.

Sawchenko, P.E., Swanson, L.W., 1982. Immunohistochemical identification of neurons in the paraventricular nucleus of the hypothalamus that project to the medulla or to the spinal cord in the rat. J. Comp. Neurol. 205, 260–272.

Selye, H., 1976. Stress in Health and Disease. Butterworths, Boston.

Schumacher, M., Coirini, H., Johnson, A., et al., 1993. The oxytocin receptor: a target for steroid hormones. Regul. Pept. 45, 114–119.

Sofroniew, M.V., 1983. Morphology of vasopressin and oxytocin neurones and their central and vascular projections. Prog. Brain Res. 60, 101–114.

Stachowiak, A., Macchi, G., Nussdorfer, G.G., Malendowicz, L.K., 1995. Effects of oxytocin on the function and morphology of the rat adrenal cortex: in vitro and in vivo investigations. Res. Exp. Med. 195, 265–274.

Stock, S., Uvnäs-Moberg, K., 1988. Increased plasma levels of oxytocin in response to afferent electrical stimulation of the sciatic and vagal nerves and in response to touch and pinch in anaesthetized rats. Acta Physiol. Scand. 132, 29–34.

Stock, S., Fastbom, J., Björkstrand, E., Ungerstedt, U., Uvnäs-Moberg, K., 1990. Effects of oxytocin in vivo release of insulin and glucagon studied by microdialysis in the rat pancreas and autoradiographic evidence for [3H]oxytocin binding sites within the islets of Langerhans. Regul. Pept. 30, 1–13.

Stoeckel, M.E., Freund-Mercier, M.J., 1989. Autoradiographic demonstration of oxytocin-binding sites in the macula densa. Am. J. Physiol. 257, F310–F314.

Swanson, L.W., Sawchenko, P.E., 1980. Paraventricular nucleus: a site for the integration of neuroendocrine and autonomic mechanisms. Neuroendocrinology 31, 410–417.

Swanson, L.W., Sawchenko, P.E., 1983. Hypothalamic integration: Organization of the paraventricular and supraoptic nuclei. Annu. Rev. Neurosci. 6, 269–324.

Szeto, A., Nation, D.A., Mendez, A.J., Dominguez-Bendala, J., Brooks, L.G., Schneiderman, N., et al., 2008. Oxytocin attenuates NADPH-dependent superoxide activity and IL-6 secretion in macrophages and vascular cells. Am. J. Physiol. Endocrinol. Metab. 295, E1495–E1501.

Törnhage, C.J., Serenius, F., Uvnäs-Moberg, K., Lindberg, T., 1996. Plasma somatostatin and cholecystokinin levels in preterm infants during the first day of life. Biol. Neonat. 70, 311–321.

Tsuchiya, T., Nakayama, Y., Sato, A., 1991. Somatic afferent regulation of plasma corticosterone in anesthetized rats. Jpn. J. Physiol. 41, 169–176.

Uvnäs-Moberg, K., 1996. Neuroendocrinology of the mother–child interaction. Trends Endocrinol. Metab. 7, 126–131.

Uvnäs-Moberg, K., 1997. Oxytocin-linked antistress effects – the relaxation and growth response. Acta Physiol. Scand. 161 (Suppl. 640), 38–42.

Uvnäs-Moberg, K., 2003. The oxytocin factor. Tapping the hormone of calm, love and healing. A Merloyd Lawrence Book. Da Capo Press.

Uvnäs-Moberg, K., 2004. Massage and wellbeing, an integrative role for oxytocin?. In: Field, T. (Ed.), Touch in Labour and Infancy. J&J Publishing.

Uvnäs-Moberg, K., Lundeberg, T., Bruzelius, G., Alster, P., 1992. Vagally mediated release of gastrin and cholecystokinin following sensory stimulation. Acta Physiol. Scand. 146, 349–356.

Uvnäs-Moberg, K., Bruzelius, G., Alster, P., Lundeberg, T., 1993. The antinociceptive effect of non-noxious sensory stimulation is mediated partly through oxytocinergic mechanisms. Acta Physiol. Scand. 149, 199–204.

Uvnäs-Moberg, K., Alster, P., Lund, I., Lundeberg, T., Kurosawa, M., Ahlenius, S., 1996a. Stroking of the abdomen causes decreased locomotor activity in conscious male rats. Physiol. Behav. 60, 1409–1411.

Uvnäs-Moberg, K., Alster, P., Petersson, M., 1996b. Dissociation of oxytocin effects on body weight in two variants of female Sprague–Dawley rats. Integr. Physiol. Behav. Sci. 31, 44–55.

Uvnäs-Moberg, K., Björkstrand, E., Hillegaart, V., Ahlenius, S., 1999. Oxytocin as a possible mediator of SSRI-induced antidepressant effects. Psychopharmacology 142, 95–101.

Uvnäs-Moberg, K., Eklund, M., Hillegaart, V., Ahlenius, S., 2000. Improved conditioned avoidance learning by oxytocin administration in high-emotional male Sprague–Dawley rats. Regul. Pept. 88 (1), 27–32.

Uvnäs-Moberg, K., Arn, I., Magnusson, D., 2005. The psychobiology of emotion: the role of the oxytocinergic system. Integr. Physiol. Behav. Sci. 12, 59–65.

Vallbo, A.B., Olausson, H., Wessberg, J., 1999. Unmyelinated afferents constitute a second system coding tactile stimuli of the human hairy skin. J. Neurophysiol. 81, 2753–2763.

Van Oers, H.J., de Kloet, D., Whelan, T., Levine, S., 1998. Maternal deprivation effect on the infant's neural stress markers is reversed by tactile stimulation and feeding but not by suppressing corticosterone. J. Neurosci. 18, 10171–10179.

Von Knorring, A.L., Söderberg, A., Austin, L., Arinell, H., Uvnäs-Moberg, K., 2009. Massage induces decrease of aggressive behavior in pre-school children. A long-term pilot study. Acta Paediatr. Scand. (in press).

Widström, A.M., Ransjö-Arvidson, A.B., Christensson, K., Matthiesen, A.S., Winberg, J., Uvnäs-Moberg, K., 1987. Gastric suction in healthy newborn infants. Effects on circulation and developing feeding behaviour. Acta Paediatr. Scand. 76, 566–572.

Wright, D.M., Clarke, G., 1984. Inhibition of oxytocin secretion by μ and δ receptor selective enkephalin analogues. Neuropeptides 5, 273–276.

Yazawa, H., Hirasawa, A., Horie, K., Saita, Y., Iida, E., Honda, K., Tsujimoto, G., 1996. Oxytocin receptors expressed and coupled to Ca2+ signaling in a human vascular smooth muscle cell line. Br. J. Pharmacol. 117, 799–804.

Viscerosensory pathways in the brain

Lisa E Goehler

Introduction

Health and wellness depend on coordinated responses to disturbances in the body (injury, disease) as well as to challenges from the environment (stress, threat). The brain closely monitors conditions within the body (e.g., metabolic and cardiovascular status, pain, infection and inflammation), and this information is propagated from primary sensory processing regions in the brainstem and spinal cord via *viscerosensory* projections to other brain regions that coordinate physiological, neuroendocrine and behavioral adjustments to ongoing internal conditions. This information is integrated with signals related to psychological functions as well. In this way the brain serves as the "mastermind" controlling bodily functions related to disease, healing and recuperation.

In addition to providing the critical information necessary for homeostatic functions, viscerosensory signals can potently affect cognitive and emotional functioning. For instance, we remember emotionally arousing events better than things that are routine, and this is dependent upon vagal sensory neurons detecting the levels of stress hormones (epinephrine) circulating in the body (Miyashita & Williams 2004). Vagal sensory neurons in turn drive brain pathways related to stress and arousal that enhance memory formation. In addition, infections in the body can cause symptoms of depression and anxiety (Dantzer 2004, Lyte et al. 2006). Whereas somatosensory information from joints, skin, muscles provide us with a sense of where we are in space, viscerosensory information contributes not only to emotional states (Wiens 2005), including fear, anxiety, excitement etc. but also may contribute to the perception of our core "selves" (Damasio 2003). The demands of regulating our bodily functions are intimately tied into our ability to cope with both physiological and psychological challenges. Successful resolution of such challenges is critical to survival, thus homeostatic systems must be able to influence psychological aspects of motivation. In this way, by providing information about the bodily states, viscerosensory systems constitute a principal conduit for mind and body interactions. However, perturbations in balance/interactions of homeostatic and psychological states contribute to functional disorders, such as irritable bowel syndrome and chronic pain syndromes (Bonaz 2003, Mayer, Naliboff & Craig 2006). Targeting therapeutic interventions toward restoring optimal functioning of viscerosensory systems could improve outcomes of these disorders.

It is becoming increasingly clear that manual therapies (MT) exert actions beyond the specific joints and spinal segments stimulated (Schmid et al. 2008), likely involving supraspinal (brain) and neuroendocrine components. Indeed, MT can influence autonomic functions (heart rate and respiration) and induce analgesia at body sites away from site of MT (reviewed in Schmid et al. 2008), and these actions likely contribute significantly to MT efficacy. However, the specific mechanisms and pathways that mediate the effects of MT on autonomic and pain-related functions are not well-established. As Bialosky et al. (2008) point out, understanding mechanisms of MT is critical to targeting of treatment, predicting outcome, and increasing acceptance by health care providers. Thus, delineating

brain mechanisms influenced by MT will provide important insights and enhance efficacy of these modalities.

The integration of psychological states and viscerosensory signaling involves a complex choreography of brain activation patterns that ultimately influence autonomic functions. Current research using functional neuroimaging in humans is clarifying the picture of how different brain systems collaborate to maintain health, but it is still not complete. This chapter will highlight current ideas about the multiple pathways viscerosensory information takes in the brain, and how this information interfaces with other systems related to psychological functions such as emotion and decision-making. This information is relevant to brain substrates affected in disorders associated with functional impairment (e.g., functional gastrointestinal disorders, fibromyalgia, chronic pain) and can serve as a starting point for understanding how MT can improve functioning in individuals with these disorders.

Outcome studies of interventions with humans typically use measures of autonomic functions, such as cardiovagal tone (presumed a measure of parasympathetic activity) and galvanic skin response (GSR), an index of sympathetic activity, that are useful because they are non-invasive and can be used in many patients economically. However, it needs to be acknowledged that these measures do not reflect the complex interaction and collaboration of the parasympathetic and sympathetic systems in regulating bodily functions. They can provide general indications of autonomic activity that can be useful as initial probes of central nervous system (CNS).

Organization of ascending viscerosensory pathways

Origins of viscerosensory pathways

Parallel pathways originating in the spinal cord and brain stem collect information from all of the tissues of the body and propagate the signals to brain regions involved in homeostasis. Traditionally, viscerosensory pathways have been conceptually limited to those derived from the nerves innervating thoracic, abdominal, or pelvic organs and tissues. However, it has recently been pointed out by Craig (2002, 2003) that nerve fibers innervating skin and blood vessels, etc. are functionally and anatomically more similar to viscerosensory nerve fibers (also called 'interoceptive') than somatosensory fibers such as touch, which provide 'exteroceptive' information. For instance, all of these fibers, regardless of their target of innervation, are thinly myelinated or unmyelinated, and most if not all respond to inflammatory signals, including prostaglandins, bradykinins, and cytokines. Thus, signals from all bodily tissues contribute to the representation in the brain of 'condition of the body' (e.g., health, damaged tissues, etc.), and converge at multiple levels of the neuraxis (Cameron 2001, Craig 2003). In this chapter, the terms viscerosensory or interoceptive will refer to pathways derived from neurons in spinal lamina 1, the spinal trigeminal nucleus, or the dorsal vagal complex and ventrolateral medulla (Fig. 10.1).

Lamina 1 of the spinal cord

Lamina 1 of the spinal cord collects information from small-diameter primary sensory neurons that signal tissue damage and/or inflammation, temperature, and itch, in all tissues of the body except the head, where analogous fibers run with the trigeminal cranial nerve and terminate in the spinal trigeminal nucleus (Sessle 2005). These fibers project to the autonomic nuclei of the spinal cord and ascend to terminate in the thalamus, while giving off collaterals to the several nuclei in the brain stem, including the nucleus of the solitary tract, the ventrolateral medulla, and the parabrachial nucleus (reviewed in Craig 2003).

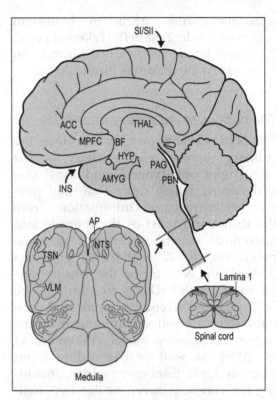

Figure 10.1 Locations of the primary viscerosensory nuclei in the spinal cord and medulla, and the major targets of the viscerosensory pathways in the brain. ACC, anterior cingulate cortex; AMYG, amygdala; AP, area postrema; BF, basal forebrain; HYP, hypothalamus; INS, insula; MPFC, medial prefrontal cortex; NTS, nucleus of the solitary tract; PAG, periaquiductal gray; PBN, parabrachial nucleus; SI/SII, somatosensory cortex; THAL, thalamus; TSN, trigeminal sensory nuclei; VLM, ventrolateral medulla.

Trigeminal sensory nuclei

The trigeminal sensory nuclei monitor pain and immune/inflammatory signals from tissues of the head: tooth pulp, mucosal surfaces of the mouth (including the tongue) and nose, salivary glands, mouth, and skin of the head. The nucleus caudalis of the spinal trigeminal nucleus has many features in common with spinal lamina 1, and serves as the principal – but not the only – site for pain processing (Sessle 2005). Pain-related and viscero-sensory signals from the trigeminal nuclei are propagated via ascending neural projections in the trigeminothalamic tracts to brainstem regions, including the NTS (Takemura et al. 2006) and lateral parabrachial nucleus, on their way to the thalamus (Sessle 2005).

The nucleus of the solitary tract (NTS)

The NTS is best known for its role as the primary sensory relay nucleus for the vagus, glossopharyngeal, and facial cranial nerves, which carry taste and general viscerosensory information from the throat and most of the thoracic and abdominal structures, as well as some pelvic organs. With the area postrema (below), the NTS forms the sensory *dorsal vagal complex* (DVC). In addition, the NTS receives ascending input from spinal lamina 1 ('bottom up') and from the trigeminal sensory nuclei (Takemura et al. 2006), as well as descending input from multiple forebrain regions, including the cortex, paraventricular hypothalamus, and central extended amygdala ('top down'). Information available to the NTS is not limited to neural input, as it contains receptors for glucocorticoids (Roozendaal et al. 1999) and, via the area postrema and the vagus nerve, senses circulating catecholamines and other hormones that signal psychological stress (Roozendaal et al. 1999) or visceral challenge. Viscerosensory information reaching the NTS is processed locally and appropriate reflexes are generated, and information is relayed to more rostral regions of the brain. The NTS contributes to the mediation of sickness symptoms, notably those associated with sickness behavior, including fatigue (Marvel et al. 2004), modulates cardiovascular and gastrointestinal functions, and plays a critical role in the pathway by which peripheral arousal facilitates memory (Williams & McGaugh 1993). Thus, the NTS operates as a clearing house for a wide variety of viscerosensory signals.

The area postrema

The area postrema is one of the circumventricular organs (CVOs), which are sensory structures located within the brain at various places adjacent to ventricular spaces. In CVOs the blood–brain barrier is weak, allowing cells within them access to substances in the blood that are excluded from the rest of the brain. Such substances include hormones and products of inflammation such as cytokines, which are large lipophobic molecules that do not readily pass the blood–brain barrier, as well as pathogens or pathogen products such as lipopolysaccharide (LPS). CVOs harbor immune cells that produce cytokines during infection or inflammation (Goehler et al. 2006), which are important for the induction of sickness behavior (Dantzer 2004). Unlike the other circumventricular organs, however, the area postrema receives direct viscerosensory input via the vagus nerve, which terminates extensively throughout it (Shapiro & Miselis 1985). This arrangement allows the area postrema access to a uniquely wide variety of peripheral signals: those present in the general circulation, in the cerebrospinal fluid, and, carried by vagal sensory nerves, those arising from distant viscera, e.g., related to local tissue conditions such as inflammation. Area postrema projection neurons propagate these signals to the NTS and to the lateral parabrachial nucleus in the pons (Shapiro & Miselis 1985). Whereas the area postrema is famous as an 'emetic' center, it apparently also contributes to EEG synchronization and slow-wave sleep (Bronzino et al. 1976). Thus, signals transduced by the area postrema contribute to ascending viscerosensory pathways and may play a role in brain and behavioral arousal.

The ventrolateral medulla

The ventrolateral medulla (VLM) refers to large neurons that express catecholamines or other substances, including glutamate and neuropeptides, within the reticular formation, an extensive network of large interconnected neurons that tend to form columns rather than well-defined nuclei. The VLM is driven by input from the dorsal vagal complex and spinal lamina 1, and modulates pulmonary and cardiovascular function. Like the NTS, neurons in the VLM projecting to more rostral brain regions contribute to responses to immune and other visceral challenges (Dayas et al. 2001, Gaykema et al. 2007, Sawchenko et al. 2000). In particular, the catecholaminergic neurons that target the hypothalamus respond to circulating cytokines, and provide the primary drive on hypothalamic neuroendocrine systems under conditions of sickness (Sawchenko et al. 2000) and other viscerosensory challenges, such as hypotension or pain (Pan et al. 1999).

Ascending viscerosensory pathways in the brain

Ascending projections from the VLM/DVC derive from at least two neurochemically distinct groups of neurons. The largest group comprises the noradrenergic and adrenergic neurons that innervate structures distributed more rostrally along the neuraxis, in particular the parabrachial, periaqueductal, and dorsal raphe nuclei, hypothalamus, and basal forebrain, including the amygdala and bed nucleus of the stria terminalis (Gaykema et al. 2007, Hajszan & Zaborszky 2002, Herbert & Saper 1992, Peyron et al. 1996), discussed in the following section. Along with the DVC, the VLM seems to provide most of the noradrenergic and all of the adrenergic innervation of the hypothalamus, including the paraventricular nucleus (PVN; contains corticotrophin-releasing hormone, CRH, neurons driving corticosteroid responses) and tuberomammillary neurons (histaminergic neurons), as well as most of the innervation to the basal forebrain (including cholinergic neurons) (Gaykema et al. 2008, Hajszan & Zaborszky 2002, Peyron et al. 1996). Based on these

connections, VLM and DVC neurons serve as links between visceral challenges, arousal, and thus potentially affective states. Many of these adrenergic and noradrenergic neurons located in the VLM and DVC become strongly activated by systemic challenge with immune stimulants (Dayas et al. 2001, Gaykema et al. 2007, Sawchenko et al. 2000) and other potentially dangerous viscerosensory challenges, including pain (Pan et al. 1999). Thus, they can be thought of as constituting a specific 'danger pathway'.

The other group of ascending projection neurons resides in the DVC and expresses a variety of peptides (e.g., glucagon-like peptide-1, cholecystokinin, galanin; Herbert & Saper 1990, Rinaman 2004). These nerve fibers project primarily to the parabrachial nucleus and hypothalamic structures. Although there is less information available on the functional aspects of the non-catecholamine projections than on the catecholamine neurons, they probably contribute to propagation of viscerosensory challenges (because non-catecholamine cells respond to challenges) as well as to other types of homeostatic stimuli.

Targets of viscerosensory projections

Viscerosensory information is represented preferentially along midline structures near the cerebral ventricles, following from the developmental subdivisions of the embryo in which viscerosensory structures differentiate from neurons in the region dorsolateral and adjacent to the neural tube and visceromotor structures derive from around the ventrolateral region surrounding the neural tube. This area can be thought of as the 'visceral core' of the central nervous system, and is concerned with homeostasis and regulatory behavior (drinking, feeding, aggression, sexual behavior, defensive responses, recuperative responses).

Principal viscerosensory targets integrate physiological adjustments associated with mood and physiological or behavioral challenges

In contrast to other sensory systems, which are characterized by well-defined projection patterns to a limited number of targets and feature relatively sequential processing, viscerosensory projections are highly collateralized and target a large number of nuclei at multiple levels of the neuraxis, from the brain stem to the telencephalon. The targets of ascending projection from the DVC and VLM are briefly described below.

Brainstem

Parabrachial nucleus (PBN)

The PBN is located in the rostral pons and receives massive projections from all levels of the NTS, including both taste and viscerosensory information. It also receives many projections from the AP and VLM, from the trigeminal sensory nuclei and lamina 1 spinal viscerosensory fibers. Neurons are organized in the PBN according to functional specificity, such that viscerosensory fibers terminate in the lateral subdivisions, and taste fibers terminate in the medial ones. Viscerosensory information seems to be mapped further in the lateral subdivisions, in that dangerous or stress-related information, such as immune activation, targets the external lateral region. Similarly, submodalities of viscerosensory information are propagated to different targets from the PBN. For instance, gustatory and general viscerosensory information is relayed to the ventrobasal complex of the thalamus, whereas immune-related signals also target the amygdala and midline thalamic nuclei.

Periaqueductal gray (PAG)

The PAG forms a cell-rich area surrounding the cerebral aqueduct in the midbrain. A major function of the PAG involves responses to danger or threats, and it is organized topographically in columns of cells according to specific behavioral and cardiovascular responses to such threats (Green & Paterson 2008). In addition, the PAG contributes to descending pain-modulating pathways targeting the spinal dorsal horn. In the context of real threat of danger (fear), activation of PAG neurons inhibits pain transmission. Interestingly, in the context of anxiety, however, another PAG-derived pathway acts to enhance pain (Lovick 2008). This mechanism may mediate psychological contributions to anticipatory pain, as well as to enhanced pain perceptions in conditions such as fibromyalgia and irritable bowel syndrome.

Diencephalon

Hypothalamus

The hypothalamus, located in the ventral basal part of the forebrain, serves as a principal integrator for psychological 'top-down' and viscerosensory 'bottom-up' signals controlling physiological regulation (Herman et al. 2005, Sawchenko et al. 2000). The hypothalamus contains populations of neurons that control neuroendocrine aspects of reproductive behavior, responses to physiological and behavioral challenges, and fluid balance via their influence on the pituitary gland. Hypothalamic control over neuroendocrine stress responses is effected via the release of corticotrophin-releasing hormone (CRH), which induces the pituitary gland to release adrenocorticotropic hormone (ACTH), which in turn induces the adrenal gland to release the stress hormone cortisol. Via this HPA axis the brain controls systemic stress responses. In addition to direct control of the endocrine system, hypothalamic neurons contribute top-down control over both branches of the autonomic nervous system, as well as on brainstem neurocircuitry controlling motor aspects of ingestive behavior. As noted previously, ascending viscero-sensory pathways derived from both the NTS and VLM project heavily to the hypothalamus, providing the critical information necessary for induction of appropriate hypothalamic output.

Thalamus

The thalamus constitutes a major link between viscerosensory pathways originating in the spinal cord and brain stem, and the cortical regions associated with viscerosensory perception and integration of viscerosensory input with mood and cognition. Vicerosensory information targets two regions of the thalamus, the ventrobasal complex, and the midline thalamus (Krout & Loewy 2000). The functional specificity observed between projections to the ventrobasal complex and the midline thalamic nuclei continues in their patterns of projections. The ventrobasal complex projects to the insula, a region of cortex located on the inner side of the temporal lobe. These cortical areas seem to be involved in taste and viscerosensory perception, and thus these pathways can be considered as part of the primary sensory pathways for these modalities. In contrast, the dorsomedial nucleus and midline nuclei project to brain regions such as the medial prefrontal cortex, striatum, nucleus accumbens, hippocampus, and amygdala that are involved in integrative functions (discussed below). Thus the thalamus disseminates viscerosensory information to widespread areas of the cortex, as well as to subcortical areas.

Telencephalon

Amygdala

The amygdala is located ventrally and rostrally in the temporal lobe. It is highly heterogeneous, in that it processes information from all sensory systems (with particularly notable input from the olfactory system), as well as from cortical and thalamic regions. Functions of the amygdala include induction of visceromotor adjustments to emotional and behavioral situations carried out primarily by the central nucleus of the amygdala (CEA), as well as processing of

information necessary for the manifestations of emotional states such as fear and anxiety (Walker et al. 2003). The NTS and VLM both target the CEA, as does the PBN. The amygdala is extensively connected with the hippocampus and cortical regions involved in emotion and interoception, and thus provides one of the pathways by which viscerosensory information can influence emotions. As the hippocampus is involved in memory processes, the amygdala also provides a pathway for bodily conditions, such as arousal, to influence memory and cognition. In addition, the amygdala provides significant input to the ventromedial prefrontal cortex.

Bed nucleus of the stria terminalis – (BNST)

The BNST is located anterior to the amygdala, in the vicinity of the anterior commissure. The BNST and the amgydala are closely related functionally and are extensively interconnected via the stria terminalis. Like the amygdala, the BNST is implicated in the regulation of emotion (Walker et al. 2003). Interestingly, catecholamine drive on BST seems to control the negative effective components of pain and opiate drug withdrawal. In addition, the BNST projects directly to the hypothalamic PVN, and seems to constitute a major final pathway by which psychological (top-down) stressors influence the HPA axis (Herman et al. 2005).

Basal forebrain

Ascending viscerosensory projections target ventral brain regions anterior to the hypothalamus, including the nucleus accumbens and the nucleus basalis of Meynert (Hajszan & Zaborszky 2002). The nucleus accumbens plays a role in motivation and reward, via connections with the lateral hypothalamus. It is topographically organized according to hedonic quality, such that the rostral nucleus accumbens responds to situations that are aversive, whereas the caudal nucleus accumbens is active during positive motivational conditions, such as in the context of palatable food (Reynolds & Berridge 2002). The nucleus basalis contains cholinergic neurons that target the hippocampus and have been implicated in mechanisms of learning and memory. Vicerosensory inputs into the basal forebrain provide a direct pathway by which signals from the body modulate motivation and cognition.

Arousal systems are viscerosensory targets

Appropriate and effective responses to circumstances and challenges from the external world (e.g., stress), as well as internal tissues, require the brain to be physiologically prepared in a systematic and coordinated way. Collections of neurons distributed throughout the brain stem, midbrain, hypothalamus, and basal forebrain function as 'arousal' systems directed towards coordinating sleep/wake cycles, de/synchronization of thalamocortical discharges (EEG), behavioral arousal,

vigilance, and responses to exteroceptive challenges (Fig. 10.2). These arousal nuclei include the dorsal raphe nucleus (DRN) in the midbrain that provides most of the neuro-transmitter serotonin to the forebrain, the locus ceruleus in the rostral pons, which supplies most of the norepinephrine to the forebrain (with the notable exception of the hypothalamus, where the norepinephrine is derived from viscerosensory projections), the histaminergic neurons of the tuberomammillary nuclei of the caudal hypothalamus, the orexin neurons of the lateral hypothalamus, and the cholinergic neurons of the basal forebrain. All of these receive direct viscerosensory projections from the DVC and VLM (Espana & Berridge 2006, Gaykema et al. 2008, Hajszan & Zaborszky 2002, Peyron et al. 1996). In this way, information regarding conditions within the body can powerfully influence the ability of the brain to respond to cognitive or behavioral challenges, and, conversely, aid in the suppression of arousal necessary for sleep and recuperation.

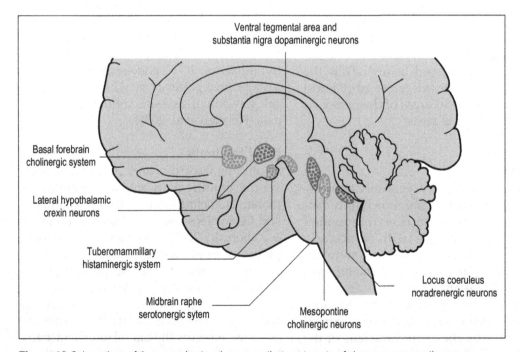

Figure 10.2 Locations of the arousal network neurons that are targets of viscerosensory pathways.

Viscerosensory information is processed in frontal and temporal cortical areas

Tracing studies in animals, functional neuroimaging and assessment of the effects of brain injuries in humans have indicated that representation of viscerosensory information occurs in frontal and temporal brain regions. For instance, epilepsy patients with viscerosensory auras showed enhanced activity in these areas concomitant with the auras (di Bonaventura et al. 2005). In particular, the insula in the temporal lobe and the anterior cingulate, medial and orbital prefrontal cortex process information necessary for 'interoceptive awareness' and the induction of appropriate autonomic and behavioral responses to ongoing conditions. Interestingly, cortical processing of viscerosensory information seems to be somewhat lateralized (reviewed in Craig 2005), such that the right hemisphere processes situations relevant to sympathetic activation (such as pain), whereas the left hemisphere seems to be active in the context of positive emotion, affiliation, and coping, and drives increases in parasympathetic activity, including cardiac vagal tone.

Insula

The insula is located in the temporal lobe, within the lateral fissure. It is typically divided into anterior and posterior subregions divided by the middle cerebral artery. The insula has been termed 'interoceptive cortex' or 'primary viscerosensory cortex' based on the fact that it receives viscerosensory input from both the spinal laminal 1 and DVC pathways (Craig 2003). Activation seems to be associated with conscious visceral perception, such as monitoring heartbeat (Wiens 2005). Viscerosensory information initially targets the posterior insula, followed by 're-representations' in the anterior insula and other regions (Craig 2003). In addition to a role in visceral perception,

the anterior insula, especially the right anterior insula, responds to viscerosensory challenges such as pain (Craig 2005), and thus probably serves as the principal target of the spinal lamina 1 system. In contrast, the insula responds bilaterally to vagus nerve stimulation (Narayanan et al. 2002). In this way, contributions from the different pathways are represented in discrete regions of the insula.

Anterior cingulate cortex (ACC)

The cingulate cortex surrounds the corpus callosum, with the anterior part (ACC) being associated with the prefrontal area (Brodmanns areas 24, 32). The ACC consistently responds to viscerosensory challenges, especially those related to pain stimuli and immune challenge (Capuron et al. 2005, Craig 2003), suggesting that the ACC constitutes part of the cortical representation of the viscerosensory 'danger' pathway. Bilateral damage to the ACC produces a state of akinetic mutism, in which individuals are awake but indifferent to pain, thirst, or hunger, and show a lack of behavioral initiative (apathy) (Tekin & Cummings 2002). Symptoms of apathy occur with damage to some of the inputs to the ACC, including dorsomedial thalamus, nucleus accumbens, and ventromedial caudate nucleus. This network of brain regions (medial prefrontal network, Price 1999) thus seems to be involved in organizing motivated responses to interoceptive challenges.

Subgenual medial prefrontal cortex (sgmPFC)

This area includes the part of the ACC ventral to the genu of the corpus callosum (areas 24 and 32) along with the subjacent ventral area of the medial prefrontal cortex (area 25). The ventromedial prefrontal cortex (vmPFC) has traditionally been conceptualized as 'visceromotor' cortex, based on its extensive output to all areas of the hypothalamus and autonomic premotor areas, including the PAG (reviewed in Price 1999). However, the mPFC receives relatively few cortical inputs (primarily from orbitofrontal and anterior insula); rather, it receives signals from the amygdala, the subiculum of the hippocampus, and the medial thalamus. Thus, the mPFC seems to integrate limbic, emotion-related information and translate this into modulation of autonomic and behavioral outflow. In particular, functional studies in humans indicate that the mPFC contributes to vagal tone in humans and rodents (Ter Horst & Postema 1997, Thayer & Brosschot, 2005, Wong et al. 2007). In addition to its role in control of autonomic function, the sgmPFC plays a role in regulation of mood. Neuroimaging studies have found this area to be reduced in volume and metabolism during episodes of depression, and normalized following effective treatment (Linden 2008). Electrical stimulation of the area (deep brain stimulation) in depressed patients can improve symptoms (Drevets et al. 2008). Taken together, these findings emphasize the close association between viscerosensory function and emotion. This may account, at least in part, for the findings that depression is associated with poor health outcomes (Drevets et al. 2008, Thayer & Brosschot 2005).

In addition to a role in the regulation of emotion, the mPFC contributes to neurological aspects of coping with stress. One factor that seems to strongly influence coping is the controllability of the stressor. When stress is perceived as uncontrollable, behavioral deficits occur, termed 'learned helplessness'. In these situations, animals and people no longer attempt to cope with the stressor, even if the stressor becomes controllable. Neurological correlates of learned helplessness involve excessive release of the neurotransmitter serotonin in the dorsal raphe nucleus (DRN) of the rostral brain stem. The DRN provides most of the serotonin to the forebrain, and is recognized to play a role in stress responses and control of mood. One of the mechanisms by which controllability protects against behavioral deficits (helplessness) involves activation of the medial prefrontal cortex (mPFC) (Amat et al. 2006). The mPFC projects directly to inhibitory interneurons on the DRN, which in turn reduce serotonin release. If activation of the mPFC is prevented, however, even controllable stress leads to helplessness. Thus, the mPFC functions as one pivotal point where factors that affect coping with stressors can act, suggesting that interventions that influence the mPFC could be efficacious in mitigating behavioral effects of stress.

Orbitofrontal cortex

The orbitofrontal cortex forms the concave part of the rostral prefrontal cortex. It receives projections from sensory areas of the cortex, including visual cortex, and the ventrobasal complex of the thalamus. It connects with the medial prefrontal cortex, and is thought to be the major conduit of sensory (as opposed to 'limbic') information to the mPFC (Drevets et al. 2008, Price 1999).

Viscerosensory contribution to stress and pain syndromes

Stress

One of the critical functions of the brain is to coordinate responses to behavioral and physiological challenges, which are often referred to as 'stressors'. 'Stressors' are usually conceptualized as belonging to two categories (Dayas et al. 2001, Sawchenko et al. 2000). Viscerosensory/interoceptive pathways signaling physiological or 'bottom-up' challenges to our *internal* bodily function include dehydration, hunger, infection, inflammation, and pain. In contrast, psychological 'top-down' stressors involve challenges in our *external* or mental environment, and range from social or cognitive (e.g., mental math) to fear of future consequences. Neural signals resulting from bottom-up and top-down stressors finally converge in the hypothalamic paraventricular nucleus, which activates endocrine (hypothalamopituitary–adrenal responses leading to elevated cortisol levels) and autonomic responses (e.g., elevated blood pressure or glucose). Brainstem autonomic 'premotor' areas, including the periaqueductal gray area of the midbrain and raphe nuclei of the ventromedial medulla, also integrate information regarding threats and drive sympathetic cardiac responses. 'Defensive' behavioral responses are coordinated in the PAG, as noted previously. In addition, recent findings support the idea that forebrain areas (e.g., mPFC and CEA) that function to coordinate emotional responses with autonomic function project directly to the caudal brain stem, and thus may be important for modulating parasympathetic – especially vagal – outflow.

Numerous studies in humans and rodents have shown that mood or behavioral symptoms follow from the effects of cytokines or other products of inflammation, induced by infection or inflammation ('bottom-up' immune and viscerosensory mediated; Anisman & Merali 2002, Dantzer 2004, Reichenberg et al. 2001). Thus, in the context of acute or chronic illness such symptoms can manifest from the direct effects of peripheral inflammation, and not solely from the stress of dealing with a medical condition, or personality factors ('top-down' brain mediated). This principle is particularly relevant for the anxiety and depressive symptoms that are often concomitant with chronic inflammation in heart disease, Crohn's disease/inflammatory bowel disease, and in functional gastrointestinal disorders such as irritable bowel syndrome. Viscerosensory signals arising from inflammation in coronary arteries, bowel symptoms such as constipation or diarrhea, pain, from altered immune function, or microbial population in the gut can drive brain regions that respond to stress. Because stress may potentiate peripheral inflammatory conditions, this increased drive might be predicted to exacerbate ongoing inflammation in the gastrointestinal tract, or other peripheral tissues. In this way, a feedforward loop could maintain and exacerbate both peripheral and neurological symptoms.

Visceral pain syndromes

Irritable bowel syndrome (IBS) and fibromyalgia represent visceral and somatic pain syndromes that seem to follow from a convergence of top-down stress reactivity and peripheral signals derived from the spinal viscerosensory pathways (Bonaz 2003, Mayer et al. 2006). IBS is diagnosed in people with abdominal pain associated with changes in bowel frequency, but in the absence of abnormalities indicating a physical cause, such as an obstruction (Lydiard 2001). Thus it is a functional, as opposed to a structural, gastrointestinal disorder. It is more common among women, is exacerbated by stress, and is associated with activation of mucosal immune cells (Chadwick et al. 2002). In as many as 30% of patients, symptoms follow a bout of food poisoning, often with *Campylobacter jejuni* (Spiller 2002). This condition is termed 'postinfective IBS', and symptoms can persist for a year or more. IBS is associated with a high prevalence of psychiatric symptoms, including depression, panic disorder, generalized anxiety, and post-traumatic stress disorder (Lydiard 2001). Functional neuroimaging studies of IBS patients using a rectal distension stimulus have indicated that peripheral pain pathways do not seem to be abnormal in such individuals, but that the enhanced perception of pain derives from altered brain processes, including increased attention to the stimulus and a failure to activate pain inhibitory pathways (Mayer et al. 2006).

Viscerosensory influences on mood and cognition

In the late 1800s William James, a psychologist at Harvard University, published a provocative theory of emotion: that the perception of emotions follows from perception of our physical responses to cognitive apprehension of external threats (or more pleasant stimuli). That is, the experience of emotion is integrated with signals from the body that result from cognitively driven motor, neuroendocrine, or autonomic responses, in a kind of brain–body–brain 'loop' communication sequence. He further predicted that, when emotions were mapped in the brain, rather than existing as separate centers (e.g., anxiety center, happiness center), the neural representations of emotion would be integrated with those of the body (James 1890). Although James is usually remembered for the assertion that bodily sequelae of emotion-inducing stimuli 'are' the emotions, this corollary prediction regarding brain substrates of emotions has proved prescient.

Although details of the 'James–Lange Theory of Emotion' have been criticized over the years (e.g., Berntsen et al. 2003), based partly on the fact that human emotional experiences can result from learned associations, and thus do not induce or rely upon the induction of physiological responses (Damasio 1996), recent findings have tended to support the idea that a full experience of emotion is blunted when somato- or viscerosensory signals do not reach the brain (Critchley et al. 2001). Findings from neuroanatomical, neuropsychological, and functional neuroimaging studies support James' contention that the brain's representations of emotions would be co-represented with information derived from internal tissues (Craig 2003, Dalgleish 2004, Nauta 1971, Price 1999). Regions implicated in both emotion and interoception include the medial and orbital prefrontal and anterior cingulate cortex, insula, hypothalamus, amygdala, and bed nucleus of the stria terminalis, as noted previously.

The integral relationship between bodily states and emotion was not really a new idea: indeed, belief in an inseparable relationship between bodily states and emotions is ancient, a well-known example being the theory of the four humors, which correlated observable bodily secretions with health and personality, and dominated medical thinking for over

1000 years (Sternberg 2001). Although modern medical practice has progressed beyond this, the idea that observable physical states (melancholic, sanguine, etc.) reflect emotion lives on in the English language.

Depression associated with a medical condition

Depression is often seen in chronic illness, including heart disease (Artinian et al. 2004), in which peripheral inflammation is present, and these symptoms probably represent responses to this viscerosensory challenge. Consistent with this idea, current evidence supports a pivotal role for brain systems responsible for coping with stressors and the induction of recuperative behaviors in the etiology of dysphoric symptoms concomitant with medical illness. In depressed patients, altered or dysregulated activity occurs in the constellation of brain regions associated with interoception, including limbic areas of the cortex, notably temporal and anterior cingulate, insular and frontal cortex, and in conjunction with subcortical regions including basal forebrain/basal ganglia, hippocampus, amygdala, hypothalamus, and medial thalamus (Drevets 2001, Drevets et al. 2008). Imaging studies in patients undergoing immunotherapy have revealed a similar pattern (Capuron et al. 2005, Matthews et al. 2004). As noted previously, together these regions have in common participation in cognitive, emotional, and/or autonomic responses to stress.

Some types of depression (melancholia) involve a suppression of arousal and the occurrence of mood symptoms and behavior similar to that of illness, for instance a loss of interest in social activity, food, and increases or changes in sleep (Drevets et al. 2008). In the context of illness, this behavioral syndrome is thought to promote recuperation. The overlap of symptoms and brain activation patterns in depression and illness suggests that, in depression, interoceptive brain regions become engaged, and that from a neurological point of view melancholic depression recapitulates a viscerosensory or interoceptive challenge.

Viscerosensory signaling can enhance anxiety

Anxiety is usually conceptualized as a response to a possible threat. Experimentally, these typically take the form of *exteroceptive* threats, i.e., those arising from the environment, notably potential predators in the form of predator scents, or of open spaces where predators may lurk. However, recent findings show that *interoceptive* threats, such as infection, allergy, or systemic immune challenge, also can engage behaviors typical of threat avoidance, and increase drive in brain regions that process threat-related information (Basso et al. 2003; Castex et al. 1995, Lacosta et al. 1999, Lyte et al. 2007, Rossi-George et al. 2005). These areas also contribute to neurocircuitry that support stress responses.

In addition to influencing stress-related brain regions, 'subclinical' infections in mice – that is, infections that do not lead to inflammation or classic sickness symptoms – lead to increases in anxiety-like behavior. The infected animals engage in more 'risk assessment' behaviors and spend more time in 'safe' areas of the behavior-testing apparatus (Lyte et al. 1998, 2007). In mice challenged with peroral live bacteria, these stimuli seem to use a vagal pathway to signal the brain, based on the lack of circulating cytokines and the expression in vagal sensory neurons of the activation marker protein c-Fos (Goehler et al. 2005, Lyte et al. 2006). In the brain, the activation pattern was consistent with viscerosensory challenge, indicating strong responses in the DVC and VLM of the caudal brain stem, PBN, and locus ceruleus in the pons, hypothalamus, thalamus, amygdala, BNST, and insula. In animals challenged with bacteria and exposed to an anxiogenic behavioral challenge there was additional activation in brain regions involved in behavioral defense, including the PAG, as well as in the mPFC. In particular, the immune challenge seemed to enhance responses in the hypothalamic PVN, amygdala, and mPFC, and activity in the BNST seemed to contribute more specifically to the enhanced anxiety-like behavior. These findings provide strong evidence that viscerosensory pathways contribute to changes in mood by influencing brain regions that coordinate defensive behavior and responses to stress.

Viscerosensory contributions to decision-making

Damasio (1996) adapted the James–Lange theory of emotion to the issue of decision making. Based on studies of humans with damage to the mPFC and/or amygdala, Damasio proposed that the mPFC encodes memories of physical (somatovisceral) responses to rewards or punishments, and when faced with the need to make a decision, the mPFC reactivates brain regions, including the amygdala, to reinstate either the actual physiological state (e.g., arousal), or neural representations of the physiological states associated with the previous situation. In this way, viscerosensory consequences of previous situations bias responses to new ones. Patients with damage to the mPFC show no intellectual impairment but consistently perform poorly on 'gambling' tasks, involving the evaluation of contingencies, and tend to make poor decisions in real-life situations. Recent studies have now shown that lesions of the insula (as noted earlier, also a principal interoceptive cortical region) are also associated with deficits in decision making that are somewhat different from those associated with mPFC damage (Clark et al. 2008). Taken together, the observations indicate that brain regions that process viscerosensory information contribute to decision making, probably by providing information about the possible consequences, positive or negative, based on the physiological feedback of a given choice.

Summary

Optimal mental and physical health is dependent upon the integration of information about the condition of the body with that concerning psychological states and challenges (e.g., stress). Functioning across the brain regions involved in this integration needs to be balanced and regulated, to prevent or ameliorate pathology. Primary viscerosensory regions (spinal lamina 1, the trigeminal sensory nuclei, and the dorsal vagal complex) propagate information concerning the physiological status of bodily tissues to brain regions that control physiology, behavior, and emotion. The information is conveyed in parallel pathways to the parabrachial nucleus, thalamus, arousal network nuclei, and subcortical regulatory nuclei in the periaquiductal grey, hypothalamus, amydala, and basal forebrain (Fig. 10-3). These regions collate viscerosensory signals such that information relevant to viscerosensory perception and ingestive behavior take different trajectories through the brain than information related to viscerosensory challenges such as pain, inflammation, or hypotension. Signals derived from potentially dangerous situation target the subcortical regions that control physiological adjustments to these challenges (e.g., PAG, hypothalamus, amygdala, medial

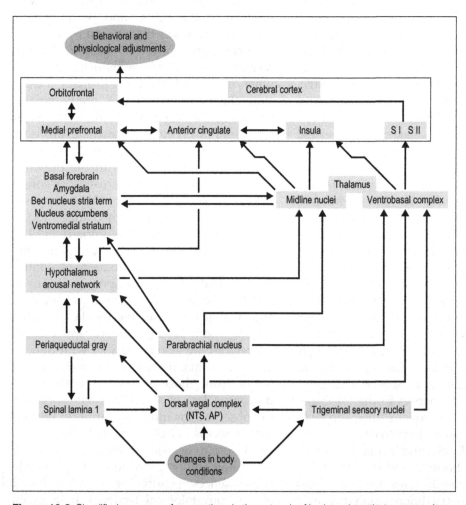

Figure 10.3 Simplified summary of connections in the network of brain regions that process viscerosensory information.

thalamus) and drives networks associated with the medial prefrontal cortex (including anterior insular cortex and ACC) that coordinate autonomic responses to emotion. Together these networks mediate the physiological, behavioral and effective responses to changes in bodily conditions.

In functional pain disorders (such as IBS and fibromyalgia) emotional responses and perception of discomfort is heightened, and is exemplified by enhanced activation of brain regions, notably the ACC, mPFC, insular cortex, amygdala and hypothalamus, that integrate viscerosensory information with stress-related signals. The difficulty in treating these disorders may follow from learning-like enhancement of viscerosensory pathways in the brain, (perhaps secondary to repeated or persistent activation) leading to exaggerated or persistent brain responses to body-related stimuli. Modulation of viscerosensory input to the brain by MT modalities could provide a means for re-balancing the interactions of viscerosensory/autonomic function with emotion/stress-related processes in the brain, thereby providing relief from symptoms and facilitating functional improvement. Research into specific brain contributions to the mechanisms of MT modalities could provide important information relevant to treatment of functional somatic disorders.

References

Amat, J., Paul, E., Zarza, C., Watkins, L.R., Maier, S.F., 2006. Previous experience with behavioral control over stress blocks the behavioral and dorsal raphe nucleus activating effects of later uncontrollable stress: role of ventral medial prefrontal cortex. J. Neurosci. 26 (51), 13264–13272.

Anisman, H., Merali, Z., 2002. Cytokines, stress, and depressive illness. Brain Behav. Immun. 16 (5), 513–524.

Artinian, N.T., Artinian, C.G., Saunders, M.M., 2004. Identifying and treating depression in patients with heart failure. J. Cardiovasc. Nurs. 19, S47–S56.

Basso, A.S., Costa Pinto, F.A., Russo, M., et al., 2003. Neural correlates of IgE-mediated food allergy. J. Neuroimmunol. 140, 69–77.

Berntsen, G.G., Sarter, M., Cacioppo, J.T., 2003. Ascending visceral regulation of cortical affective information processing. Eur. J. Neurosci. 18, 2103–2109.

Bialosky J.E., Bishop M.D., Price D.D., et al., 2009. The mechanisms of manual therapy in the treatment of musculoskeletal pain: A comprehensive model. Manual Therapy14, 531–538.

Bonaz, B., 2003. Visceral sensitivity perturbations in the brain-gut axis in functional digestive disorders. J. Physiol. Pharmacol. 54 (Suppl. 4), 27–42.

Bronzino, J.D., Stern, W.C., Leahy, J.P., Morgane, P.J., 1976. Sleep cycles in cats during chronic electrical stimulation of the area postrema and the anterior raphe. Brain Res. Bull. 1, 235–239.

Cameron, O.G., 2001. Interoception: The inside story – A model for psychosomatic processes. Psychosom. Med. 63, 697–710.

Capuron, L., Pagnoni, G., Demetrashvili, M., et al., 2005. Anterior cingulate activation and error processing during interferon-alpha treatment. Biol. Psychiatry 58, 190–196.

Castex, N., Fioramonti, J., Fargeas, M.J., et al., 1995. c-fos expression in specific rat brain nuclei after intestinal anaphylaxis: involvement of 5-HT3 receptors and vagal afferent fibers. Brain Res. 688, 149–160.

Chadwick, V.S., Chen, W., Shu, D., et al., 2002. Activation of the mucosal immune system in irritable bowel syndrome. Gastroenterology 120, 1778–1783.

Clark, L., Bechara, A., Damasio, H., et al., 2008. Differential effects of insular and ventromedial prefrontal cortex lesions on risky decision-making. Brain 131, 1311–1322.

Craig, A.D., 2002. How do you feel? Interoception: the sense of the physiological condition of the body. Nat. Rev. Neurosci. 3, 655–666.

Craig, A.D., 2003. Interoreception: the sense of the physiological condition of the body. Curr. Opin. Neurobiol. 13, 500–505.

Craig, A.D., 2005. Forebrain emotional asymmetry: a neuroanatomical basis? Trends Cogn. Sci. 9, 566–571.

Critchley, H.D., Mathias, C.J., Dolan, R.J., 2001. Neuroanatomical basis for first- and second-order representations of bodily states. Nat. Neurosci. 4, 207–212.

Dalgleish, T., 2004. The emotional brain. Nat. Rev. Neurosci. 5, 582–589.

Damasio, A.D., 1996. The somatic marker hypothesis and the possible functions of the prefrontal cortex. Philos. Trans. R. Soc. Lond. 351, 1413–1420.

Damasio, A.D., 2004. Mental self: the person within. Nature 423, 227.

Dantzer, R., 2004. Cytokine-induced sickness behavior: a neuroimmune response to activation of innate immunity. Eur. J. Pharmacol. 500, 399–411.

Dayas, C.V., Buller, K.M., Crane, J.W., et al., 2001. Stressor categorization: acute physical and psychological stressors elicit distinctive recruitment patterns in the amygdala and in medullary noradrenergic cell groups. Eur. J. Neurosci. 14, 1143–1152.

Di Bonaventura, C.D., Giallonardo, A.T., Fottouch, J., 2005. Symptoms in focal sensory seizures: Clinical and electroencephalographic features. Seizure 14, 1–9.

Drevets, W.C., 2001. Neuroimaging and neuropathological studies of depression: implications for the cognitive–emotional features of mood disorders. Curr. Opin. Neurobiol. 11, 240–249.

Drevets, W.C., Price, J.L., Furey, M.L., 2008. Brain structural and functional abnormalities in mood disorders: implications for neurocircuitry models of depression. Brain Structure and Function 213, 93–118.

Espana, R.A., Berridge, C.W., 2006. Organization of noradrenergic efferents to arousal-related basal forebrain structures. J. Comp. Neurol. 496, 668–683.

Gaykema, R.P.A., Chen, C.C., Goehler, L.E., 2007. Organization of immune-responsive medullary projections to the bed nucleus of stria terminalis, central amygdala, and paraventricular nucleus of the hypothalamus: Evidence for parallel viscerosensory pathways in the rat brain. Brain Res. 1140, 130–145.

Gaykema, R.P.A., Park, S.M., McKibbin, C.R., Goehler, L.E., 2008. Lipopolysaccharide suppresses activation of the tuberomammillary histaminergic system concomitant with behavior: a novel target of immune-sensory pathways. Neurosci. 152, 273–287.

Goehler, L.E., Gaykema, R.P.A., Opitz, N., et al., 2005. Activation in vagal afferents and central autonomic pathways: early responses to intestinal infection with *Campylobacter jejuni*. Brain Behav. Immun. 19, 334–344.

Goehler, L.E., Erisir, A., Gaykema, R.P.A., 2006. Neural-immune interface in the area postrema. Neurosci. 140, 1415–1434.

Green, A.L., Paterson, D.J., 2008. Identification of neurocircuitry controlling cardiovascular function in humans using functional neurosurgery: implications for exercise control. Exp. Physiol. 93, 1022–1028.

Hajszan, T., Zaborszky, L., 2002. Direct catecholaminergic–cholinergic interactions in the basal forebrain. III. Adrenergic innervation of choline acetyltransferase-containing neurons in the rat. J. Comp. Neurol. 449, 141–157.

Herbert, H., Saper, C.B., 1990. Cholecystokinin-, galanin-, and corticotropin-releasing factor-like immunoreactiveprojections from the nucleus of the solitary tract to the parabrachial nuclei in the rat. J. Comp. Neurol. 293, 581–598.

Herbert, H., Saper, C.B., 1992. Organization of medullary adrenergic and noradrenergic projections to the periaqueductal gray matter in the rat. J. Comp. Neurol. 315, 34–52.

Herman, J.P., Ostrander, M.M., Mueller, N.K., et al., 2005. Limbic system mechanisms of stress regulation: hypothalamo-pituitary–adrenocortical axis. Prog.

Neuropsychopharmacol. Biol. Psychiatry 29, 1201–1213.

James, W., 1890. Chapter XXV: The Emotions. The Principles of Psychology, vol. II. Henry Holt & Co., New York.

Krout, K.E., Loewy, A.D., 2000. Parabrachial nucleus projections to the midline and intralaminar thalamic nuclei of the rat. J. Comp. Neurol. 428, 475–494.

Lacosta, S., Merali, Z., Anisman, H., 1999. Behavioral and neurochemical consequences of lipopolysaccharide in mice: anxiogenic-like effects. Brain Res. 818, 291–303.

Linden, D.E.J., 2008. Brain imaging and psychotherapy: methodological considerations and practical implications. Eur. Arch. Psychiatry Clin. Psychol. 258 (Suppl. 5), 71–75.

Lovick, T.A., 2008. Pro-nociceptive action of cholecystokinin in the periaqueductal grey: A role in neuropathic and anxiety-induced hyperalgesic states. Neurosci. Biobehav. Rev. 32, 852–862.

Lydiard, R.B., 2001. Irritable bowel syndrome, anxiety, and depression: what are the links? J. Clin. Psychiatry 62, 38–45.

Lyte, M., Varcoe, J.J., Bailey, M.T., 1998. Anxiogenic effect of subclinical bacterial infection in mice in the absence of overt immune activation. Physiol. Behav. 65, 63–68.

Lyte, M., Wang, L., Opitz, N., et al., 2006. Anxiety-like behavior during initial stage of infection with agent of colonic hyperplasia *Citrobacter rodentium*. Physiol. Behav. 89, 350–357.

Marvel, F.A., Chen, C.C., Badr, N.A., et al., 2004. Reversible inactivation of the dorsal vagal complex blocks lipopolysaccharide-induced social withdrawal and c-Fos expression in central autonomic nuclei. Brain Behav. Immun. 18, 123–143.

Mayer, E., Naliboff, B.D., Craig, A.D., 2006. Neuroimaging of the brain-gut axis: From basic understanding to treatment of functional GI disorders. Gastroenterology 131, 1925–1942.

Matthews, S.C., Paulus, M.P., Dimsdale, J.E., 2004. Contribution of functional neuroimaging to understanding neuropsychiatric side effects of interferon in hepatitis C. Psychosomatics 45, 281–286.

Miyashita, T., Williams, C.L., 2004. Peripheral arousal-related hormones modulate norepinephrine release in the hippocampus via influences on brainstem nuclei. Behav. Brain Res. 153, 87–95.

Narayanan, J.T., Watts, R., Haddad, N., et al., 2002. Cerebral activation during vagus nerve stimulation: a functional MR study. Epilepsia 43, 1509–2151.

Nauta, W.J.H., 1971. The problem of the frontal lobe: A reinterpretation. J. Psychiatry Res. 8, 167–187.

Pan, B., Castro-Lopes, J.M., Coimbra, A., 1999. Central afferent pathways conveying nociceptive input to the hypothalamic paraventricular nucleus as revealed by a combination of retrograde labeling and c-fos activation. J. Comp. Neurol. 413, 129–145.

Peyron, C., Luppi, P.H., Fort, P., 1996. Lower brainstem catecholamine afferents to the rat dorsal raphe nucleus. J. Comp. Neurol. 364, 402–413.

Price, J.L., 1999. Prefrontal cortical networks related to visceral function and mood. Ann. N. Y. Acad. Sci. 383–396.

Reichenberg, A., Yirmiya, R., Schuld, A., et al., 2001. Cytokine-associated emotional and cognitive disturbances in humans. Arch. Gen. Psychiatry 58, 445–452.

Reynolds, S.M., Berridge, K.C., 2002. Positive and negative motivation in nucleus accumbens shell: Bivalent rostrocaudal gradients for GABA-elicited eating, taste 'liking'/'disliking' reactions, place preference/ avoidance, and fear. J. Neurosci. 22, 7308–7320.

Roozendaal, B., Williams, C.L., McGaugh, J.L., 1999. Glucocorticoid receptor activation in the rat nucleus of the solitary tract facilitates memory consolidation: involvement of the basolateral amygdala. Eur. J. Neurosci. 11, 1317–1323.

Rossi-George, A., Urbach, D., Colas, D., et al., 2005. Neuronal, endocrine and anorexic responses to the T-cell superantigen staphylococcal enterotoxin A: Dependence on tumor-necrosis factor-α. J. Neurosci. 25, 5314–5322.

Sawchenko, P.E., Li, H.Y., Ericsson, A., 2000. Circuits and mechanisms governing hypothalamic responses to stress: a tale of two paradigms. Prog. Brain Res. 12, 61–78.

Schmid A., Brunner F., Wright A., et al., 2008. Paradigm shift in manual therapy? Evidence for a central nervous system component in the response to passive cervical joint mobilization. Manual Therapy 13, 387–396.

Sessle, B.J., 2005. Peripheral and central mechanisms of orofacial pain and their clinical correlates. Minerva Anestesiol. 71, 117–136.

Shapiro, R.E., Miselis, R.R., 1985. The central neural connections of the area postrema. J. Comp. Neurol. 234, 344–364.

Spiller, R.C., 2002. Role of nerves in enteric infection. Gut 51, 759–762.

Sternberg, E., 2001. The Balance Within. W.H. Freeman.

Takemura, M., Sugiyoo, S., Moritani, M., et al., 2006. Mechanisms of orofacial pain control in the central nervous system. Arch. Histol. Cytol. 69, 79–100.

Tekin, S., Cummings, J.L., 2002. Frontal-subcortical neuronal circuits and clinical neuropsychiatry: An update. J. Psychosom. Res. 53, 647–654.

Ter Horst, G.J., Postema, F., 1997. Forebrain parasympathetic control of heart activity: retrograde transneuronal viral labeling in rats. Am. J. Physiol. 273 (6 Pt 2), H2926–H2930.

Thayer, J.F., Brosschot, J.F., 2005. Psychosomatics and psychopathology: looking up and down from the brain. Psychoneuroendocrinology 30, 1050–1058.

Walker, D.L., Toufexis, D.J., Davis, M., 2003. Role of the bed nucleus of the stria terminalis versus the amygdala in fear, stress, and anxiety. Eur. J. Pharmacol. 463, 199–216.

Wiens, S., 2005. Interoception in emotional experience. Curr. Opin. Neurol. 18, 442–447.

Williams, C.L., McGaugh, J.L., 1993. Reversible lesions of the nucleus of the solitary tract attenuate the memory-modulatory effects of posttraining epinephrine. Behav. Neurosci. 107, 955–962.

Wong, S.W., Masse, N., Kimmerly, D.S., 2007. Ventral medial prefrontal cortex and cardiovagal control in conscious humans. Neuroimage 35, 698–708.

The use of sham or placebo controls in manual medicine research

Michael M Patterson

Introduction

One of the key problems facing practitioners of manual therapy is to show that their treatments produce beneficial changes in their patients. Of course, practitioners of manual procedures are not alone in this, as it has long been recognized that proving the benefit of medical techniques in general, whether they be drugs, surgical procedures, or psychotherapies, is difficult. Indeed, it is only relatively recently in the history of medicine that true experimental designs have been developed to attempt to test the results of medical treatments. Perhaps the first skepticism regarding medical procedures began in the late 1700s, with doubts over such practices as 'mesmerism' (animal magnetism) and 'homeopathy' (Kaptchuk 1998). In the early 1780s what appears to be the first 'blind' test of a medical procedure, mesmerism, was used to determine whether subjects who could not see where the 'mesmeric energy' was being applied could tell the area of application. Women were either blindfolded or not blindfolded during the magnetic application (a magnet near the body surface). When they could see the application, the reported sensations were at the point of application, whereas when blindfolded, the reported sensations did not correlate with the site of application (Kaptchuk 1998). However, until the early 1940s, little was done to verify any sort of treatment effectiveness for the many 'drugs' and procedures in common use. Thus, practices such as purging, bloodletting, puking, leeching, and various surgeries continued to be used. It was not until much later, in the mid to late 1940s, that the need for some sort of proof of result became evident. The advent of antibiotics led to the beginning of the current era of medical experimental design, in it was recognized that several design factors were necessary to improve the credibility of study outcomes. With the development of the first antibiotics came the need for rigorous experimental methodology to determine the effectiveness of the new drugs. Thus, rigorous experimental pharmaceutical research design arose along with the growth of the modern pharmaceutical industry. However, one of the major questions that must be asked is whether the pharmaceutical model of medical research applies to research in manual treatments and therapies. Understanding the differences between pharmaceutical and manual procedures will allow the correct application of experimental design to the manual arts. Incorrect application of design principles will lead to false conclusions about the effectiveness of manual treatments and therapies.

In the discussion that follows, it is recognized that manual treatments are those performed by fully licensed physicians and therapies are those manual practices that are performed by other healthcare providers. The term manual procedures will be used to denote both practice types.

Types of study

Several recognized types of study can be applied to show the effectiveness of medical procedures (Patterson 2003), and they have varying levels of effectiveness in showing a causal relationship between procedure and outcome. The *case study design* is seen as the least effective model for showing effectiveness. Here, either a single or a few cases are

reported, with the treatment given and the observed outcome. Because of various factors, in case report studies it is often difficult to interpret whether the treatment given actually produced the observed outcome. A somewhat more effective design is the *prospective case study series*, in which a protocol for identifying patients, a format for collecting data about the case, and a means of clearly identifying changes in symptoms after treatment are put in place. Here, owing to the systematic process, there can be somewhat more credibility in any reported change supposedly due to treatment. However, such case studies and series do little to actually establish a cause and effect relationship between the treatment and subsequent changes in disease state or function of the patient. There are of course other types of study design, such as epidemiological, survey, and descriptive, that are very valuable in biomedicine but which do not show cause and effect. These designs can often begin to pinpoint relationships that can then be studied with experimental designs (Patterson 2010).

Indeed, proving cause and effect relationships is very difficult, especially in human medicine. Over thousands of years of evolution and development, humans have developed a huge capacity to recognize correlations between events and outcomes. The rustle in the grass on a dark night correlates well with the approach of a predator looking for a meal. The human thus links the noise in the grass with danger of being eaten and retreats to the cave. However, the rustle may be caused by a number of things, such as a non-predator, the wind, or a family member returning from a night on the savannah. The wind does not cause the hearer to be eaten. Thus, we are very good at detecting correlations, but assigning cause and effect relationships is much more difficult.

Thus in order to begin to have data that can give some indication of real cause and effect relationships between treatment and effect or outcome, there needs to be an experimental design that allows comparisons between treated and untreated patients, or between patients given one or other of two treatments. These designs have varying levels of complexity and varying levels of explanatory power, depending on factors such as numbers of subjects, what is measured, and many others.

This chapter will examine the use of control groups in experimental designs and how they apply to manual procedures. Of major interest is the meaning of changes in outcomes in control groups that are attributed to the 'placebo' effect, and how this concept applies to manual procedures.

The gold standard

We will begin the examination of experimental designs, and especially control groups, by considering the 'gold standard' for such designs and how it may or may not apply to manual procedures. The current 'gold standard' for biomedical research is the randomized, double-blind placebo-controlled (RDBPC) clinical trial. This was developed in the 1940s and 1950s to answer a very specific question stemming from the introduction of the antibiotic drugs. For all practical purposes, the question that was to be answered was: 'What is the effect of this drug on the natural course of a disease process in the human who is unaware of what drug, if any, is being given?'

The need in medical studies for the features of this design is well recognized. The necessity for randomizing subjects to the two or more arms of a study so as to have important variables such as age, gender, presenting symptoms, etc. equal in the various study groups is one of the baseline requirements of an experimental study. Randomization gives some assurance that the two or more groups of subjects are equal at the beginning of the trial on all important measures that might affect the outcome. This provides the necessary starting point for the trial. Provided that the assumptions of randomization are met and the groups are essentially identical, especially on those variables that are to be measured as outcomes, the ability to identify the effects of those drugs or procedures given to one group and not the other are more likely to be the result of the drug or procedure, and not to some underlying initial difference between the groups.

The blinding in experimental trials was established during the development of the model in order to guard against several factors other than the cause and effect relationship that could influence the outcome. First, and most importantly, the person collecting the data, in whatever form, must not know to which trial group the subject was assigned. It is readily acknowledged that even the most conscientious investigator can unwittingly affect the results of a study by judging the outcomes of a treated patient as better than those of the untreated patient (or the patient given a different treatment). In the worst case, the investigator may even consciously skew the results to favor the hoped-for outcome. Thus, in all experimental studies, the person or persons who collect the data must be blinded to patient assignment.

In drug trials the double-blind designation usually also refers to the patient and to the person administering the drug and the control substance. Here, the object is to keep the patient from knowing what substance they are receiving, and hence to avoid the possibility that this knowledge will sway the outcomes of the trial. Thus, in the typical drug study, the blinding is actually a triple blinding, with patient, drug administrator, and data collector blinded as to what is being given to the patient. It is impossible to triple blind procedure and surgical studies because the treater or surgeon must know what is being done.

The drug trial model also includes the administration of what is commonly known as a placebo. This is done so that patients do not know whether they are being given an active substance or one that has no effect on the course of the process or disease for which the drug is being tested. This inactive substance is known as the 'placebo,' and in strict form should look like, taste like, feel like, and weigh the same as the active drug. Thus, the patient and the substance administrator cannot deduce whether the patient is being given the active drug or the inactive substance. This then meets the requirements of the 'gold standard' drug trial.

As stated earlier, the goal of this design is very specific and tries to rule out or equalize all other factors that might influence the results or outcomes other than that of the active ingredient, the drug under study. Thus, for the question asked of most drug trials, the randomized, *triple*-blind placebo-controlled trial is appropriate and very useful in determining cause and effect relationships.

The issue of the placebo

Although it may seem simple to construct an acceptable placebo substance for most drug trials, problems arise almost immediately. What if the drug under consideration has certain side effects: for example causes some degree of nausea? If the placebo does not cause the nausea, the subjects in the experimental group have a different sensory experience from those in the placebo group, thereby potentially biasing the results. Thus, many drug trials in which the active ingredient causes some sensory experience for the patient attempt to mask that experience, or to create a placebo that also causes that experience but has no active effect on the process or organism causing the disease. Again, this is an attempt to keep the subject from knowing to which group he/she has been assigned. Thus, even in the best of circumstances, the design of a placebo-controlled study can be quite difficult.

However, the issue of placebo is much more than this. In 1955, Beecher (1955) published his famous article that set the stage for the debate about the effects of placebos

that continues to this day. Based on his analysis of 15 studies, he claimed that in several diseases, 35% of patients could be successfully treated by the administration of a placebo alone (Kiene 1996a,b, Kienle & Kiene 1996). This shifted the concept of a placebo and its effects from something that was an inert substance and hence did nothing, to something that produced some effect on the patient. The placebo effect in the response to a given disease has been estimated to range from 0% to almost 100% of the total effect seen during treatment (Kienle & Kiene 1996). What has changed? The placebo as originally defined was an inert substance having no effect on the disease being studied. Suddenly, it is seen as having anything from none to almost curative effects. How can an inert substance have an effect on anything? The answer lies in a shift in thinking about the meaning of placebo and a shift in emphasis from the placebo to the placebo response. As originally stated, a placebo was given to keep the subject from knowing the group assignment and thus from providing information that would please the investigator (placebo-to-please) and thus bias the outcome measures. However, it is apparent that, given the definition of placebo – i.e., an inert substance with no effect – the placebo response cannot be caused by the placebo but must be caused by the patient. Benedetti (2009) has recently summarized this concept well by stating that the placebo response is '...a psychobiological phenomenon occurring in an individual or in a group of individuals.' Thus, the emerging understanding of the patient's response to a placebo that is effectively an inert substance having no effect is that the response is caused by the patient's expectations, beliefs, and ideations, and not by the active treatment.

The literature on the placebo and the placebo response is huge. In 2006, Moerman indicated that a PubMed database search for just reviews of placebo yielded 10062 articles. In May 2009 a search for placebos yielded 28385 articles (Patterson search,

31 May 2009). It is evident that most of these articles are studies using placebo controls in one form or another, but many are attempts to define the characteristics of the placebo response itself. However, there is little agreement on what the response is, or how large it may be. Indeed, in their seminal article on the placebo concept, Kienle and Kiene (1996) argued that much of the so-called placebo response that has been reported can well be accounted for by such effects as the natural course of the disease process, regression to the mean, concomitant treatments, patients attempting to please, methodological defects in the studies, and misquotes, among other things. In their discussion, Kienle and Kiene suggest that psychosomatic phenomena are not to be considered placebo responses if they are not elicited by a specific placebo treatment (the administration of a placebo substance). They readily admit to the power of psychosomatic events on physiological function, but state that 'When psychosomatic events are indiscriminately labeled "placebo effects," both are shown in a false light: The placebo effect is given undue status, whereas psychosomatic effects are undeservedly discredited' (Kienle & Kiene 1996). Thus, there is obviously no real agreement among major authors on the issue about what comprises a placebo response. Kienle and Kiene's definition ties it to a specific circumstance, whereas Benedetti's definition is much broader. In any event, it seems to entail effects that are not directly tied to the active ingredient being given in a drug trial.

To be fair, there are many more aspects to the placebo response than have been touched on here. Benedetti's book and many of his articles (e.g., Benedetti 2008) discuss placebos in relation to specific circumstances and disease processes. In fact, one especially interesting study that Benedetti carried out involved the administration of pain-reducing drugs (Benedetti et al. 2003). The study used administration of narcotics either by a doctor at the bedside injecting the substance in an overt manner, or by a 'hidden' injection

done mechanically without the patient's knowledge that the drug was being injected. The results showed a marked increase in effectiveness with the overt administration (or, conversely, a decreased effect with the hidden administration). This is clearly a psychobiological effect that is a combination of the patient's knowledge and the drug itself. Presumably the effect is mediated by the psychological knowledge influencing endogenous opioids that enhance the effects of the drug. Besides an interesting discussion of placebo effects, Benedetti also provides a discussion of the opposite effect, nocibos, which enhance pain and distress (Benedetti 2009, Enck et al. 2008).

The meaning response

Another interpretation of the placebo effect has been put forward by Moerman (Moerman 2002, 2006, Moerman & Jonas 2000, 2002). In his essays and studies, Moerman has looked at the placebo response in a different way: as a response to the meaning of the situation. Here, the patient is responding to the interactions with the doctor, to the delivery of a drug or a procedure, to the cultural aspects of the situation, in a way that can be either beneficial or detrimental to function and consequent symptoms. Thus, he accepts the definition of a placebo as an inert substance or even ineffective procedure, and places the response directly on the meaning of the situation to the patient. Thus, the patient responds to the placebo, the situation, the doctor, etc. by producing actual changes in function, such as Parkinson's patients producing dopamine (de la Fuente-Fernandez et al. 2001) or pain patients producing endorphins (Moerman 2006). Moerman points out that some types of problems may be unresponsive to such meaning responses, for example liver function, but even this may be influenced in some circumstances. Thus, the outcome of a study comparing an active ingredient with a true placebo can still be influenced by the meaning to the patient of the whole or parts of the situation. The meaning response is always there and active in some degree. He also cites studies such as Branthwaite and Cooper (1981) on effectiveness of aspirin on headaches, which used real aspirin, but in one group it was given a brand name and in the other no brand name. The effect was greater with the brand name. As he points out, no placebo was used – only the meaning of the name differed between the groups.

Another aspect of the meaning of placebo is a holdover from cartesian dualistic thinking. The usual thought about placebo responses is that they are simply the product of the mind in the form of expectations, responses to sensory input (hands-on effect) and so forth, but do not represent anything that can change actual function and hence the course of health or disease. Besides the vast literature now supporting the physiological effects of massage and hands-on therapies (e.g., Diego et al. 2008, Field 2002, Field et al. 2002), there are other studies showing remarkable effects of psychological influences on structure and hence function. Pascal-Leone and his colleagues (Pascual-Leone et al. 1995, 2005) have shown that practice on the piano can lead to reorganization of the cortical areas controlling finger movement. The changes also require the attention of the individual for their formation. Such changes most likely entail synaptic growth and sprouting of dendrites in the cortex. Even more remarkable are their findings that simply thinking about practicing the piano can also lead to changes in cortical areas controlling the fingers. Such structural changes pursuant to psychological activity show the role of psychological factors in brain structure. Thus, the workings of the mind affect brain structure and hence function. The mind is not an entirely separate entity from the physical brain, but is one determinant of brain function and hence of bodily function.

From the above, it is evident that the effects of most – if not all – treatments, whether they be drugs or manual procedures, have both specific and nonspecific effects that influence the outcome of the encounter. Studies to delineate the specific effects of a drug have been called 'fastidious' (Feinstein 1983) as opposed to pragmatic, now often called outcome studies. The fastidious study attempts to limit the results to the direct effects of the active ingredient being studied and to delimit its mechanism, whereas the pragmatic or effectiveness study attempts to find how the agent responds in a more clinical setting. In the fastidious study, all nonspecific effects should be accounted for in the control group, so that only the active ingredient (usually a drug) is being studied for effect. In the effectiveness or pragmatic study, a broader approach to placebo may be taken. Also, by changing the emphasis of placebo from what has become perceived as an unimportant or even false effect, the meaning response seems to be an extremely useful way to look at the so-called nonspecific effects of any treatment encounter. How does changing the emphasis apply to manual procedures research and thinking?

Study designs in manual procedures

There are at least three general types of design that can be used for manual procedures, with subtypes within them:
1. Technique studies
2. Treatment studies
3. Care studies.

Technique studies

In technique studies, a single isolated technique (or limited number of specified techniques) is studied. Subjects must be selected carefully so as to be homogeneous for the presenting complaint. Each subject receives the same technique administered in the same way. This study can be set up essentially like the RDBPC trial. The 'active' ingredient is considered to be the single or a very limited number of techniques delivered. The control group would receive a similar movement pattern but without whatever was considered the active phase. Subjects need to be naive to manual procedures for best control, and of course randomly assigned to groups.

A very nice example of the technique study was provided by the Irvine study in the late 1970s, carried out at the College of Medicine at the University of California, Irvine (Buerger 1980, Hoehler et al. 1981). In this elegantly designed and executed study the goal was to determine the effect of a high-velocity lateral recumbent roll thrust on acute low-back pain. This procedure involves positioning the patient on one side and rotating the pelvis one way and the thorax the other. The 'active' phase is a sharp, short counter-rotational thrust designed to articulate or move the joints at a specific level of the lumbar spine. The subjects were recruited from a large back pain clinic and had very similar complaints. They were randomly assigned to experimental and control groups, were naive to manual medicine, and were given extensive tests before and after the treatment. The experimental group received the lateral recumbent roll with thrust to a specific lumbar area, whereas the control group received the positioning of the roll but were not thrust. The results showed a significant difference on several measures of the syndrome, including straight leg raising and pain. After several weeks, no differences remained between the groups, most likely due to a normal course of such acute back pain.

The study had most of the hallmarks of the gold standard study design except for one: the operator obviously could not be blinded to what was done. However, the subjects were shown to be blinded by asking whether or not they had received treatment. There was no difference between the groups in the answer. The data collectors were blinded as well. However, owing to the fact that the treater could not be blinded,

many reviews of manual medicine omit this study from consideration. This highlights one of the difficulties of designing fastidious studies of manual medicine: it is probably impossible to blind the person delivering the manual procedure – as is also the case for studies of surgical and injection procedures. This highlights the fact that manual procedure and surgical studies can only be double blind, not triple blind as drug studies can be. However, in this study, it would appear that most of the nonspecific effects of the treatment interaction were the same between the groups. Thus, it would appear that the effect was due to the specific effect of the 'active ingredient' – the thrust itself.

Treatment studies

In treatment studies, the total manual procedure that the treating doctor or therapist deems necessary is given to the patient. Other aspects of treatment are ideally constant between experimental and control groups. However, here an entirely different problem is present. One such study was conducted by Licciardone and his colleagues on the effect of osteopathic manipulative treatment (OMT) on recovery from knee or hip replacement (Licciardone et al. 2004). In this study, regular individualized OMT was provided for one group of patients while a 'sham' consisting of range of motion and light touch was provided to the control group. The results showed no differences between the groups, except for a slight but significant reduction in rehabilitation efficiency with the OMT.

What is an appropriate control group for such a study? Many attempts have been made to devise an appropriate control for the treatment study design, but none have really been satisfactory. This is due to the obvious fact that a placebo in the true sense of the word is not possible. At one end of the spectrum is a control group that simply comes into the office, receives a standard physical examination employing the usual hands-on methods of examining the body, then spends a period of time resting on a table, perhaps with the doctor or therapist sitting nearby. The other end of the spectrum would have to be a manual procedure session exactly like that the treatment group receives, which would not be a contrast control, and no information could be obtained regarding treatment. In between, controls have been used that have included stroking the control subjects with hands, detuned diathermy wands, touching with 'no intention to treat' (whatever that may be), and even having untrained people move the person's body for a while. However, for the reasons discussed above, all of these things are actually forms of treatment, as body contact, even by the untrained, produces some of the same nonspecific effects as does the actual treatment or therapy.

It is true that the 'controls' in these trials may not have identical nonspecific effect magnitude as the experimental subjects, but how can this be assessed? What is the active ingredient in manual procedures? Many would suggest that the specific movements of manual procedures are the active ingredients. However, the apparent clinical success of manual procedures given by a wide range of practitioners with a wide range of skills and movement tactics would suggest that there is more to the 'active ingredient' than specific movements of the body by the treater. In this, we agree with Benedetti when he states 'For example, how should we devise a placebo treatment that is similar to a real physiotherapeutic manipulation (e.g., a massage) of the body? As this is almost impossible, no good placebo control exists' (Benedetti 2009). If this is so, any placebo group using body contact in a manual procedure study is actually comparing one form of treatment with another and should be so designated. The problem is that the other effects are not available for comparison, such as the natural course of the symptoms, regression to the mean, etc. that are not considered either placebo or meaning responses. The only way to know whether an observed effect is made up

of nonspecific, natural effects such as normal fluctuation of symptoms or regression to the mean, or is a true treatment effect made up of response to an active ingredient plus meaning responses, is to compare the total manual procedure group with a group receiving no such contact.

Care studies

In care studies, one form of full care is compared against a community standard form of care or a proven – or at least accepted – treatment regimen. Such a study was done comparing the effects of osteopathic care to community standard care in low back pain (Andersson et al. 1999). Despite the title, the study was designed to compare osteopathic care, which included manipulative treatment, with standard care for low back pain delivered by physicians, who could not use manipulative treatment. The study found no difference in outcomes between the two types of care, although the osteopathic care group used fewer drugs and physical therapy. It is difficult to analyze such studies, but in such a case one can say that apparently the two types of care, one including manipulative treatment as a standard part, were equivalent. No statements can be made about the role of expectation or other nonspecific treatment effects.

In the three general study types discussed here there are obviously variations on the basic designs, such as within-subject designs that have their own design problems and advantages, but this will not be further elaborated here.

The role of meaning in treatment

It seems inescapable that the meaning response is an integral part of manual procedures. What are the implications of this? As noted above, what is generally considered a placebo response – that is, a response to an inert substance – when taken in context of meaning is really a measure of the patient's ability to respond to the situation and what the situation means to him/her. Owing to the fact that a true placebo cannot be constructed for manual procedures, it must be concluded that the total response of the patient, including both specific responses to the movements and the meaning response to touch, the doctor–patient interaction and the response to situation are all true responses to manual procedures.

Writing in 1991, Korr stated this concept as follows: 'Therefore, that which is regarded as nuisance and source of error from one perspective is essence and source of clinical results from the osteopathic perspective' (Korr 1991).

The osteopathic treatment, the chiropractic, massage, or the physical therapy session cannot be factored apart or taken piecemeal, but each procedure is a unified unit of treatment that includes both specific and 'nonspecific' elements inherent in any patient–provider interaction. These elements combine as a whole that depend on one another for their total effect. The patient's clinical response depends on this combination for full effect. Thus, to fully appreciate the effectiveness of a manual procedure, one must study the full treatment or therapy as it is given to the patient. It cannot be standardized or broken apart, as this makes it less than the treatment or therapy to be studied. The patient's meaning responses to the total manual procedure are an integral part of the clinical effectiveness. In other words, the 'active ingredient' in manual procedures is the total procedure.

Taken in this light, the study of manual procedures is different from the study of drug effectiveness, or even a surgical procedure. To attempt to separate what are called nonspecific effects from the specific effects of the manual procedure does not make sense, as what are called nonspecific effects in drug therapy are actually specific effects of the manual procedure. This also implies that the study of manual procedures must allow the treating practitioner to use whatever methods seem appropriate for the individual patient at the time of treatment.

Having said this, it is of course possible, as stated above, to study parts of a manual procedure, as did the Irvine study (Buerger 1980). Such a study in fact can be constructed to be very similar to the RDBPC trial that is the gold standard for drug trials. In such studies of specific movement sequences it is possible to do the same thing except for one or a few movements to both control and experimental groups, and thus to assess the effects of that part(s) of the sequence. However, this is not studying manual procedures: it is studying a specific sequence of movements for their effects. Such studies are justified and useful, but should not be confused with studying manual procedures. In studies of specific movement sequences it is important to control for patient expectations of the treatment and so forth, as it is the aim of the study to assess only the effects of certain movements. Licciardone (Licciardone & Russo 2006) provided a good explanation of this process in a recent paper on blinding and expectations.

With this understanding of manual procedures, the use of control groups is much clearer. The optimal control group would be a group given only an examination to determine what problems exist, followed by no treatment at all. This would allow the study to assess the actual effectiveness of the manual procedure against the natural course of the problem in question, and would control for regression to the mean, natural fluctuations of the disease, etc. It is true that partial procedures can be compared to the total manual procedure, as has been done in many studies. In most such studies, the control has been called a sham or placebo control, and may consist of light touch, manual procedures at parts of the body remote from the complaint, etc. In the current view, this is incorrect. These controls are actually forms of alternative or partial treatment and should be recognized as such. In this light, if such a condition is to be used as a control, it should first be compared with a no-treatment control to assess the effect of the partial treatment. Thus, should one wish to compare, for example, a light touch regimen with a full manual procedure, it may well be that the best design would be to have three arms: a non-treated group, a light touch group, and a full manual procedure group. In this way, the effects of a light touch manual procedure can be assessed against both full and no manual procedure. To have only the light touch and full manual procedure groups is to assess the effectiveness of one treatment of unknown effectiveness against another treatment of unknown effectiveness.

The importance of understanding the hypothesis

The above discussion suggests that testing the effectiveness of manual procedures is unlike that of testing the effectiveness of a drug. Likewise, the design of studies to test the pragmatic effectiveness of manual procedures should be driven by the hypothesis to be tested, not by a preconceived notion of what the study design 'must' be (Patterson 2003). The hypothesis, not the preconceived design, should drive how the study is designed. Thus, the investigator should understand whether the study is designed to examine effects of actual manual procedures or of some defined part of such a procedure, and design the study accordingly. Both study types are valuable, but only if there is a thorough understanding of what manual procedures entail in terms of what the treatment or therapy actually is. Manual procedures intrinsically include the movements generated, the interactions between patient and physician, the patient's expectations and perceptions, and the effects of all these on subsequent function. To attempt to factor these apart without first showing that the total combination produces an effect on function is not logical and indeed is counterproductive.

Conclusions

The concept of placebo in manual procedures is different from that of a drug trial. A specific active ingredient is evident in a drug trial, but not in a manual procedure study. This leads to a rethinking of what 'nonspecific' effects or placebos mean in manual medicine. By redefining such nonspecific effects as meaning effects that are an integral part of the effectiveness of manual procedures, a different appreciation for what constitutes the effect of manual procedures is gained. Studies of manual procedures should be designed to compare these treatments with no treatment, thereby taking into consideration the patient's expectations and interactions, not factoring them out or treating them as undesirable or artifacts. Studies of parts of, or differing, manual procedures can be done in much the same way as drug trials, but must not be confused with studies of the full manual procedure. Such an understanding will allow more rapid and meaningful delineations of the true effectiveness of manual procedures used by so many practitioners.

References

Andersson, G.B.J., Lucente, T., Davis, A., Kappler, R.E., Lipton, J.A., Leurgans, S., 1999. A comparison of osteopathic spinal manipulation with standard care for patients with low back pain. N. Engl. J. Med. 341, 1426–1431.

Beecher, H.K., 1955. The powerful placebo. J. Am. Med. Assoc. 159, 1602–1606.

Benedetti, F., 2008. Mechanisms of placebo and placebo-related effects across diseases and treatments. Annu. Rev. Pharmacol. Toxicol. 48, 33–60.

Benedetti, F., 2009. Placebo Effects, Understanding the Mechanisms in Health and Disease. Oxford University Press, Oxford.

Benedetti, F., Maggi, G., Lopiano, L., et al., 2003. Open versus hidden medical treatments: The patient's knowledge about a therapy affects the therapy outcome. Prev. Treat. 6 (1). ArtID 1a, Available at http://content2.apa.org/journals/pre/6/1/1

Branthwaite, A., Cooper, P., 1981. Analgesic effects of branding in treatment of headaches. Br. Med. J. 282, 1576–1578.

Buerger, A.A., 1980. A controlled trial of rotational manipulation in low back pain. Man Med. 2, 17–26.

de la Fuente-Fernandez, R., Ruth, T.J., Sossi, V., Schulzer, M., Clalne, D.B., Stoessl, A.J., 2001. Expectation and dopamine release: Mechanism of the placebo effect in Parkinsons's disease. Science 293, 1164–1166.

Diego, M.A., Field, T., Hernandez-Reif, M., 2008. Temperature increases in preterm infants during massage therapy. Infant Behav. Dev. 31, 149–152.

Enck, P., Benedetti, F., Schedlowski, M., 2008. New insights into the placebo and nocebo responses. Neuron 59, 195–206.

Feinstein, A.R., 1983. An additional basic science for clinical medicine: II. The limitations of randomized trials. Ann. Intern. Med. 99, 544–550.

Field, T., 2002. Massage therapy. Med. Clin. North Am. 86, 163–171.

Field, T., Diego, M., Cullen, C., Hernandez-Reif, M., Sunshine, W., Douglas, S., 2002. Fibromyalgia pain and substance P decrease and sleep improves after massage therapy. J. Clin. Rheumatol. 8, 72–76.

Hoehler, F.K., Tobis, J.K., Buerger, A.A., 1981. Spinal manipulation for low back pain. J. Am. Med. Assoc. 245, 1835–1838.

Kaptchuk, T.J., 1998. Intentional ignorance: a history of blind assessment and placebo controls in medicine. Bull. Hist. Med. 72, 389–433.

Kiene, H., 1996a. A critique of the double-blind clinical trial, part 1. Altern. Ther. Health Med. 2, 74–80.

Kiene, H., 1996b. A critique of the double-blind clinical trial, part 2. Altern. Ther. Health Med. 2, 59–64.

Kienle, G.S., Kiene, H., 1996. Placebo effect and placebo concept: a critical methodological and conceptual analysis of reports on the magnitude of the placebo effect. Altern. Ther. Health Med. 2, 39–54.

Korr, I.M., 1991. Osteopathic research: The needed paradigm shift. J. Am. Osteopath. Assoc. 91, 156 161–158, 170–151.

Licciardone, J.C., Russo, D.P., 2006. Blinding protocols, treatment credibility, and expectancy: methodologic issues in clinical trials of osteopathic manipulative treatment. J. Am. Osteopath. Assoc. 106, 457–463.

Licciardone, J.C., Stoll, S.T., Cardarelli, K.M., Gamber, R.G., Swift, J.N., Winn, W.B., 2004. A randomized controlled trial of osteopathic manipulative treatment following knee or hip arthroplasty. J. Am. Osteopath. Assoc. 104, 193–202.

Moerman, D.E., 2002. The meaning response and the ethics of avoiding placebos. Eval. Health Prof. 25, 399–409.

Moerman, D.E., 2006. The meaning response: thinking about placebos. Pain Pract. 6, 233–236.

Moerman, D.E., Jonas, W.B., 2000. Toward a research agenda on placebo. Adv. Mind Body Med. 16, 33–46.

Moerman, D.E., Jonas, W.B., 2002. Deconstructing the placebo effect and finding the meaning response. Ann. Intern. Med. 136, 471–476.

Pascual-Leone, A., Nguyet, D., Cohen, L.G., Brasil-Neto, J.P., Cammarota, A., Hallett, M., 1995. Modulation of muscle responses evoked by transcranial magnetic stimulation during the acquisition of new fine motor skills. J. Neurophysiol. 74, 1037–1045.

Pascual-Leone, A., Amedi, A., Fregni, F., Merabet, L.B., 2005. The plastic human brain cortex. Annu. Rev. Neurosci. 28, 377–401.

Patterson, M.M., 2003. Foundations of osteopathic medical research. In: Ward, R.C. (Ed.), Foundations for Osteopathic Medicine, second ed. Lippincott, Williams & Wilkins, Philadelphia.

Patterson, M.M., 2010. Foundations for osteopathic medical research. In: Chila, A.G. (Ed.), Foundations for Osteopathic Medicine, third ed. Lippincott, Williams & Wilkins, Philadelphia.

Section Three
Clinical impact of manual therapy on physiologic functions and systemic disorders

Research related to clinical applications of manual therapy for musculoskeletal and systemic disorders from the osteopathic experience

Hollis H King

Introduction

Researchers in osteopathic medicine have conducted research on both the hypothesized mechanisms of action for osteopathic manipulative treatment (OMT) and the clinical outcomes of its application. For the purpose of consistency and ease of discussion, the more general term 'manual therapy' includes OMT unless specific reference is needed for clarity. This chapter deals with the research on the impact of manual therapy on musculoskeletal disorders, physiological functions, and systemic disorders from the perspective of osteopathic medicine. Also presented is further consideration of osteopathic theory on mechanisms of action for manual therapy. Last, but pertinent to the present book, some attention is given to the challenges encountered in the process of conducting manual therapy research.

The distinction between musculoskeletal and systemic disorders is fairly straightforward, though at times the two are inextricably related. Musculoskeletal disorders refer primarily to conditions of pain and restricted function of the spinal area and extremities. Systemic disorders refer to disease entities such as pneumonia, hypertension, and diabetes mellitus, which are primarily viscerally related, usually with organ-specific etiology. Related to systemic disorders is the associated interest in general physiologic functions such as heart rate, digestion, and respiratory function.

Current status of manual therapy research for musculoskeletal disorders

As briefly discussed in Chapter 1, manual therapy has succeeded in obtaining recognition by scientific and governmental entities for clinical application in patients suffering from musculoskeletal pain, which is the most common reason for a person to seek primary medical care in the US (USBJD 2009). In addition to primary care and manual therapy practitioners, a number of medical specialties, including orthopedics, rehabilitation, neurology, and rheumatology, devote much of their clinical attention to musculoskeletal disorders. However, the research emanating from the non-osteopathic medical specialties has focused on surgical, exercise, and pharmacological interventions, and relatively little on manual therapy applications.

In the current era of emphasis on evidence-based practice, it is interesting to note in relation to musculoskeletal disorders that there is no evidence-based research supporting surgery for low back pain (Palmer & Patijn 2009), and that only 13% of all medical practice is considered beneficial, with another 23% considered likely to be beneficial (BMJ Clinical Evidence Centre 2009). Traditional practices taught and handed down through postdoctoral medical training still rely greatly on expert opinion and generally accepted standards of practice for credibility.

In like manner, for over 100 years osteopathic physicians, as well as chiropractors, have provided manual therapy in accordance with techniques taught in training programs and deemed to be beneficial in clinical practice. As discussed below, the milieu for manual therapy research has faced challenges not usually encountered by conventional medical practice researchers. Despite limited resources, the manual therapy professions have produced an evidence base for the treatment of musculoskeletal disorders. Before describing the much less well established clinical applications of manual therapy in systemic disorders, which was the focus of the symposium (see Preface) upon which this book is based, it may be of interest to provide some perspective for the reader unfamiliar with research in this area.

Based on the osteopathic concepts presented in Chapter 1, osteopathic research has reached the level of established benefit of OMT for chronic low back pain. Licciardone (Licciardone et al. 2005) conducted a systematic review and meta-analysis of the randomized controlled clinical trials of OMT applied to patients with chronic low back pain. This analysis was favorable for benefit of OMT in these patients.

Based primarily on chiropractic research, practice guidelines published in 1994 (Bigos et al. 1994) accepted the clinical application of spinal manipulation in the care of low back pain if there were no other contraindications. Such contraindications included the presence of cancer or infection around the spine, or conditions such as cauda equina syndrome, which involve compromise of the L3–S2 nerve roots, rendering spinal manipulation too dangerous owing to the possibility that the condition could be exacerbated. A Cochrane Review (Assendelft et al. 2004) found that spinal manipulation was more effective in reducing pain and improving the ability to perform everyday activities than sham (fake) therapy and therapies already known to be unhelpful. However, it was no more or less effective than medication for pain, physical therapy, exercises, back school, or the care given by a general practitioner. Other systematic reviews give qualified conclusions: typical is that of Cherkin (Cherkin et al. 2003), who concluded that spinal manipulation has small clinical benefits that are equivalent to those of other commonly used therapies.

Subsequent to the reviews reported above, other clinical trials of manual therapy applied to patients with low back pain have been reported. Geisser et al. (2005) reported a single-blind (because the treatment provider knew whether they were administering real or sham manual therapy) randomized controlled clinical trial of manual therapy for low back pain with adjuvant exercise. In this trial the patients did not know whether they received real or sham therapy, and the data gatherer was also blind to the patient's treatment. The researchers found that patients receiving manual therapy with specific exercise significant improvements in pain when controlling for pretreatment levels of pain. No significant changes in disability were observed, with the exception that the sham manual therapy-specific exercise group displayed a significant increase in disability over the 6 weeks of the study. Based on reports such as those reported above, the medical literature in primary care includes manual therapy in management plans for low back pain (Patel & Ogle 2000).

The osteopathic structure–function concept may have its greatest relevance to healthcare benefit when considered in relation to the axial skeleton and related neurovascular structures, which is a focus of this book. However, there are well-designed studies, too numerous to detail in this chapter, that report benefit for manual therapy in a variety of musculoskeletal conditions not necessarily directly related to spinal dysfunction. Three representative examples of such areas of study from the osteopathic literature are presented here:

- Knebl et al. (2002) reported a randomized controlled trial which found significantly improved function in the elderly when OMT was applied in a specific manner to dysfunctional shoulders. This study confirmed many case reports in which similar benefits were reported.
- In a series of studies, Sucher (Sucher 1993, Sucher & Hinrichs 1998, Sucher et al. 2005) demonstrated a decrease in carpal tunnel syndrome pain and an increase in carpal tunnel/wrist range of

motion and function by the application of OMT in techniques designed to correct anatomic derangement and increase the diameter in the carpal tunnel area. These OMT techniques are now widely taught and utilized in clinical practice, and are a part of research protocol in an NIH–NCCAM-funded clinical trial on the treatment of carpal tunnel syndrome.

- Gamber et al. (2002) conducted a clinical trial on fibromyalgia patients and found that standard care plus OMT produced significant relief of pain compared to standard care only.

The Knebl and Sucher studies also illustrated the osteopathic structure–function concept, in that the OMT was specifically formulated to treat fascial and muscular restrictions in the shoulder and wrist that limited mobility.

As set forth in the Preface, the focus of this book is the nature of the research on viscerosomatic interactions and related concepts that may pertain to the mechanisms of action for manual therapy. Our focus must, however, be seen in the context of the traditional and usual clinical application of manual therapy and related research, which is devoted mainly to conditions of the musculoskeletal system. The above brief review is intended to make the point that there is evidence-based research supportive of the benefit of manual therapy in certain musculoskeletal conditions, primarily low back pain. There is also an emerging body of research supportive of benefit for manual therapy in a variety of musculoskeletal conditions, based primarily on the structure–function relationship between anatomic structures and the function of nerve and vascular structures possibly affected by the dysfunctional anatomic structures. For further discussion of these and other studies supportive of the benefit of manual therapy, the reader is referred to *Evidence-Based Manual Medicine* (Seffinger & Hruby 2007).

Impact of manual therapy on systemic disorders and physiologic functions

As demonstrated by references to AT Still's reported experience and Louisa Burns' (1907) original formulation and research on viscerosomatic reflexes, the manual therapy professions have long reported impact of their manual applications for systemic disorders. This is still a controversial field of inquiry, with only a few systemic disorders and physiologic functions receiving more than one published research report. There have been a number of case reports that have served to support and maintain clinical application of OMT in these conditions during the past 100 years, and these are not reviewed here. It is acknowledged from the outset that there are relatively few large-scale studies, and no claims of 'proof' are made. However, the breadth and unique nature of topics and findings are potentially valuable from a heuristic perspective in so far as the development of future larger well-designed studies is concerned.

In most of the studies reported in this section, the assumption was made and described in various ways that the clinically applied OMT benefit, if any, resulted from the restoration of neuromusculoskeletal structures to a more normal motion and anatomic position, which then aided natural healing and physiologic regulation processes. Some authors even developed and reported specific OMT protocols designed to affect autonomic nerve pathways, vascular channels, and the surrounding myofascial structures in areas related to the visceral organs involved in the systemic disorder under consideration.

Pulmonary and immune system function

The area of manual therapy's impact on physiological functions and systemic disorders that has received the most attention is in pulmonary system disease and immune system function in general. Because of the inextricable combination of the impact of spinally oriented and lymphatic system-oriented OMT on pulmonary disease and function, these two topics are discussed together.

One of the important events in the establishment of the osteopathic medical profession in the public eye was the benefit of OMT in the 1918–1919 influenza pandemic. In the USA, 500 000 people died of the influenza in 1917–1918, and between 50 and 100 million more died worldwide. From survey data collected at the time, it appeared that patients treated osteopathically during 1917–1918 had a 0.25% mortality rate, compared to the national average of 6%, and 10% for pneumonia patients, and compared to 33–75% for the national average (Smith 1920).

The traditional spinal and appendicular skeleton manipulation techniques of the day were apparently effective. Normalized spinal alignment and function were, and are, thought to enhance the efficiency of nervous system and vascular system functions. For example, the rib-raising technique (manipulation at the costovertebral junction) was thought to improve functional capacity that might have been restricted by strain in ribs brought about by coughing or trauma, and which might have adversely affected the excitability of the sympathetic chain underlying this area on the inner surface of the body cavity. This was presumed to bring the best possible coordination of the body's self-regulatory and self-healing functions.

In the past 10 years well-designed clinical trials have investigated the effects of rib raising and other OMT techniques on pulmonary disease, particularly pneumonia in the elderly. These studies are summarized in Table 12.1. After the experience derived from the 1918–1919 influenza pandemic, the OMT armamentarium for the treatment of pulmonary disease was increased to include lymphatic pump techniques (Miller 1923, 1927), which have now been studied

Table 12.1 Comparison-group studies investigating osteopathic manipulative treatment in pulmonary disease and immune system function (immunity)

Citation	Study design	Sample size	Experimental intervention*	Comparison group intervention	Study duration or endpoint(s)	Physiological outcomes
Pneumonia						
Noll et al. 2009	RCT	306	OMT MFR, rib raising, lymphatic pumps	Light touch	Hospital discharge or death	Those aged 50–75 and who received OMT twice daily had 25% reduction in hospital stay which was statistically significant. Both OMT and light touch reduced hospital mortality
Noll et al. 2000	RCT	58	OMT MFR, rib raising, lymphatic pumps	Light touch	Hospital discharge	Statistically significant shorter duration of IV antibiotics and a shorter hospital stay
Noll et al. 1999	RCT	21	OMT MFR, rib raising, lymphatic pumps	Light touch	Hospital discharge	Statistically significant shorter duration of oral antibiotic use
COPD						
Noll et al. 2008	RCT	35	OMT MFR, rib raising, lymphatic pumps	Light touch	2 days	OMT group significantly decreased FEV1and ERV and increased RV, TLC
Immunity						
Breithaupt et al. 2001	RCT	97	OMT TLP	No OMT	4 weeks	No significant increase in antigen-specific antibody count
Jackson et al. 1998	RCT	31	OMT TLP, SP	No OMT	2 weeks for OMT 13 weeks F/U for titers at 6 weeks and 13 weeks	Significantly higher antibody titers for OMT group at 6 weeks and 13 weeks
Mesina et al. 1998	Case control	12	OMT TLP, SP, PTT	No OMT	6 hours	Significantly higher basophil count with OMT
Paul et al. 1986	Clinical series SOC	12	OMT TLP		1 day	No increase in Interferon levels 24 hours after OMT
Measel 1982	Clinical series SOC	24	OMT TLP		14 days for titer analysis	Statistically significant increased antigen-specific antibody titers

*OMT, osteopathic manipulative treatment; SOC, subject own control; MFR, myofascial release; COPD, chronic obstructive pulmonary disease; TLP, thoracic lymphatic pump; SP, splenic pump; PTT, pectoral traction technique; IV, intravenous; FEV1, forced expiratory volume at one second; ERV, expiratory reserve volume; RV, residual volume; TLC, total lung capacity.

extensively in both human and animal models. As described below, increased lymphatic flow is related to increases in immune system cell counts (Hodge et al. 2007), but it is important to distinguish between effleurage – a stroking of the skin which acts superficially to move fluids, including lymph – and the osteopathic lymphatic pump techniques, which involve manually guided forces over the ribs and abdominal area, or through leg motion generated from the feet with enough force to move lymph centrally. While the emphasis has been on techniques directed toward an impact on centrally situated structures, vertebral and paravertebral bone, nerve, muscular, and connective tissue, these techniques are often combined with lymphatic pump techniques directed at structures involved in lymph circulation, such as the respiratory diaphragm and chest muscles.

Using an OMT protocol (Noll et al. 2008b) directed toward an impact on axial skeleton structures and lymphatic pump techniques, Noll conducted two preliminary studies (Noll et al. 1999, 2000) which found significant reductions in the use of intravenous antibiotics and duration of hospital stay in elderly pneumonia patients. Based on these studies, a multisite clinical trial using OMT on elderly patients hospitalized with pneumonia was carried out. At the time of writing of this chapter, the results of this clinical trial were in review for publication. However, some results were presented at the 2008 meeting of the Infectious Disease Society of America (Noll 2009) and confirm the preliminary study findings of reduced hospital stay associated with the OMT protocol.

The findings from the pneumonia studies highlight one of the major features in the results of manual therapy delivery: not only are healthcare outcomes improved, but also significant cost savings are derived by utilization of fewer healthcare resources. This finding is particularly pertinent when hospitalization is required, and this cost reduction

benefit theme is echoed in manual therapy research studies described below.

Not all findings were positive, but even these negative studies have implications for understanding the optimal application of manual therapy, especially as related to mechanism of action. A COPD study which used the osteopathic lymphatic pump technique (Noll et al. 2008a) found evidence of worsened alveolar air trapping. The authors speculate that the 'active' component of the thoracic lymphatic pump technique was primarily responsible for the increase in residual volume because the activation portion of the technique promotes a sudden rush of air into the lungs. This air may not be fully exhaled in the context of airway resistance in COPD. If this is found to be the case, the authors recommend elimination of this OMT technique in cases of COPD. However, the authors also pointed out that this study did not deal with long-term effects, which could be quite different.

Five studies that used OMT on human subjects had outcome measures related to immune system function. Three showed immune system enhancement in the form of increased antigen-specific antibody titers (Measel 1982), increased basophil count (Mesina et al. 1998), and increased vaccine antibody titers (Jackson et al. 1998) following OMT. Authors of the other two studies, which showed no immune system enhancement (Breithaupt et al. 2001, Paul et al. 1986), speculated that time from OMT to laboratory testing and host response issues mitigated their findings. Nevertheless, with improved technology, research design, and sufficient funding, the likelihood that further clinical research would demonstrate benefit of OMT for immune system function appears promising. Similar results from the massage therapy literature (see Chapter 15) support this view, and together constitute an emerging consensus on the benefit of manual therapy for immune system function.

Equally important is the basic science, animal model work, demonstrating the effects of manual therapy on lymphatic and immune system functions. After the 1918–1919 pandemic, the lymphatic pump techniques were developed. Albeit demonstrated in clinical practice to be beneficial, there was no evidence that these techniques actually affected lymphatic flow.

The lymph flow stimulation question was answered in a study on instrumented conscious, non-anesthetized dogs. Eight minutes of lymphatic pump technique adapted to dogs produced measurable increases in thoracic duct flow (Knott et al. 2005). Building on this research, Hodge et al. (2007) replicated the enhanced lymph flow finding and found that the lymphatic pump treatment (LPT) also significantly increased leukocyte count and flux. Leukocyte flux is the combination of lymph flow and leukocyte count, giving a more complete picture of the total impact on the body of the LPT, and provides a mechanism of action for the benefits seen in human clinical applications of such techniques. Research by Hodge (2009) indicates that the source of most of the leukocytes stimulated by the LPT is gastrointestinal-associated lymphoid tissue (GALT). These results are yet to be replicated in humans, but certainly suggest the likely mechanism of action for humans as well.

In summary, human and animal model investigations have provided some insight into the mechanism of action for manual therapy effects in pulmonary disease, which appear to be related, at least in part, to humoral factors in immune system enhancement (Licciardone 2010). According to research reported so far, there are no data to support any autonomic effects, though the idea of nervous system involvement is suggested by osteopathic concepts (see Chapter 1).

Pregnancy and reproductive system function

Another area where the application of OMT has received much attention is its impact during pregnancy and with reproductive system disorders. Table 12.2 summarizes the studies cited in this section. Two studies (Guthrie & Martin 1982, Licciardone et al. 2010) showed significant reduction of low back pain during pregnancy when OMT was provided. One investigation (King et al. 2003) found that pregnant women who received OMT had significantly fewer preterm deliveries and instances of meconium-stained amniotic fluid. A physiological study on women in the third trimester showed improved vagal control of heart rate after just one OMT treatment (Hensel 2009). The Hensel study continues and will also assess birth outcomes.

OMT applied during pregnancy is another application which may have very significant healthcare benefits and cost savings. The cost to society of preterm deliveries alone is in the billions (King et al. 2003), and if OMT reduces this cost then further study should be a high priority. Spinal manipulation in pregnancy and related conditions has been systematically reviewed (Khorsan et al. 2009) and described as an 'emergent' field of study.

The two studies (Boesler et al. 1993, Holtzman et al. 2008) investigating the impact of OMT on dysmenorrhea were positive for reported pain reduction, and one (Boesler et al. 1993) even showed reduced EMG activity after OMT. Taken together with the chiropractic studies on the treatment of dysmenorrhea (Chapter 14), a case can be made for greater clinical application of manual therapy for dysmenorrhea, as long as there are no contraindications for a particular patient.

Indeed, the results of OMT applied in pregnancy, as well as OMT and chiropractic applied in the treatment of dysmenorrhea, may be just the beginning of broader applications in women's health. The mechanism of action in pregnancy and dysmenorrhea appears to be improved musculoskeletal alignment and balance, as suggested by Hensel (2009). If this is further delineated by her ongoing research, then overall female reproductive system function improvement

Table 12.2 Comparison-group studies investigating osteopathic manipulative treatment for pregnancy and reproductive system conditions in women

Citation	Study design	Sample size	Experimental intervention*	Comparison group intervention	Study duration or endpoint	Physiological outcomes	Patient-reported outcomes
Pregnancy							
Hensel 2009	RCT	60	OMT OCF ME, myofascial release	Sham sub-therapeutic ultrasound	1 wk	Improved vagal control of heart rate and lowered heart rate	
Licciardone et al. 2009	RCT	146	OMT myofascial release, ME, articulatory	Sham sub-therapeutic ultrasound	8 wks	Deterioration of back-specific functioning halted during the third trimester of pregnancy	
King et al. 2003	Retrospective case control	321	OMT cranial ME, HVLA SCS, myofascial release articulatory	Matched group received no OMT	Case review	OMT group had significantly fewer instances of meconium-stained amniotic fluid and fewer preterm deliveries	
Guthrie & Martin 1982	Matched groups	209	OMT L spine pressure	Sham OMT light pressure T spine	Pre- and post delivery	L spine OMT significantly less pain medication	L spine OMT group reported back labor pain reduced by OMT, Sham OMT group reported no pain relief
Dysmenorrhea							
Holtzman et al. 2008	Prospective case series	14	Drop table		2 menstrual cycles	Statistically significant less EMG activity after OMT	VAS and severity ratings decreased
Boesler et al. 1993	Prospective case series	12	OMT – HVLA		2 menstrual cycles		Reports of reduced low back pain corresponded with reduced EMG activity

*OMT, osteopathic manipulative therapy; HVLA, high-velocity, low-amplitude; ME, muscle energy technique; OCF, osteopathy in the cranial field; Articulatory, range of motion; SCS, strain–counterstrain technique; VAS, visual analog scale; C, cervical vertebrae; T, thoracic vertebrae; L, lumbar vertebrae.

may be a realistic expectation for manual therapy, especially OMT. This author's clinical experience with improved menstrual regularity and reduced dysmenorrhea also supports this possible outcome. The likely mechanism of action for OMT in pregnancy and reproductive system functions is impact innervation of these organs, with some possible lymphatic flow enhancement.

OMT in the hospital and surgical setting

Osteopathic physicians who do surgery and who care for hospitalized patients have also contributed to the research literature on the effects of OMT. Table 12.3 summarizes the studies described in this section. In the USA, osteopathic physicians have the 'full scope of medical practice' licence. Many osteopathic physicians are surgeons, and this has facilitated research on the application of OMT to hospitalized patients. The OMT protocols utilized in these studies were directed toward axial skeletal areas where somatic dysfunction could affect autonomic nervous system function, as well as peripheral areas that could affect vascular flow. Such areas were the occipito-atlanto and sacral areas possibly influencing functions related to the parasympathetic nervous system (i.e., gastrointestinal tract, heart, lung, pelvic organs) and T1–L5 segments targeting somatic dysfunctions and function related to the sympathetic nervous system.

One study on women who had had a hysterectomy found that preoperative OMT significantly reduced the need for postoperative analgesia (Goldstein et al. 2005). Unfortunately, due to insufficient hospital record keeping it was not possible to evaluate the subjective impression that these same patients also recovered faster.

In a dramatic study on outcomes in coronary artery bypass graft surgery (CABG), investigators found that the application of postoperative OMT significantly improved drainage from the operative site (Yurvati et al. 2005). Postoperative oxygen saturation and cardiac efficiency were also significantly improved in the patients who received OMT compared to those who did not. The OMT protocol utilized cervical spine and upper thoracic techniques to reduce the strains caused by prolonged anesthesia and open chest surgery.

In a substantial chart review study, patients who had had abdominal surgery and also had the diagnosis of postoperative ileus were examined (Crow & Gorodinsky 2009). In this particular hospital, OMT service was available to inpatients. Those who received OMT postoperatively had significantly shorter hospital stays than those patients who did not. This study supported the clinical experience that postoperative OMT improved bowel function and reduced the duration of ileus symptoms.

Another postoperative complication studied was atelectasis (Sleszynski & Kelso 1993). The results of the application of OMT did not reduce the occurrence of atelectasis, but the OMT was correlated with a faster return to preoperative respiratory function. Patients hospitalized with pancreatitis were also studied (Radjieski et al. 1998): those who received OMT had significantly shorter hospital stays.

In the hospital and surgical areas the application of OMT as a cost-saving application can be especially appreciated. Although the main concern is the optimization of healthcare outcomes, the matter of cost saving by fewer medications and resources consumed and shorter hospital stays is certainly a compelling reason to consider offering OMT in these types of conditions where it can be applied to the hospitalized patient. The OMT used in these studies was directed toward spinal and skeletal structures as well as viscera. This is suggestive of OMT's impact on central innervation (including spinal processing and supraspinal control) as well as local effects due to somatic dysfunction.

Table 12.3 Comparison-group studies investigating osteopathic manipulative treatment as adjunctive treatment patients requiring hospitalization or surgical case management

Citation	Study design	Sample size	Experimental intervention*	Comparison group intervention	Study duration or endpoint(s)	Physiological outcomes
Crow & Gorodinsky 2009	Retrospective case review	331 patients who had abdominal surgery	172 received OMT-US but based on diagnosis of somatic dysfunction	139 did not receive OMT	Chart review	Statistically significant shorter hospital stay for OMT group
Yurvati et al. 2005	Prospective clinical trial	29 patients who received CABG surgery	10 received OMT MFR, gentle lymphatic pumb	19 did not receive OMT	Discharge from hospital	OMT patients had statistically significant improved thoracic impedance, oxygen saturation, and cardiac index
Goldstein et al. 2005	RCT	39 patients who received TAH surgery	20 received OMT ST, MFR	19 received sham OMT light touch to unrelated area	Discharge from hospital	Pre-Op OMT decreased pre- and post-op analgesia following TAH
Radjieski et al. 1998	RCT	14 patients hospitalized with pancreatitis	6 received OMT MFR, SCS, PTT, TL, IL	8 received standard care only	Discharge from hospital	Statistically significant reduced hospital stay by 3.5 days
Sleszynski & Kelso 1993	RCT	42 patients hospitalized for gall bladder surgery	21 received OMT LPT	21 received incentive spirometry	Discharge from hospital	No difference in occurrence of atelectasis. OMT group returned to preoperative FVC and FEV1 values faster

*OMT, osteopathic manipulative therapy; ST, soft tissue technique; MFR, myofascial release; PTT, pectoral traction technician; SCS, strain–counterstrain technique; LPT, lymphatic pump technique; TL, thoraco-lumbar mobilization; IL, iliosacral mobilization; CABG, coronary artery bypass surgery; TAH, total abdominal hysterectomy; FVC, forced vital capacity; FEV1, forced expiratory volume in one second; US, unspecified.

OMT in pediatrics

Another area receiving substantial clinical and research attention is OMT applied in children. Table 12.4 summarizes the studies cited in this section. Most OMT applied in pediatric cases is gentle and directed at correcting somatic dysfunction, which may cause disturbed function of cranial nerve impulse flow possibly underlying conditions such as infantile colic and cranial structure compression, which could derange temporal bone position and disturb eustachian tube drainage, leading to recurrent otitis media. The presumed effect of OMT in cognitive function is the correction of cranial nerve functions for auditory and visual reception and processing that have been disturbed by biomechanical pressures due to birth trauma or other head injuries.

Otitis media is a common childhood condition which can have serious adverse effects if not treated effectively. The application of OMT in otitis media has been examined in two published reports (Degenhardt & Kuchera 2006, Mills et al. 2003). The findings were that the children who received OMT had significantly fewer episodes of acute otitis media and improved tympanogram results. These findings supported decades of clinical experience and further research on this topic, which is now under way.

A common neonatal condition is colic. In its worst manifestation, intractable vomiting can result in death. Clinical experience was once again confirmed by research (Hayden & Mullinger 2006) which showed significantly reduced colic symptoms and increased sleep in infants who received OMT. In slightly older children, sleep apnea symptoms were significantly reduced during a 4-week period when OMT was applied; however, after OMT was terminated there was no difference between OMT and control patients.

There is also evidence that OMT improves cognitive function (Lassovetskaia 2005) and neurological development (Frymann et al. 1992) in children. In Lassovetskaia's study, children in a special education program achieved significantly higher test scores and teacher ratings on behavior when OMT was applied, and the effects appeared to be long lasting. Using the Houle Profile of Neurological Development, children who received OMT had significantly higher scores than a matched group of children on the waiting list for treatment (Frymann et al. 1992).

Although so far there have not been many studies on the application of OMT to pediatric disorders, those that have been done corroborate decades of clinical experience. The mechanism of action for benefit, as suggested above, is the return of deranged neuromusculoskeletal structures to normal anatomic configuration and function, which in turn may restore normal functions such as viscerosomatic interactions. 'As the twig is bent, so inclines the tree' is a phrase applicable in the application of OMT in pediatric disorders. The idea is that OMT attempts to straighten the 'bent twigs' so that normal structure may produce normal function.

Hemodynamic functions, peripheral artery disease, and heart rate variability

Exploration of the impact of OMT has also been extended to vascular and cardiac functions. Table 12.5 summarizes the studies cited in this section. OMT has been shown to increase diastolic blood pressure (Rivers et al. 2008), increase vertebral basilar artery perfusion (Huard 2005), and increase digital pulse contour (Purdy et al. 1996). Each of these studies was carried out from a 'proof of concept' perspective, that is, there was no specific diagnosed disease process under consideration. These investigations were done to assess the possible impact of OMT on hemodynamic function; however, little can be said as to mechanism of action, and they are reported here as suggestions for possible further investigation.

Table 12.4 Comparison-group studies investigating osteopathic manipulative treatment in pediatric patients diagnosed with otitis media, colic, apnea or cognitive disorders

Citation	Study design	Sample size	Experimental intervention	Comparison group intervention	Study duration or endpoint(s)	Physiological outcomes
Otitis media						
Mills et al. 2003	RCT	57	Routine care plus OMT, BMT, ME, SCS myofascial release	Routine care only	9 visits 3 weekly 3 biweekly 3 monthly	Statistically significant fewer episodes of AOM, surgery for ear tubes, and more normal tympanograms
Degenhardt & Kuchera 2006	Pilot cohort study	8	OMT based on finding of somatic dysfunction		3 weekly visits for OMT, then 1 year F/U	5 of 8 had no documented episodes of AOM at one year follow-up
Colic						
Hayden & Mullinger 2006	RCT	28	OMT – OCF, soft tissue	No OMT, physical exam only	4 weeks	Statistically significant decrease in crying and increase in time spent sleeping. All 14 who received OMT improved and 10 required no OMT after 3 weeks
Apnea						
Vandenplas et al. 2008	RCT	28	OMT FT based on somatic dysfunction present	Sham OMT standard mobilization of extremities	2 weeks	Statistically significant decreased episodes of obstructive apnea during time OMT received. No difference between groups after OMT stopped
Cognitive & Neurological						
Lassovetskaia 2005	Cohort study	96	OMT based on finding of somatic dysfunction	Compared to children in special education program not receiving OMT	6–12 weeks	Statistically significant improved academic performance in children who received OMT compared to those who did not
Frymann et al. 1992	Cohort study	118	OMT based on finding of somatic dysfunction	Compared to children on wait list for treatment	6–8 weeks	Statistically significant improvement on Houle's Profile of Development

OMT, osteopathic manipulative therapy; BMT, balanced membrane tension; ME, muscle energy technique; OCF, osteopathy in the cranial field; SCS, strain–counterstrain technique; FT, functional techniques; AOM, acute otitis media; US unspecified.

Table 12.5 Comparison-group studies investigating osteopathic manipulative treatment effects on hemodynamic functions, peripheral artery disease, heart rate variability

Citation	Study design	Sample size	Experimental intervention	Comparison group intervention	Study duration or endpoint(s)	Physiological outcomes
Hemodynamic						
Rivers et al. 2008	Random cross over	15	OMT myofascial release, rib raising, lymphatic pump	Rest supine	2 hours	Statistically significant decrease in hemoglobin platelet count and increase in diastolic BP
Huard 2005	RCT	117	OMT – VST	Light touch	2 hours	Statistically significant increase in vertebral basilar artery perfusion
Purdy et al. 1996	Random cross over	25	OMT sub-occipital guided manual force	Light touch no pressure in sub-occipital area	2 hours	Statistically significant increase in digital pulse contour in both total pulse amplitude and height from dicrotic notch to peak
Peripheral artery disease						
Lombardini et al. 2009	Case Control	30	OMT: MFR SCS, ME, ST, HVLA, CST, TLP	Rest, supine	6 months	Statistically significant Increase in vasodilation, ankle/brachial pressure index, time to first claudication pain
HR variability						
Henley et al. 2008	Random cross over	17	C spine MFR	Sham OMT touch	2 days	Statistically significant increase in HRV in OMT group in tilt position which increased SNS tone compared to horizontal position
Giles 2006	Random cross over	24	OMT – OA decompression C-spine soft tissue stretching and kneading	Sham OMT touch	2 hours	Statistically significant increase in HRV for OMT condition
Zhang et al. 2006	Cohort subject own control	111	CMT	Sham impulse over scapulae	1 and 4 weeks	Statistically significant increase in HRV sustained at 4 weeks
Budgell & Polus 2006	Random cross over	20	TSM HVLA	Sham CV – 4	1 week	Statistically significant increase in HRV

OMT, osteopathic manipulative therapy; CST, cranial sacral therapy; VST, venous sinus technique; MFR, myofascial release; CV-4, compression of the forth ventricle; CMT, spinal manipulative therapy delivered by chiropractor; ME, muscle energy technique; ST, soft tissue technique; SCS, strain–counterstrain technique; TSM, thoracic spinal manipulation; HVLA, high velocity, low amplitude; HR, heart rate; BP, blood pressure.

In a case–control study on a population of men with peripheral artery disease, the effects of OMT were found to significantly increase brachial flow-mediated vasodilation, ankle/brachial pressure index, time to first claudication in, and the physical health component of quality of life (Lombardini et al. 2009). In this study there was also a significant negative correlation between changes in brachial flow-mediated vasodilation and IL-6 levels: the lower the IL-6 level, the higher the brachial flow-mediated vasodilation. Albeit limited in generalizability by the study design, the changes in levels of cardiac function-related biomarkers and quality of life ratings are illustrative of possible hormonal and neurohumoral mechanisms of action related to viscerosomatic interaction effects of manual therapy in cardiac and vascular function.

Chapter 5 deals in greater depth with heart rate variability (HRV) as a possible measure of autonomic activity in the context of manual therapy research. In the context of this chapter, it is suggested that the HRV findings are consistent with the previously described formulation of improved autonomic nervous system function as a result of the OMT or spinal manipulation, which appeared to return musculoskeletal structures to a more normal anatomic position and function – another way of describing the 'structure–function' concept of osteopathy.

Four studies (Budgell & Polus 2006, Giles 2006, Henley et al. 2008, Zhang et al. 2006) showed increased HRV variability with OMT or chiropractic spinal manipulation, a beneficial outcome in itself. A reasonable explanation for these results is changes in autonomic control of circulatory function. In these four studies the OMT or chiropractic manipulation was to the cervical and thoracic areas.

Urinary dysfunction in multiple sclerosis

A recent study in Israel evaluated the impact of OMT on urinary tract function and quality of life in outpatients with multiple sclerosis. Summarized in Table 12.6, the results of OMT using craniosacral therapy (CST) were statistically significant reductions in postvoid residual volume, urinary frequency, urinary urgency, and improvement in quality of life. The nature of CST suggests that an impact on parasympathetic centers in the lower brain stem and the sacral spinal cord may be the likely mechanism of action in this study.

Table 12.6 Patient as own control study of effect of OMT on urinary tract signs and symptoms in outpatients with multiple sclerosis

Citation	Study design	Sample size	Experimental intervention	Comparison group intervention	Study duration or endpoint(s)	Physiological outcomes
Raviv et al. 2009	Subject as own control	28	OMT: CST		4 weeks	Statistically significant reduction in post voiding residual volume, urinary frequency, urinary urgency, and improvement in quality of life

OMT, osteopathic manipulative therapy; CST, cranial sacral therapy.

Research on viscerosomatic interactions and implications for manual therapy

Beal (1985) catalogued over 100 separate published reports in the osteopathic literature of patients with verified disease (e.g. cardiac, pulmonary, gastrointestinal, renal, and reproductive) in which the patients were examined structurally and demonstrated specific vertebral-level somatic dysfunction. An example was the finding that patients with heart disease had somatic dysfunction at T1–T5. Beal also reviewed the extant neuroanatomic literature for segmental sympathetic activity and described the near-perfect correlation of the osteopathic clinical reports with the neuroanatomic data.

Subsequent to her initial research in 1907, Burns carried out a number of studies on viscerosomatic interactions. One was titled 'Qualities distinguishing muscles affected by primary vertebral lesions from those affected by viscerosomatic nerve reflexes' (Burns 1928), and others dealt with treatment implications in pulmonary disease (Burns 1933) and cardiac disease (Burns 1944). Work was done by Hix (1972, 1976) with rats in the Denslow–Korr laboratory specifically on musculoskeletal reactions to renal and urological viscera stimulation.

Contemporary research focusing specifically on viscerosomatic interaction tested the hypothesis that myocardial ischemia induces increased paraspinal muscular tone localized to the T2–T3 region that can be detected by palpation. The subjects were 15 conscious, instrumented dogs who were examined before, during, and after experimentally induced myocardial ischemia. Electromyographic (EMG) analysis and blinded manual palpatory assessments (MPA) of the tissue over the transverse spinal processes at segments T2–T3 and T11–T12 (control) were performed. Findings were that myocardial ischemia is associated with significant paraspinal increased muscle tone localized to the left-side T2–T5 myotomes in neurally intact dogs. Left ventricular sympathectomy, which interrupted the visceral afferents from the heart, stopped previously palpated and EMG-measured changes at T2–T5 on the left that had been induced by myocardial ischemia (Gwirtz et al. 2007). In Chapter 7 data suggestive of a mechanism of action for Gwirtz et al.'s findings are presented and interpreted.

Gwirtz et al.'s (2007) results, along with many other studies, including those cited in this book, support the viability of viscerosomatic interactions as a scientific concept, as well as part of the explanation of the mechanism of action for OMT and other manual therapies. The relationship between viscerosomatic interactions and the concept of facilitated segments may be somewhat more suppositional, but if seen as a long-term or chronic effect of visceral pathology has explanatory value and heuristic implication.

Further considerations of the facilitated area concept

As described in Chapter 1, the palpatory finding of somatic dysfunction and any associated pain or discomfort may be due to what is called a facilitated segment or area. In the osteopathic literature, a facilitated area may be due to visceral disease via the viscerosomatic reflex route or musculoskeletal injury which causes malalignment of the vertebral structures, or functional problems such as motion restrictions of the vertebral and associated structures (Ward 2003). Are facilitated segments indicative of visceral disease? This is still an open question, but the possibility of validity would serve to provide even greater understanding of the impact of manual therapy on systemic disorders.

Many controlled studies – too numerous to mention – on animals demonstrating viscerosomatic interactions have been carried out, many by researchers who have written chapters (Chapters 2–4, 7, 8) in this book and/or have presented in the International Symposia leading to this book (Cervero 1985, Gebhart & Randich 1992, Jänig & Morrison 1986, Patterson & Howell 1992). A significant number of human clinical and animal studies support the position that visceral disease can cause spinal and peripheral neuromusculoskeletal changes, not otherwise attributable to musculoskeletal trauma. From the osteopathic perspective, the concept of facilitated areas proposed by Korr (Chapter 1) is viable and has received much attention.

Beal (1985), in his extensive review of viscerosomatic reflexes, stated: 'The strength and duration of the visceral afferent stimulus necessary to effect a somatic response is not known. It is recognized that visceral afferents may be reinforced by somatic stimuli from skin and muscle, as well as by impulses from higher centers, which may lower the threshold for visceral afferents or facilitate their action at a specific spinal cord level. Prior facilitation of a cord segment or cord learning may enable a weaker visceral afferent stimulus to affect a somatic response.' The formulation of viscerosomatic interactions and facilitated areas are clearly linked in osteopathic research and theory.

Beal found significant correlation between cardiovascular disease and somatic dysfunction in segments T1–T7 (Beal 1982). He also found a correlation between pulmonary disease and somatic dysfunction in segments T2–T7 (Beal & Morlock 1984). Beal then took the correlation a step further and found that palpation predicted the presence of coronary artery disease in 79% of patients scheduled for cardiac catheterization (Beal & Kleiber 1985). Somatic dysfunction was generally found in segments T1–T4. Similar findings were reported in a series of studies by Johnston (1988, 1992) which addressed the issue of how to identify somatic findings of visceral reflex origin, and then went on to examine spinal palpatory findings in patients with hypertension (Johnston et al. 1980, 1982, Johnston & Kelso 1995) and renal disease (Johnston et al. 1987).

In more recent research a study on the palpatory findings in 92 patients with type 2 diabetes mellitus consistently found tissue changes, including tenderness at T12–L2 on the right. This was consistent with the kidney viscerosomatic distribution of renal diabetic pathophysiology (Licciardone et al. 2007). There is older osteopathic research, consistent with facilitated segment(s)/viscerosomatic reflex findings, which suggested that OMT directed at T12–L2 affected blood glucose levels (Bandeen 1948).

Bandeen's research has recently been reviewed and reanalyzed (Licciardone 2008), and it was suggested that, along with OMT to T12–L1, the addition of OMT for pancreatic stimulation directed at ribs 2–5 also significantly affected blood glucose levels (Bandeen 1949). In 121 patients Bandeen's OMT to both areas produced rapid decreases in blood glucose levels in the range of 40 mg/dl within 30 minutes, and in 86 patients an even greater reduction within 60 minutes. No data were reported on the duration of such changes. Bandeen's hypothesis, which reflected the fact that very little was known about diabetes mellitus in 1949, was that his treatment somehow restored normal function to the pancreas's islets of Langerhans. However, much more study is required before Bandeen's OMT protocol can be considered as a viable treatment modality for blood glucose disorders.

OMT utilizing stimulation to the T11 vertebral segment intended to affect adrenal function was found to be statistically significant at lowering aldosterone levels in hypertensive patients, but not at lowering blood pressure itself (Mannino 1979).

A practical application of the concept of viscerosomatic interactions has been the practice of osteopathic physicians to consider visceral disease if somatic dysfunction does not resolve in a timely manner after appropriate treatment including OMT. In a novel study, osteopathic physicians in an emergency department reported a case series of 177 patients who were treated in the conventional manner for musculoskeletal pain, including OMT (Lucas et al. 2009). Of these 177 patients, 38 returned to the emergency department within 2 weeks with the same or worse pain. Further evaluation revealed a visceral etiology for their complaint in four of these 38 patients, including pneumonia, ventral hernia, endometriosis with adhesions, and focal lung infection. From the perspective of these emergency department physicians, their rule was to consider the possibility of visceral disease or disorder when treating musculoskeletal complaints, especially if the complaint persisted.

At present there are only a few studies with enough data to suggest support for the concept that specific segments or segmental areas subjected to manual therapy of any kind may affect a systemic disorder. In these cases specific vertebral segments, consistent with the target viscera innervation, appeared to produce measurable effects. There is not enough evidence to support the idea that OMT at a specific vertebral level can affect a disease process. There are also not enough data to establish the mechanism of action of facilitated areas, but the ability to palpate somatic dysfunction may assist osteopathic physicians in evaluating for the presence of a visceral disorder contrasted with a musculoskeletal disorder. However, the idea of a process such as the facilitated area is intriguing and worthy of further consideration as one of the explanations for the mechanism of action for manual therapy. To better understand viscerosomatic interactions and clinical application, more research is needed. However, such research faces significant obstacles, which are discussed next.

The research milieu for osteopathic and manual therapy research

Historically, all of the manual therapy professions have to a greater or lesser degree developed and been sustained by providing the public with a service for which they are willing to pay, regardless of any reimbursement benefit. However, to survive in a medical–scientific world, research to support this form of healthcare is required. To some extent this has been done as reported above. Certain areas of clinical interest, such as musculoskeletal pain, have received attention from all the manual therapy professions represented in this book: chiropractic (Chapter 13), physical therapy (Chapter 14), massage therapy (Chapter 15), and osteopathic medicine (this chapter).

It is outside the scope of this chapter to discuss the 'active ingredients' of manual therapy, whether these be the placing on of hands, the actual manipulation or mobilization, or higher center processes such as perceptions or situational cues. Chapter 12 addresses this issue, as do Chapters 15 and 9.

Despite the decades of public patronage for osteopathic manual therapy services, there has been a significant increase during the last 20 years in demands to demonstrate that manual therapy provides benefit. These demands may in part be related to the increase in the last 20 years of the public's use of complementary and alternative medicines (CAM) (Eisenberg et al. 1993, 1998). Despite the evidence that manual therapies have been a part of contemporary healthcare practices for millennia, as witnessed by depictions of such techniques in ancient Egyptian and Greek art and writing (Porter 1999, Smith 2007), the current medical perspective places manual therapy in the CAM arena, which in some medical–scientific circles has pejorative implications.

The pressure to provide proof of benefit for manual therapy is usually framed in the context of reimbursement by insurance companies, national health programs, and to a lesser extent hospitals, which have to grant a practitioner the privilege of providing manual therapies in their institution. Whether based on legitimate concerns, or possibly reflecting an attempt to deny reimbursement to reduce healthcare costs in general, the manual therapy professions have all mounted research efforts to provide the evidence for proof of concept and clinical efficacy.

Unfortunately, funding for manual therapy research has been quite limited in comparison with conventional medical – especially pharmacologic – research. Up until the last 20 years, manual therapy research has been funded primarily by individual professional institutions and organizations, with only occasional governmental support. This profession-provided support was sufficient to accomplish the body of research that led to the Agency for Health Care Policy and Research (now called the Agency for Healthcare Research and Quality) 1994 practice guidelines (Bigos et al. 1994), which included spinal manipulation for low back pain. Relatively few, generally small, grants for research have been made by the National Institutes of Health (NIH), especially the National Institute for Neurological Disorders and Stroke (NINDS), since the 1960s. For example, some of the research by Denslow and Korr cited in Chapter 1 received NINDS funding.

At present, most manual therapy research in the US is funded by the National Center for Complementary and Alternative Medicine (NCCAM), but it is still relatively a very small amount. To give some perspective, the 2008 NIH budget was US$29.3 billion; of this amount, NCCAM received $122 million (US Department of Health and Human Services 2009). NCCAM funding for research on manual therapy in 2008 was approximately $7.3 million, or 6% of the NCCAM budget for research (Langevin et al. 2009, personal communication with office of NCCAM Office of Communications). The author's estimate is that ongoing research in manual therapy funded by professional institutions and private foundations for 2008 may be half the NCCAM amount (King 2010). To those familiar with the cost of both basic science and clinical research, these are sparse resources to meet the demands for proof of

mechanism of action and benefit. Probable reasons for the generally low levels of funding support include lack of research grant applications of sufficient merit to justify funding; attracting 'talent and interest' to this area of research has been difficult, owing to the perceived low status of such practices by conventional medical practitioners and basic scientists already committed to other areas of research; the low priority of manual therapy research in the light of scientific community perception that genomic and pharmacology research holds a greater likelihood of meeting healthcare needs.

Despite these and other challenges, there has been sufficient research published to begin to outline the potential for the impact of manual therapy on physiologic functions and systemic disorders. As suggested above and in Chapter 1, there have been Cochrane Reviews (Assendelft et al. 2004) and other systematic review and meta-analyses (Cherkin et al. 2003, Licciardone et al. 2005) describing the benefit of manual therapy for low back pain. Most research projects related to the impact of manual therapy on physiological functions and systemic disorders described in this chapter were not sufficiently powered or designed clinical trials that would provide material for systematic review. However, the number and quality of research projects in basic science and the clinical arena in this area merit examination, and demonstrate the potential to answer questions of mechanism of action and clinical efficacy.

Summary

The studies discussed in this chapter, as well as others that were not discussed, lend support to the idea that from the osteopathic perspective manual therapy (OMT) may have an impact on physiological function and systemic disorders through increasingly understood mechanisms of action and health benefits. The discussion on the concepts of facilitated segment(s) and viscerosomatic interactions underlies another overriding osteopathic concept that must be mentioned here: the concept that OMT itself is often not a 'push-button' type of intervention that can have the type of specific outcome that can be often identified by research on pharmaceutical agents. Rather, its impact is to restore the neuromusculoskeletal system to optimal alignment and function, so that normal healing and self-regulatory processes can operate optimally. Stated in another way, OMT is often not the treatment of a specific disease or state, but rather a means of removing impediments to optimal function of the naturally occurring body resources that provide for and maintain health. Despite being stated explicitly in the osteopathic literature, this benefit appears to be presumed in almost all manual therapy theories and applications, and forms the basis for the likely mechanisms of action involving various neurobiological mechanisms, which include neuroanatomical, neurophysiological, neuroendocrine, and humoral processes.

References

Assendelft, W.J., Morton, S.C., Yu, E.I., et al., 2004. Spinal manipulative therapy for low-back pain. Cochrane Database Syst. Rev. (1), CD000447. DOI: 10.1002/14651858.CD000447.pub2.

Bandeen, S.G., 1948. Pancreatic stimulation and blood chemical changes, vol. 48. American Academy of Osteopathy Yearbook, Indianapolis, IN, pp. 78–99.

Bandeen, S.G., 1949. Diabetes: report covering twenty-five years research on stimulation of pancreas, blood changes. Osteopath. Prof. 17, 11–15, 38, 40, 42, 46–47.

Beal, M.C., 1982. Palpatory testing for somatic dysfunction in patients with cardiovascular disease. J. Am. Osteopath. Assoc. 82, 822–831.

Beal, M.C., 1985. Viscerosomatic reflexes: a review. J. Am. Osteopath. Assoc. 85, 786–801.

Beal, M.C., Kleiber, G.E., 1985. Somatic dysfunction as a predictor of coronary artery disease. J. Am. Osteopath. Assoc. 85, 302–307.

Beal, M.C., Morlock, J.W., 1984. Somatic dysfunction associated with pulmonary disease. J. Am. Osteopath. Assoc. 84, 179–183.

Bigos, S.J., Bowyer, O.R., Braen, G.R., et al., 1994. Acute low back problems in adults: assessment and treatment. Clinical practice guideline number 14. Publication no. 95-0643, US Department of Health and Human Services, Public Health Services, Agency for Health Care Policy and Research, Rockville, MD. December, 1994.

BMJ Clinical Evidence Centre, 2009. How much do we know? Online: Available http://clinicalevidence.bmj.com/ceweb/about/knowledge.jsp, 30 Aug, 2009.

Boesler, D., Warner, M., Alpers, A., et al., 1993. Efficacy of high-velocity low amplitude manipulation technique in subjects with low-back pain during menstrual cramping. J. Am. Osteopath. Assoc. 93, 203–214.

Breithaupt, T., Harris, K., Ellis, J., et al., 2001. Thoracic lymphatic pumping and the efficacy of influenza vaccination in healthy young and elderly populations. J. Am. Osteopath. Assoc. 101, 21–25.

Budgell, B., Polus, B., 2006. The effects of thoracic manipulation on heart rate variability: a controlled crossover trial. J. Manipulative Physiol. Ther. 29, 603–610.

Burns, L., 1907. Viscerosomatic and somatovisceral spinal reflexes. J. Am. Osteopath. Assoc. 7, 51–57.

Burns, L., 1928. Qualities distinguishing muscles affected by primary vertebral lesions from those affected by viscerosomatic nerve reflexes. J. Am. Osteopath. Assoc. 27, 542–545.

Burns, L., 1933. Osteopathic case reports of pulmonary disease: a review. J. Am. Osteopath. Assoc. 33, 1–5.

Burns, L., 1944. Principles governing the treatment of cardiac conditions. J. Am. Osteopath. Assoc. 43, 231–234.

Cervero, F., 1985. Visceral nociception: peripheral and central aspects of visceral nociception. Philos. Trans. R. Soc. B 308, 325–337.

Cherkin, D.C., Sherman, K.I., Deyo, R.A., et al., 2003. A review of the evidence for the effectiveness, safety, and the cost of acupuncture, massage therapy, and spinal manipulation for low back pain. Ann. Intern. Med. 138, 898–906.

Crow, W.T., Gorodinsky, L., 2009. Does osteopathic manipulative treatment (OMT) improve outcomes in patients who develop postoperative ileus: a retrospective chart review. Intern. J. Osteopath. Med. 12, 32–36.

Degenhardt, B.F., Kuchera, M.L., 2006. Osteopathic evaluation and manipulative treatment in reducing the morbidity of otitis media: a pilot study. J. Am. Osteopath. Assoc. 106, 327–334.

Eisenberg, D.M., Kessler, R.C., Foster, C., et al., 1993. Unconventional medicine in the United States – prevalence, costs and patterns of use: results of a national survey. N. Engl. J. Med. 328, 246–252.

Eisenberg, D.M., Davis, R.B., Ettner, S.L., et al., 1998. Trends in alternative medicine use in the United States, 1990–1997: results of a follow-up national survey. J. Am. Med. Assoc. 280, 1569–1575.

Frymann, V.M., Carney, R.E., Springall, P., 1992. Effect of osteopathic medical management on neurological development in children. J. Am. Osteopath. Assoc. 92, 729–744.

Gamber, R.G., Shores, J.H., Russo, D.P., et al., 2002. Osteopathic manipulative treatment in conjunction with medication relieves pain associated with fibromyalgia syndrome: results of a randomized clinical pilot project. J. Am. Osteopath. Assoc. 102 (6), 321–326.

Gebhart, G.F., Randich, A., 1992. Vagal modulation of nociception. American Pain Society Journal 1, 26–32.

Geisser, M.E., Wiggert, E.A., Haig, A.J., et al., 2005. A randomized, controlled trial of manual therapy and specific adjuvant exercise for chronic low back pain. Clin. J. Pain 21, 462–470.

Giles, P.D., 2006. Effects of cervical manipulation on autonomic control. Unpublished Master's Thesis University of North Texas Health Science Center, Fort Worth, TX.

Goldstein, F.J., Jeck, S., Nicholas, A.S., et al., 2005. Preoperative intravenous morphine sulfate with postoperative osteopathic manipulative treatment reduces patient analgesic use after total abdominal hysterectomy. J. Am. Osteopath. Assoc. 105, 273–279.

Guthrie, R.A., Martin, R.H., 1982. Effect of pressure applied to the upper thoracic (placebo) versus lumbar areas (osteopathic manipulative treatment) for inhibition of lumbar myalgia during labor. J. Am. Osteopath. Assoc. 82, 247–251.

Gwirtz, P.A., Dickey, J., Vick, D., et al., 2007. Viscerosomatic interaction induced by myocardial ischemia in conscious dogs. J. Appl. Physiol. 103, 511–517.

Hayden, C., Mullinger, B., 2006. A preliminary assessment of the impact of cranial osteopathy for the relief of infantile colic. Complement. Ther. Clin. Pract. 12, 83–90.

Henley, C.E., Ivins, D., Mills, M., et al., 2008. Osteopathic manipulative treatment and its relationship to autonomic nervous system activity as demonstrated by heart rate variability: a repeated measures study. Osteopathic Medicine and Primary Care 2, 7.

Hensel, K.L., 2009. Osteopathic manipulative medicine in pregnancy: acute physiological and biomechanical effects. Unpublished doctoral dissertation. University of North Texas Health Science Center, Fort Worth, TX.

Hix, E.L., 1972. A visceral influence on the cutaneorenal receptive field. J. Am. Osteopath. Assoc. 72, 72–158.

Hix, E.L., 1976. Reflex viscerosomatic reference phenomena. Osteopathic Annals 4, 496–503.

Hodge, L.M., King, H.H., Williams, A.G., et al., 2007. Abdominal lymphatic pump treatment increases leukocyte count and flux in thoracic duct lymph. Lymphat. Res. Biol. 5, 127–132.

Hodge, L.M., Bearden, M.K., Schander, A., et al., 2009. Abdominal lymphatic pump treatment mobilizes leukocytes from the gastrointestinal associated lymphoid tissue into lymph. Lymphatic Research and Biology [in review].

Holtzman, D.A., Petrocco-Napuli, K.L., Burke, J.R., 2008. Prospective case series on the effects of lumbosacral manipulation on dysmenorrhea. J. Manipulative Physiol. Ther. 31, 237–246.

Huard, Y., 2005. Influence of the venous sinus technique on cranial hemodynamics. In King, H.H. (Ed.), Proceedings of international research conference: Osteopathy in Pediatrics at the Osteopathic Center for Children in San Diego, CA 2002. American Academy of Osteopathy, Indianapolis, IN, pp. 32–36.

Jackson, K.M., Steele, T.F., Dugan, E.P., et al., 1998. Effect of lymphatic and splenic pump techniques on the antibody response to hepatitis B vaccine: a pilot study. J. Am. Osteopath. Assoc. 98, 155–160.

Jänig, W., Morrison, J.F.B., 1986. Functional properties of spinal visceral afferents supplying abdominal and pelvic organs, with special emphasis on visceral nociception. Prog. Brain Res. 67, 87–114.

Johnston, W.L., 1988. Segmental definition: part III Definitive basis for distinguishing somatic findings of visceral reflex origin. J. Am. Osteopath. Assoc. 88 (3), 347–353.

Johnston, W.L., 1992. Osteopathic clinical aspects of somatovisceral interaction. In Patterson, M.M., Howell, J.N. (Eds), Central connection: somatovisceral/viscerosomatic interaction. American Academy of Osteopathy, Indianapolis, IN, pp. 30–46.

Johnston, W.L., Kelso, A.F., 1995. Changes in presence of a segmental dysfunction pattern associated with hypertension: part II. A long-term longitudinal study. J. Am. Osteopath. Assoc. 95 (5), 315–318.

Johnston, W.L., Hill, J.L., Sealey, J.W., Sucher, B.M., 1980. Palpatory findings in the cervicothoracic region: variations in normotensive and hypertensive subjects. A preliminary report. J. Am. Osteopath. Assoc. 79 (5), 55–63.

Johnston, W.L., Hill, J.L., Elkiss, M.L., Marino, R.V., 1982. Identification of stable somatic findings in hypertensive subjects by trained examiners using palpatory examination. J. Am. Osteopath. Assoc. 81 (2), 59–66.

Johnston, W.L., Kelso, A.F., Hollandsworth, D.L., Karrat, J.J., 1987. Somatic manifestations in renal disease: a clinical research study. J. Am. Osteopath. Assoc. 87 (1), 61–74.

Khorsan, R., Hawk, C., Lisi, A.J., et al., 2009. Manipulative therapy for pregnancy and related conditions: a systematic review. Obstet. Gynecol. Surv. 64 (6), 416–427.

King, H.H., 2010. Development and support of osteopathic research. In: Chila, A. (Ed.), Foundations for osteopathic medicine, third ed. Lippincott, Williams & Wilkins, Philadelphia (in press).

King, H.H., Tettambel, M.A., Lockwood, M.D., et al., 2003. Osteopathic manipulative treatment in prenatal care: A retrospective case control design study. J. Am. Osteopath. Assoc. 103, 577–582.

Knebl, J.A., Shores, J.H., Gamber, R.G., et al., 2002. Improving functional ability in the elderly via the Spencer technique, an osteopathic manipulative treatment: a randomized, controlled trial. J. Am. Osteopath. Assoc. 102 (7), 387–396.

Knott, E.M., Tune, J.D., Stoll, S.T., et al., 2005. Increased lymphatic flow in the thoracic duct during manipulative intervention. J. Am. Osteopath. Assoc. 105, 447–556.

Langevin, H., Goertz, C., King, H.H., Khalsa, P., Dryden, T., Woodhouse, L.J., 2009. Synergistic research goals for manual treatments of musculoskeletal and soft tissue disorders. Symposium presented at North American Research Conference on Complementary and Integrative Medicine, Minneapolis, MN, May 12–15, 2009.

Lassovetskaia, L., 2005. Applications of the osteopathic approach to school children with delayed psychic development of cerebro-organic origin. In: King, H.H. (Ed.), Proceedings of international research conference: Osteopathy in Pediatrics at the Osteopathic Center for Children in San Diego, CA 2002. American Academy of Osteopathy, Indianapolis, IN, pp. 52–59.

Licciardone, J.C., 2008. Rediscovering the classic osteopathic literature to advance contemporary patient-oriented research: a new look at diabetes mellitus. Osteopathic Medicine and Primary Care 2, 9.

Licciardone, J.C., Brimhall, A., King, L.N., 2005. Osteopathic manipulative treatment for low back pain: a systematic review and meta-analysis of randomized controlled trials. BMC Musculoskelet. Disord. 6, 43–54.

Licciardone, J.C., Fulda, K.G., Stoll, S.T., et al., 2007. A case control study of osteopathic palpatory findings in type 2 diabetes mellitus. Osteopathic Medicine and Primary Care 1, 6.

Licciardone, J.C., Buchanan, S., Hensel, K., et al., 2010. Osteopathic manipulative treatment of back pain and related symptoms during pregnancy: a randomized controlled trial. Am J Obstet Gynecol 202 (43), e1–8.

Lombardini, R., Marchesi, S., Collebrusco, L., et al., 2009. The use of osteopathic treatment as adjuvant therapy in patients with peripheral arterial disease. Man Ther. 14, 439–443.

Lucas, C.A., Bradford, J.C., Kyriakedes, C.G., 2009. Osteopathic manipulation for somatic dysfunction: can visceral dysfunction mimic somatic dysfunction? A case series J. Am. Osteopath. Assoc. (in review).

Mannino, J.R., 1979. The application of neurologic reflexes to the treatment of hypertension. J. Am. Osteopath. Assoc. 79, 225–231.

Measel, J., 1982. The effect of the lymphatic pump on the immune system response: I. Preliminary studies on the antibody response to pneumococcal polysaccharide assayed by bacterial agglutination and passive hemagglutination. J. Am. Osteopath. Assoc. 82, 28–31.

Mesina, J., Hampton, D., Evans, R., et al., 1998. Transient basophilia following the application of lymphatic pump techniques: A pilot study. J. Am. Osteopath. Assoc. 98, 91–94.

Miller, C.E., 1923. The mechanics of lymphatic circulation; lymph hearts. J. Am. Osteopath. Assoc. 22, 397–398, 415–416.

Miller, C.E., 1927. The specific cure of pneumonia. J. Am. Osteopath. Assoc. 27, 35–38.

Mills, M.V., Henley, C.E., Barnes, L.L., et al., 2003. The use of osteopathic manipulative treatment as adjuvant therapy in children with recurrent acute otitis media. Arch. Pediatr. Adolesc. Med. 157, 861–866.

Noll, D.R., 2009. Pneumonia study presented in Washington, DC. Aging Well Newsletter 1 (1), 4.

Noll, D.R., Shores, J.H., Bryman, P.N., et al., 1999. Adjunctive osteopathic manipulative treatment in the elderly hospitalized with pneumonia: a pilot study. J. Am. Osteopath. Assoc. 99, 143–144.

Noll, D.R., Shores, J.H., Gamber, R.G., et al., 2000. Benefits of osteopathic manipulative treatment for hospitalized elderly patients with pneumonia. J. Am. Osteopath. Assoc. 100, 776–782.

Noll, D.R., Degenhardt, B.F., Johnson, J.C., et al., 2008a. Immediate effects of osteopathic manipulative treatment in elderly patients with chronic obstructive pulmonary disease. J. Am. Osteopath. Assoc. 108, 251–259.

Noll, D.R., Degenhardt, B.F., Fossum, C., et al., 2008b. Clinical and research protocol for osteopathic manipulative treatment of elderly patients with pneumonia. J. Am. Osteopath. Assoc. 108, 508–516.

Palmer, R., Patijn, J., 2009. Thoughts regarding evidence based medicine. Fédération Internationale de Médecine Manuelle. Online: Available http://www.fimm-online.com 30 Aug 2009.

Patel, A.T., Ogle, A.A., 2000. Diagnosis and management of acute low back pain. Am. Fam. Physician. Online: Available http://www.aafp.org/online/en/home.html 30 Aug 2009.

Patterson, M.M., Howell, J.N., 1992. The central connection: Somatovisceral/viscerosomatic interaction 1989 International Symposium. American Academy of Osteopathy, Indianapolis, IN.

Paul, R.T., Stomel, R.J., Broniak, F.F., et al., 1986. Interferon levels in human subjects throughout a 24-hour period following thoracic lymphatic pump manipulation. J. Am. Osteopath. Assoc. 86, 92–95.

Peterson, B., (Ed.), 1979. The collected papers of Irvin M. Korr. American Academy of Osteopathy, Indianapolis, IN.

Porter, R., 1999. The greatest benefit to mankind: a medical history of humanity. WW Norton & Co, New York.

Purdy, W.R., Frank, J.J., Oliver, B., 1996. Suboccipital dermatomyotomic stimulation and digital blood flow. J. Am. Osteopath. Assoc. 96, 285–289.

Radjieski, J.M., Lumley, M.A., Cantieri, M.S., 1998. Effect of osteopathic manipulative treatment on length of stay for pancreatitis: a randomized pilot study. J. Am. Osteopath. Assoc. 98, 264–272.

Raviv, G., Shefi, S., Nizani, D., et al., 2009. Effects of craniosacral therapy on lower urinary tract signs and symptoms in multiple sclerosis. Complement. Ther. Clin. Pract. 15 (2), 72–75.

Rivers, W.E., Treffer, K.D., Glaros, A.G., et al., 2008. Short-term hematologic and hemodynamic effects of osteopathic lymphatic techniques: a pilot crossover trial. J. Am. Osteopath. Assoc. 108, 646–651.

Seffinger, M.A., Hruby, R.J., 2007. Evidence-Based Manual Medicine. Saunders Elsevier, Philadelphia.

Sleszynski, S.L., Kelso, A.F., 1993. Comparison of thoracic manipulation with incentive spirometry in preventing postoperative atelectasis. J. Am. Osteopath. Assoc. 93, 834–836.

Smith, A.R., 2007. Manual therapy: the historical, current, and future role in the treatment of pain. Scientific World Journal 7, 109–120.

Smith, R.K., 1920. One hundred thousand cases of influenza with a death rate of one-fortieth of that officially reported under conventional medical treatment. J. Am. Osteopath. Assoc. 20, 172–175.

Sucher, B.M., 1993. Myofascial manipulative release of carpal tunnel syndrome: documentation with magnetic resonance imaging. J. Am. Osteopath. Assoc. 93, 1273–1278.

Sucher, B.M., Hinrichs, R.N., 1998. Manipulative treatment of carpal tunnel syndrome: biomechanical and osteopathic intervention to increase the length of the transverse carpal ligament. J. Am. Osteopath. Assoc. 98, 679–686.

Sucher, B.M., Hinrichs, R.N., Welcher, R.L., et al., 2005. Manipulative treatment of carpal tunnel syndrome: biomechanical and osteopathic intervention to increase the length of the transverse carpal ligament: part 2. Effect of sex differences and manipulative priming. J. Am. Osteopath. Assoc. 105, 135–143.

United States Bone and Joint Decade. 2009. Burden of musculoskeletal diseases in the United States. Online: Available http://www.boneandjointburden. org/ 30 Aug 2009.

US Department of Health & Human Services, National Institutes of Health. 2009. The NIH Almanac-Appropriations, http://www.nih.gov/about/almanac/appropriations/index.htm. Accessed August 22.

Vandenplas, Y., Denayer, E., Vandenbossche, T., et al., 2008. Osteopathy may decrease obstructive apnea in infants: a pilot study. Osteopathic Medicine and Primary Care 2, 8.

Ward, R.C., (Ed.), 2003. Foundations for Osteopathic Medicine, second ed. Lippincott, Williams & Wilkins, Philadelphia.

Yurvati, A.H., Carnes, M.S., Clearfield, M.B., et al., 2005. Hemodynamic effects of osteopathic manipulative treatment immediately after coronary artery bypass graft surgery. J. Am. Osteopath. Assoc. 105, 475–481.

Zhang, J., Dean, D., Nosco, D., et al., 2006. Effect of chiropractic care on heart rate variability and pain in a multisite clinical study. J. Manipulative Physiol. Ther. 29, 267–274.

Chiropractic practice, experience, and research related to somatovisceral interactions

Cheryl Hawk

Introduction

The broadest definition of chiropractic is that it is a healthcare profession providing non-drug, non-surgical treatment of conditions related to the neuromusculoskeletal system. Its approach to care is concerned with the relationship of structure – chiefly the musculoskeletal system – to function, as mediated chiefly through the nervous system (Christensen et al. 2005). The chiropractic healthcare model has traditionally emphasized the body's natural recuperative power through a patient-centered and holistic approach emphasizing the relationship between structure and function, with manual procedures playing a central role.

In fact, chiropractic is often viewed as being synonymous with spinal manipulative therapy (SMT). Certainly SMT has been the cornerstone of the chiropractic approach to care, and 94% of SMT in the US is performed by chiropractors. However, SMT is not used solely by Doctors of Chiropractic (DC): references to its use are found in many cultures, including ancient Greece, where it is recorded that Hippocrates practiced manipulation (Gatterman 2004). Historical references to 'bone setting' show this form of traditional medicine to be learned through observation of functional movement of the human body and passed on through an apprenticeship model (Meeker & Haldeman 2002). Osteopathy and chiropractic arose from this tradition in the late 1800s, along with incorporation of the concept of vitalism – life force – that was current in the late 19th century. The original rationale for chiropractic treatment was that areas of joint dysfunction called *subluxations* caused interference to the nervous system and imbalance of *innate intelligence,* or vital force, and that SMT corrected this imbalance, thus allowing the body's natural recuperative ability to restore normal function and health (Masarsky & Todres-Masarsky 2001).

SMT continues to play a central role in modern chiropractic practice. However, chiropractic is a profession, not a procedure, and chiropractors provide not only SMT, but a number of other conservative therapies, including soft tissue treatment and counseling on physical activity, diet and lifestyle (Meeker & Haldeman 2002). In clinical practice it is impossible to separate the effects of SMT from the other aspects of the clinical encounter, including not only various procedures and counseling, but also difficult-to-measure constructs such as patient and doctor expectations, the therapeutic effect of touch, and psychological effects of positive affect and belief (Cherkin & MacCornack 1989, Coulehan 1985, Coulter 1990, Oths 1994).

Further complicating assessment of the clinical effects of chiropractic care is the broad array of procedures used by different chiropractors, or even by the same chiropractor within a given clinical encounter. US DCs use an average of six different SMT techniques, as well as additional manual soft tissue treatment (Christensen et al. 2005) (Table 13.1).

Table 13.1 Manual procedures most commonly used by US chiropractors*

Procedure	Description	% of US DCs
Manual technique		
Diversified manipulation	High velocity, low amplitude	96
Trigger point therapy (myofascial release)	Soft tissue technique for muscle tension; not SMT[1]	91
Massage therapy	Soft tissue technique; not SMT	85
Mobilization	Low velocity, low amplitude	76
Activator method technique	Instrument-assisted adjusting protocol; small amount of biomechanical force delivered	70
Acupressure	Soft tissue technique for muscle tension; not SMT	58
Flexion–distraction manipulation	Low-velocity mobilization of spine with use of specialized table; no or minimal rotation and extension	57
Sacro-occipital technique	Use of padded wedges to lever spinal segments into position with no direct application of biomechanical forces, rotation, or extension	50
Cranial technique	Low force manual procedure	38
Logan basic technique	Very low-force 'reflex' technique to correct vertebral misalignment/fixation	26
Counseling		
Corrective exercise	Instruction to patient	98
Physical activity	Instruction to patient	98
Rehabilitation exercise	Instruction to patient	88

*Source: Christensen et al. 2005.
[1]SMT, spinal manipulative therapy.

Furthermore, DCs use an average of 12 adjunctive procedures in addition to SMT. These include not only manual procedures such as massage (85%), trigger point therapy (91%) and acupressure (58%), but also nutritional counseling and supplement advice (89%), electrical stimulation (77%), ultrasound (66%), and homeopathy (46%). Most US DCs also report using active procedures such as therapeutic exercise (98%) or rehabilitation exercise (89%) (Christensen et al. 2005).

'Spinal manipulation' refers to the application of biomechanical force to a spinal joint for the purpose of correcting joint dysfunction. In the array of SMT techniques they use, most DCs include techniques with varying amounts and applications of force, as summarized in Table 13.1. A high-velocity, low-amplitude (HVLA) procedure is most commonly used, to the extent that it is often considered to be synonymous with SMT. The biomechanical forces in the spectrum of SMT, for the more commonly used techniques, range approximately from 70 to 890 N (Fuhr 2005, Pickar et al. 2007). SMT may be applied manually or by means of instruments, specially designed tables, or padded wedges.

Chiropractic theory holds that SMT enhances function and promotes the body's self-healing capacity (Hawk 2007). However, to date theoretical constructs have not arisen to address possible differential effects of different modes of application of the biomechanical forces involved in SMT. Such theories might best be developed empirically, through both observational and experimental research. In the past 10 years, basic science investigations have begun to examine such effects (Cramer et al. 2006, Khalsa et al. 2006). Better knowledge of which specific protocols for delivering biomechanical force are most effective would greatly advance patient care. This would be an excellent application of translational research, which 'refers to the "bench-to-bedside" enterprise of harnessing knowledge from basic sciences to produce new treatment options for patients' (Woolf 2008).

However, the 'bench-to-bedside' approach might be enhanced by the addition of the 'bedside-to-bench' direction (Marincola 2003). Manual therapies were not developed by bench research, but, as described above, grew from observation and experience. Lessons learned in the clinical application of manual therapies can inform the direction and focus of bench research, just as discoveries in the laboratory can inform and refine clinical applications.

This chapter will summarize the current clinical literature on chiropractic care for the management of somatovisceral complaints, focusing on the issues particularly relevant to bench research.

Issues affecting interpretation of results

Profession vs procedure

It must be recognized that *chiropractic* is not identical to *SMT*, and that investigations may or may not be limited to examining the effects of SMT alone. For the purposes of assessing treatment effects, one might categorize chiropractic clinical research as investigating either 1) chiropractic management – the 'total package' of the chiropractic clinical encounter, or 2) spinal manipulation only, performed either by chiropractors, osteopaths, physical therapists, or other manual therapists.

Both are important perspectives, but they investigate different factors and combinations of factors, and are likely to yield different outcomes. The findings in many chiropractic clinical research studies and case reports have often been difficult to interpret, or actually misinterpreted, because these two categories have not been recognized.

Applications and treatment effects of biomechanical force are diverse

Biomechanical forces differ not only in the speed, pressure, and angle of application, but also in the exact area, frequency, and duration of application. It is imperative that treatment procedures and protocols, as well as patient characteristics and symptoms, be described in detail, to provide preliminary information on which ones are more effective for specific patient populations, as well as which ones may be associated with adverse events.

Manual therapies affect patients through diverse mechanisms

Manual therapies affect patients through diverse and complex mechanisms, of which the physiological level is only one component. When treating humans, it is difficult to tease out the effects of biomechanical forces from those of touch, belief, expectation, and other largely psychological factors often considered to be 'nonspecific' or 'placebo.' Discounting such effects as extraneous does not advance our knowledge; rather, they should be examined and quantified wherever possible.

It is also important to consider that chiropractic care and/or SMT may have systemic or unexpected beneficial effects as well as the targeted local ones, in keeping with chiropractic theory as well as the limitations of current knowledge (Leboeuf-Yde et al. 2005). Therefore, it is helpful to include global measures of health and, where possible, detailed qualitative information on patient outcomes.

Summary of chiropractic clinical research

Musculoskeletal conditions

Approximately 8% of Americans use chiropractic annually, and well over 90% of their chief complaints involve musculoskeletal pain, usually spine-related back pain, neck pain, and headache (Christensen et al. 2005). Whether as cause or effect of the prevalence of musculoskeletal complaints

in chiropractic practice, the preponderance of chiropractic research relates to these. Most of this large body of research is related to SMT rather than chiropractic care in general. Many SMT studies involved osteopathic or manual medicine practitioners, and sometimes physical therapists, as well as chiropractors. SMT now has a substantial body of evidence for its effectiveness in relieving musculoskeletal complaints, especially spine-related pain (Bronfort et al. 2008, Hurwitz et al. 2008).

Non-musculoskeletal (somatovisceral) conditions

Prevalence in chiropractic practice

Chiropractors do not commonly treat patients for non-musculoskeletal – or as they are often called, somatovisceral – conditions. According to the Job Analysis of Chiropractic, the profession's largest and most authoritative survey on practice characteristics, conducted by the National Board of Chiropractic Examiners, in 1998, 5.3% and in 2003 2.5% of chiropractic patients' chief complaints were non-musculoskeletal. All somatovisceral conditions were reported to be treated 'rarely' except for the following, which were reported to be treated 'sometimes' (on a 5-point scale from 'never' to 'routinely'): allergies, diabetes, hypertension, menstrual problems, sinus problems, and vertigo/dizziness (Christensen et al. 2005).

A 2001 practice-based research study of 7527 chiropractic patients actively recruited DCs who felt they saw higher-than-average numbers of patients with non-musculoskeletal complaints, in order to investigate factors associated with seeking chiropractic for such complaints (Hawk et al. 2001). Table 13.2 details these complaints; similar results in terms of the most commonly reported complaints were found in a 2005 international practice-based research study (Leboeuf-Yde et al. 2005). The 2001 study's results indicated that factors associated

Table 13.2 Non-musculoskeletal chief complaints reported by at least 20 (0.3%) chiropractic patients in a practice-based research study (n=7527) (Hawk et al. 2001)

Musculoskeletal complaints	78.3%
Health maintenance	9.9%
Missing or unclassifiable	1.6%
All non-musculoskeletal	10.2%
Gastrointestinal	1.1%
Upper respiratory complaint	0.9%
Allergies	0.7%
Migraines*	0.6%
Sinus problems	0.6%
Fatigue	0.4%
Cardiovascular/circulatory (including hypertension)	0.4%
Dizziness/vertigo	0.3%
Ear infection	0.3%
Asthma	0.3%
All other non-musculoskeletal†	4.6%
	100.0%

*Migraines were considered non-musculoskeletal since they have vascular and other components. Other types of headaches were classified as musculoskeletal.
†Complaints listed by 15–19 patients (> 0.2%, < 0.3%): ADHD (attention deficit/hyperactivity disorder), lower respiratory infection/COPD (chronic obstructive pulmonary disease), urinary tract infection and sleep disorders.

with seeking chiropractic care for non-musculoskeletal complaints were: age under 14 years; female gender; small town or rural resident; multiple complaints; under concurrent medical care for their complaint; and first experiencing chiropractic care prior to 1960. Factors associated with chiropractic practices with a higher proportion of patients with non-musculoskeletal complaints were: use of more uncommon chiropractic techniques and use of additional non-manual procedures, particularly diet, nutrition and supplement counseling, herbs, naturopathy and homeopathy. They were also less likely to accept insurance.

The key point for the current discussion is that chiropractors seeing a greater proportion of patients with non-musculoskeletal conditions tended to use less common chiropractic manipulative techniques and to use more non-manipulative techniques, such as counseling on diet and supplements. This emphasizes the difficulty of attributing clinical effects to any single portion of the intervention, such as SMT, especially SMT as represented by the most commonly used manipulative techniques.

Clinical research related to the effect of chiropractic care and/or SMT on somatovisceral conditions

A 2007 systematic review of chiropractic care for non-musculoskeletal conditions, covering literature published up until mid-2005, identified 179 articles addressing treatment outcomes of either chiropractic care, which included manual procedures, or other types of care (such as osteopathy) which included spinal manipulation or mobilization (Hawk et al. 2007). The review included randomized controlled trials (RCTs), systematic reviews (SRs), cohort and case–control studies, other controlled studies including pilot and small randomized or nonrandomized studies, quasi-experimental, and pre-experimental case series and case reports.

Conditions addressed in clinical studies

According to the 2007 systematic review, the 179 articles identified addressed a plethora of conditions. Table 13.3 details the types of studies addressing each condition. Fifteen conditions were addressed by at least one designed study; for this purpose, 'designed study' refers to not only randomized controlled trials (RCTs) but also to cohort studies, quasi-experimental (non-randomized) studies, pre-experimental, pilot studies, and other small experimental or pre-experimental designs. Over 30 different conditions were

Table 13.3 Articles addressing outcomes of chiropractic care and/or spinal manipulation for patients with non-musculoskeletal conditions, by condition and type of article*

Condition addressed	Systematic review	Designed study[1]	Case series/case report	Total
Total	9	48	122	179
Vision		1	17	18
Asthma	1	8	5	14
Hypertension		8	4	12
Vertigo	1	4	6	11
Dysmenorrhea/PMS	2	6	2	10
Infantile colic	1	3	4	8
Otitis media		2	6	8
ADHD/learning disabilities		1	5	6
Chronic pelvic pain		2	4	6
Dysfunctional nursing		1	5	6
Nocturnal enuresis	1	2	2	5
Phobia		1		1
Crohn's		1		1
Jet lag		1		1
Ulcer		1		1
Multiple conditions[2]	3	2	11	
All other conditions[3]			51	51

*Source: (Hawk et al. 2007). This systematic review included literature to May 2005, including both chiropractic and osteopathic studies of spinal manipulation.
[1]This category includes randomized controlled trials, pilot studies, quasi-experimental (non-randomized) designs, single-group interventions and other small experimental or pre-experimental designs.
[2]Conditions addressed in these systematic reviews were: asthma, chronic pelvic pain, dysmenorrhea, infantile colic, otitis media and phobia.
[3]Conditions for which there were case reports or case series only, with no other types of study addressing treatment outcomes: two case reports:

Anxiety	Diabetes	Parkinson's
Aphasia	Diabetic polyneuropathy	Psoriasis
Arrhythmia	Down's syndrome	Rett syndrome
Autism	Dysphonia	Seizures
Bowel/bladder dysfunction	Eczema	Sleep disorder
Cancer pain	Encopresis	Tinnitus
Cerebral palsy	Erb's palsy	Tourette's syndrome
Chronic obstructive pulmonary disease	Hearing loss	Upper respiratory infection
Constipation	Infertility/amenorrhea	Urinary tract infection
Cystic hygroma	Multiple sclerosis	Vertebrobasilar ischemia

addressed by case series or case reports only. In general, case reports far outweighed designed studies, with 122 case series/reports, 48 designed studies, and nine systematic reviews. This situation illustrates the difficulty of making inferences about causation.

Treatment effects of chiropractic care with spinal manipulation

The 2007 systematic review of chiropractic care for non-musculoskeletal conditions took a whole systems research approach, rather than looking at the effects of SMT divorced from the entire clinical encounter. 'Whole systems research' is a burgeoning approach to complementary and alternative medicine (CAM) which emphasizes that, especially in CAM practice, the whole (of the clinical encounter) may be greater than the sum of its parts (individual procedures). Thus conducting research on a procedure isolated from the complexities of the doctor–patient interaction may not actually represent the reality (Institute of Medicine 2005, Verhoef et al. 2005). The systematic review summarized the evidence related to chiropractic care for patients with non-musculoskeletal conditions from this perspective as follows:

1. *The adverse effects reported for SMT for all age groups and conditions were rare and, when they did occur, transient and not severe.*
2. *Evidence from both controlled studies and usual practice is adequate to support the 'total package' of chiropractic care, including SMT, other procedures, and unmeasured qualities such as belief and attention, as providing benefit to patients with asthma, cervicogenic vertigo, and infantile colic.*
3. *Evidence was promising for the potential benefit of manual procedures for children with otitis media and for hospitalized elderly patients with pneumonia.*
4. *Evidence did not appear to support chiropractic care for the broad population of patients with hypertension, although it did not rule out the possibility that there may be subpopulations of hypertensive patients who might benefit.*
5. *Evidence was equivocal regarding chiropractic care for dysmenorrhea and PMS; it is not clear as to the level of biomechanical force most appropriate for patients with these related conditions. It does appear that an extended duration of care – over at least three menstrual cycles – is more likely to be beneficial.*
6. *There is insufficient evidence to make conclusions about chiropractic care for patients with other conditions (Hawk et al. 2007, p. 506).*

The focus of this book is on manual procedures, especially the physiologic mechanisms through which such procedures may affect somatovisceral conditions. As demonstrated by the small number of controlled experimental studies published to date in this area, it is difficult to draw conclusions about such effects from the literature. However, clinical studies can pose interesting questions to help guide bench research (that is, 'bedside to bench'), if viewed with such a task in mind.

In order to attempt to assess outcomes to manipulative procedures, and exclude as much as possible the complexity of factors also present in the clinical encounter, it is most useful to consider clinical studies which include a comparison group to at least partially isolate the effects attributable to SMT. Tables 13.4–13.9 detail the conditions addressed in at least one study employing a comparison group, which provides some measure of control for these complex factors.

Asthma

Table 13.4 summarizes the studies with comparison groups investigating the effect

Table 13.4 Comparison-group studies investigating spinal manipulation for treatment of patients with asthma

Citation	Study design	Sample size	Experimental intervention*	Comparison group intervention	Study endpoint(s)	Physiological outcomes	Patient-reported outcomes
(Guiney et al. 2005)	RCT	140	OMT including mobilization of ribs and myofascial release	Light contact on areas of spine, without OMT	Immediately post-intervention	PEF mean improvement 13 L in OMT group, 0.3 in comparison group	
(Bockenhauer et al. 2002)	Cross-over	10	OMT, including mobilization of ribs	Sham (pressure to paraspinal area and range-of-motion of arms)	Immediately post-intervention	PEF mean improvement 14 L in OMT, 2.5 L in sham	Subjective improvement in both, but greater with OMT
(Bronfort et al. 2001)	Pilot RCT	36	CMT HVLA	Sham (manual pressure on contact point on spine with no thrust)	12 wks	Groups not compared. No changes in lung function, including PEF	Active group: QOL and severity substantially improved
(Balon J 1998)	RCT	80	CMT full spine HVLA and soft tissue massage	Simulated CMT (low amplitude, low-velocity contact) and soft tissue massage	8 and 16 wks	PEF improved 7–12 L in both groups; no significant difference between groups	B-agonist medication use and QOL improved in both groups
(Nielsen et al. 1995)	Crossover	31	CMT (full spine) drop-assisted HVLA	Sham drop-assisted manual pressure	4 wks	PEF and other lung function measures unchanged except for improvement of bronchial hyperreactivity, in both groups	Symptom severity improved in both groups

*CMT, chiropractic spinal manipulative therapy; OMT, osteopathic manipulative therapy; HVLA, high-velocity, low-amplitude manipulation procedure; PEF, peak expiratory flow; QOL, quality of life.

of spinal manipulation on asthma. These included both chiropractic and osteopathic manipulation. Although the studies varied a good deal in terms of quality, outcome measures, design, and sample size, it is still possible to formulate some research questions based on their findings. In all these studies a common physiological outcome measure, peak expiratory flow (PEF), was used. In three of the five studies, PEF improved in the groups receiving SMT; in one study (chiropractic) it improved by 7–12 L (Balon et al. 1998), and in the other two (both osteopathic) by 13 L (Guiney et al. 2005) and 14 L (Bockenhauer et al. 2002). In the three chiropractic studies the experimental groups received HVLA SMT, whereas in the osteopathic studies the experimental groups received OMT involving mobilization of the ribs, with no HVLA. The comparison groups in four of the five studies (Bockenhauer et al. 2002, Bronfort et al. 2001, Guiney et al. 2005, Nielsen et al. 1995) used light contact on or near the spine. The Balon study (Balon et al. 1998) used low-amplitude, low-velocity 'sham' manipulation with additional soft tissue massage as a comparison treatment, to control for the HVLA SMT. In two of three studies using HVLA SMT, physiological outcomes did not improve. In the one study in which they did improve, soft tissue massage was used in both groups, and the PEF improved in both groups, with no significant difference between groups. In all the studies measuring patient-reported outcomes such as quality of life or medication use, these outcomes improved in both groups.

From these somewhat complex results, it might be inferred that manual procedures that reduce tension in the intercostal muscles of the ribs, as well as the trapezius and other muscles in the shoulders and neck which are accessory muscles of respiration, may contribute to better physiological function in asthmatics. HVLA of the cervical spine alone did not appear to exhibit a significant physiological effect.

Hypertension

In most of the studies investigating SMT for hypertension, manual procedures were applied to the cervical and thoracic areas (Table 13.5). The Goertz RCT (Goertz et al. 2002) was a pragmatic trial which was highly generalizable, especially as it used the most commonly employed SMT procedure, diversified technique (which uses HVLA force). It did not show a clinically important effect on blood pressure. The treating chiropractors used usual and customary procedures, including not only full-spine SMT but also modalities such as heat, ultrasound, and soft tissue massage. Another chiropractic study (Yates et al. 1988) used instrument-assisted SMT, which usually involves somewhat less biomechanical force than manual SMT – perhaps less than half as much, depending on the practitioner and other factors (Fuhr 2005).

Of the six studies with comparison groups, three showed significant improvements in blood pressure; for two of these, the assessment demonstrating improvement was done immediately following the intervention, and so conclusions about longer-term clinical improvement cannot be made (Fichera & Celander 1969, Yates et al. 1988). The 2007 Bakris study (Bakris et al. 2007) stands out from the others both in its results, in which the mean differences in BP between groups were large, and in its intervention, which used a very low-force chiropractic upper cervical manipulation technique (NUCCA, National Upper Cervical Chiropractic Association).

Although the other studies tend to support a conclusion that SMT is very likely not effective in normalizing BP, for the general population of hypertensives the Bakris study, although a pilot, demonstrated clinically important effects. This would suggest that the area of application (upper cervical, just under the occiput) and the type of biomechanical force (very low force applied in a vector determined by the doctor's analysis of the individual patient's needs)

Table 13.5 Comparison-group studies investigating spinal manipulation for treatment of patients with hypertension

Citation	Study design	Sample size	Experimental intervention	Comparison group intervention	Study endpoint(s)	Physiological outcomes	Patient-reported outcomes
(Bakris et al. 2007)	Pilot RCT	50	CMT very low force C1 (NUCCA)	Sham CMT (misplaced contact point to avoid realignment of C1)	8 wks	mean between-groups difference in decrease in systolic BP, 14.0 mm; diastolic 8.4 mm	
(Goertz et al. 2002)	RCT	140	CMT HVLA, physical modalities and diet intervention by DC	Diet intervention by dietician	4 wks	No significant difference between groups; small decreases in BP in both	
(Yates et al. 1988)	RCT (3 groups)	21	Instrument-assisted CMT to thoracic spine	Sham group (instrument set on zero) and no-treatment group	Immediately post-intervention	Significant decrease, systolic and diastolic BP immediately post-treatment in treatment group compared to sham and control	Anxiety* significantly decreased in both groups, no significant between-groups difference
(Wagnon et al. 1988)	Cross-over	18 high-aldosterone hypertensive	CMT HVLA of C2, T9, L5	No treatment	1 and 4 wks	Significant drop in serum aldosterone after HVLA; no significant change in BP	
(Morgan et al. 1985)	Cross-over	29	OMT mobilization of C1/occiput; T1–5 and T11–L1	Soft tissue massage (by DO)	6 wks	No significant change in either group	
(Fichera & Celander 1969)	Non-equivalent comparison group	57	Soft tissue OMT to C and T paraspinal musculature to hypertensive group (22)	Same intervention to normal BP group (35)	Immediately post-intervention	Greater decrease in BP in hypertensive group	

*Anxiety measured by State-Trait Anxiety Inventory (STAI).
CMT, spinal manipulative therapy delivered by chiropractor; OMT, osteopathic manipulative therapy; HVLA, high-velocity, low-amplitude; FS, full spine; C, cervical vertebrae; T, thoracic vertebrae; L, lumbar vertebrae; BP, blood pressure; US, unspecified.

are important considerations for investigating manual therapies for hypertension.

Vertigo

A 2003 systematic review of cervicogenic vertigo – defined as vertigo induced by changes in position of the neck, or vertigo caused by dysfunction of the movement of the cervical vertebrae – found that there is level 3 (limited) evidence to support the effectiveness of manual therapy (Reid & Rivett 2005). As shown in Table 13.6, three of the four studies with comparison groups used SMT to the cervical spine (Galm et al. 1998, Heikkila et al. 2000, Rogers 1997), while the fourth used cervical mobilization and other physical therapy procedures (Karlberg et al. 1996).

All patients receiving SMT and/or mobilization of the cervical spine improved more than the comparison groups in terms of dizziness. Two comparison group studies (Heikkila et al. 2000, Rogers 1997) and an observational non-treatment study (Grod & Diakow 2002) assessed cervical kinesthesia by measuring head repositioning. Rogers found that it improved more with SMT, and Heikkila found that both SMT and acupuncture improved cervical repositioning. Grod's study found that individuals with neck pain demonstrated a significantly greater error in their perception of verticality than those without neck pain. Karlberg found that patients with postural sway improved more with mobilization and physical therapy than did a no-treatment waiting list group.

These studies suggest the mechanism of cervicogenic vertigo may be disturbed cervical proprioception, thus making a link to the possible effect of SMT on cervicogenic vertigo (Karlberg et al. 1996).

Dysmenorrhea

The comparison procedure in all four identified studies (Table 13.7) was a sham manipulation which differed in the location where it was applied and in the amount of biomechanical force (Hondras et al. 1999, Kokjohn et al. 1992, Snyder & Sanders 1996, Thomason 1979). Two of the studies (Hondras et al. 1999, Kokjohn et al. 1992) measured primary outcomes immediately (1 hour) post intervention; however, the Hondras study also followed the study patients over time, where there appeared to be a trend toward improvement in symptoms that was not detected when considering immediate post-intervention change only. The other two studies (Snyder & Sanders 1996, Thomason 1979) measured outcomes after at least three menstrual cycles (12–16 weeks).

It appears that patients in these studies who were treated with some type of manual procedure, regardless of the amount of biomechanical force – even the lesser amount of force in some of the sham treatments – reported improvement in their symptoms. Also, results suggest that it is important to follow patients with this disorder over the course of several cycles, to explore the possibility of a normalizing effect of the intervention over time.

The two studies measuring prostaglandin levels, on the theory that these were linked to dysmenorrhea symptoms, did not show results consistent with such a hypothesis. Thus, this measurement does not appear to be the most appropriate for the assessment of physiological effects. The conclusion of a Cochrane Systematic Review (Proctor et al. 2004) was that SMT did not demonstrate greater effectiveness than sham SMT, but that it was possibly more effective than no treatment.

Infantile colic

The comparison group studies (Table 13.8) as well as single group studies and case reports reported using low-force modifications of SMT for infants. Viewing the comparison group studies (Olafsdottir et al. 2001, Wiberg et al. 1999), it appears that touch and attention, especially when given by a provider who is confident and comfortable with infants, may well be factors contributing to decreased crying time in infants with colic. As stated in a systematic review

Table 13.6 Comparison-group studies investigating spinal manipulation for treatment of patients with vertigo

Citation	Study design	Sample size	Experimental intervention*	Comparison group intervention	Study endpoint(s)	Physiological outcomes	Patient-reported outcomes
(Heikkila et al. 2000)	Single-subject	14	SMT (by naprapath), acupuncture, NSAID-percutaneous	No treatment	1–2 wks per treatment with 2 wk washout	Head repositioning (kinesthetic sense) improved most with SMT and acupuncture	Dizziness VAS improved most in SMT
(Galm et al. 1998)	Non-equivalent group, pre-test/post-test	50 with dizziness	31 patients with C spine dysfunction, HVLA SMT, mobilization and PT	19 without cervical spine dysfunction, PT	12 wks		Dizziness improved in 94% SMT group; 26% PT only group
(Rogers 1997)	Nonrandomized, matched pilot study	20 with NP (age NS)	HVLA CMT to C and T spine	Stretching exercises	3–4 wks	Head repositioning improved more in CMT group	Dizziness improved more in CMT group
(Karlberg et al. 1996)	RCT	17 (all with NP and dizziness)	Soft tissue treatment; mobilization, relaxation techniques, home exercise, ergonomics)	Waiting list	5–20 wks	Trend toward less postural sway in treatment group (using dynamic posturography)	Dizziness frequency and intensity significantly reduced in treatment group compared to control

*SMT, spinal manipulative therapy delivered by chiropractor unless otherwise specified; HVLA, high-velocity, low-amplitude; FS, full spine; C, cervical vertebrae; T, thoracic vertebrae; BPPV, benign paroxysmal positional vertigo; NP, neck pain.

Table 13.7 Comparison-group studies investigating spinal manipulation for patients with dysmenorrhea

Citation	Study design	Sample size	Experimental intervention	Comparison group intervention	Study endpoint(s)	Physiological outcomes	Patient-reported outcomes
(Hondras et al. 1999)	RCT	138	CMT HVLA (>750N force to thoracolumbar spine and sacroiliac) primary outcomes 1 hour post-treatment	Low-force lumbar mimic maneuver (< 400 N force)	Immediately post-treatment, over 3 menstrual cycles	Prostaglandin decreased, both groups over time. No significant between-groups difference	Immediate decrease in VAS was not clinically meaningful and difference between groups NS; over time VAS and MDQ decreased in both groups
(Snyder & Sanders 1996)	Randomized comparison study	26	CMT low force (toftness technique, 2–32 oz mechanical force)	Sham procedure delivered to paraspinal area	12 wks with additional 12 wks followup		Treatment group only improved on MDQ; no between-groups comparisons
(Kokjohn et al. 1992)	Pilot study	45	CMT HVLA	Sham maneuver with HVLA delivered in position to minimize mechanical effect	Immediately post-treatment	Large decrease in prostaglandin in both groups	VAS decreased more in CMT group, but difference was not clinically important
(Thomason 1979)	Pilot study	11	CMT HVLA (8)	Sham with instrument (1) and no treatment (2)	12–16 wks		SMT group, symptoms improved

SMT, spinal manipulative therapy delivered by chiropractor unless otherwise specified; HVLA, high-velocity, low-amplitude; FS, full spine; C, cervical vertebrae; T, thoracic vertebrae.

Table 13.8 Comparison-group studies investigating spinal manipulation for infants with colic

Citation	Study design	Sample size	Experimental intervention	Comparison group intervention	Study endpoint(s)	Physiological effects	Patient-reported outcomes
(Olafsdottir et al. 2001)	RCT	86	CMT and mobilization	Being held by nurse	1 wk		Parent-reported improvement in crying time in both groups
(Wiberg et al. 1999)	RCT	50	CMT (specific light pressure with fingertips) and counseling	Inactive medication and counseling	2 wks		Colic diaries interpreted by blinded observer; no dropouts SMT group; 9 in control group. Parent-reported improvement in crying time in both groups, significantly greater in CMT group

CMT, spinal manipulative therapy delivered by chiropractor; HVLA, high-velocity, low-amplitude.

of this topic: 'The evidence suggests that chiropractic has no benefit over placebo in the treatment of infantile colic. However, there is good evidence that taking a colicky infant to a chiropractor will result in fewer hours of colic reported by the parents' (Hughes & Bolton 2002).

Nocturnal enuresis

Only two chiropractic studies, both using HVLA SMT, have investigated this topic (Table 13.9). A small RCT comparing HVLA SMT to a low-force sham delivered via instrument found patient-reported wet nights to be decreased in the SMT group (Reed et al. 1994). The other, larger study (Leboeuf et al. 1991) compared SMT to a no-treatment waiting-list group. Employing a more sophisticated statistical analysis with its larger sample size, it found no treatment effect for SMT after adjusting for baseline wet nights. A systematic review judged the evidence insufficient but promising (Glazener et al. 2005).

Bedside to bench: summary of issues related to basic science research

Several interesting basic science research questions, both general and condition specific, emerge from this analysis of the clinical research related to chiropractic care for patients with somatovisceral conditions. As introduced earlier in this chapter, the following issues must be kept in mind when considering physiological effects related to chiropractic care and the procedures associated with it:

- The profession of chiropractic is distinct from, and includes much more than, the procedure of spinal manipulation.
- Applications and treatment effects of biomechanical force are diverse.
- Manual therapies affect patients through varied and complex mechanisms, of which the physiological level is only one component.

What are the differential effects of different protocols of SMT?

This is a large topic, as a protocol would necessarily specify 1) mode of administration of SMT; 2) frequency with which it is applied; and 3) duration of treatments over time. Although a great deal is known about the biomechanics of manipulation (Triano 2005), there is still much more to be learned about how the application of biomechanical force may affect somatovisceral conditions. It is interesting that in the hypertension studies discussed in this chapter, different results were observed when traditional HVLA full-spine SMT was used than when a very low-force upper cervical procedure was used. Although the results were of course not definitive, they are thought-provoking.

Does SMT have a normalizing effect on abnormal physiological functions?

That is, should research be designed around an analgesic model or, for lack of a better term, a homeostatic model? The dysmenorrhea studies suggest that it may be productive to look at outcomes over time, suggesting a gradual 'balancing' of hormonal or other factors that might be contributing to dysmenorrhea, since changes were more apparent over time, rather than an hour post intervention – which would have suggested more of an analgesic effect. Of course, it is possible that both models could coexist, but testing them would require distinct research experiments.

Is there a threshold of biomechanical force below which the effect of SMT is negligible or nonspecific?

Is there such a thing as a 'sham' manipulative procedure? This issue continues to complicate chiropractic clinical research, as a 'sham' intervention which produces

Table 13.9 Comparison-group studies investigating spinal manipulation for children with nocturnal enuresis

Citation	Study design	Sample size	Experimental intervention	Comparison group intervention	Study endpoint(s)	Physiological outcomes	Patient-reported outcomes
(Reed et al. 1994)	RCT	46	CMT HVLA full spine delivered by chiropractic students	Sham (impulse instrument set on zero) delivered by chiropractic students	2 wks		Patient-reported wet nights not significantly different between groups; significantly improved within treatment group but not within control group
(Leboeuf et al. 1991)	Prospective outcome study	171	CMT, both groups; maximum of 8 treatments, all delivered by chiropractic students	One served as waiting-list group with treatment delayed for 2 weeks	Variable		After adjusting for baseline wet nights, no significant effect of treatment found with logistic regression

CMT, chiropractic spinal manipulative therapy; HVLA, high-velocity, low-amplitude.

a treatment effect is not actually a sham (Hawk et al. 2005). This results in misclassification and spuriously negative results.

A related issue is the use of active treatments such as massage or trigger point therapy as part of a control group treatment, as was done in Balon's asthma study (Balon et al. 1998). This appears to have contributed to improvement in both groups, but because the between-groups difference was non-significant, the trial was considered negative for chiropractic. However, most chiropractors and osteopaths use soft tissue techniques, and osteopathic studies such as Guiney's used soft tissue mobilization of the ribs and found significant improvements in PEF (Guiney et al. 2005). The sham SMT itself may well have been inactive, but because it was combined with an active soft tissue procedure it is difficult to tease out the difference.

Because even a Cochrane Review has found that touch therapies, which use very light touch, may have a modest pain-relieving effect (So et al. 2008), this research question might better be restated to ask: 'What are the physiological effects of different levels of biomechanical force?'

What are the physiological mechanisms of 'contextual healing'?

We have already noted that it is difficult, in clinical research, to measure independent aspects of the clinical encounter, and that in fact the whole may be greater than the sum of its parts. That is, the effects of a single aspect, such as SMT, of the chiropractic clinical encounter may not appear significant when isolated from the entire doctor–patient interaction, but when taken as a whole, the patient may show significant improvement.

Kaptchuk calls healing resulting from the entire clinical encounter 'contextual healing' (Miller & Kaptchuk 2008). Clinical research can be designed to measure these outcomes. For example, it appears that contextual healing was probably an important factor in

studies of chiropractic care for infants with colic (Olafsdottir et al. 2001, Wiberg et al. 1999). Basic sciences studies investigating the neurophysiological and other systemic mechanisms involved in contextual healing could greatly add to the knowledge base of all manual, as well as other complementary, therapies, as they tend to provide care that involves not only a number of manual procedures but also other factors such as belief and expectation.

References

Bakris, G., Dickholtz Sr., M., Meyer, P.M., et al., 2007. Atlas vertebra realignment and achievement of arterial pressure goal in hypertensive patients: a pilot study. J. Hum. Hypertens. 21, 347–352.

Balon, J., Aker, P.D., Crowther, E.R., et al., 1998. A comparison of active and simulated chiropractic manipulation as adjunctive treatment for childhood asthma. N. Engl. J. Med. 339, 1013–1020.

Bockenhauer, S.E., Julliard, K.N., Lo, K.S., Huang, E., Sheth, A.M., 2002. Quantifiable effects of osteopathic manipulative techniques on patients with chronic asthma. J. Am. Osteopath. Assoc. 102, 371–375; discussion 375.

Bronfort, G., Evans, R.L., Kubic, P., Filkin, P., 2001. Chronic pediatric asthma and chiropractic spinal manipulation: a prospective clinical series and randomized clinical pilot study. J. Manipulative Physiol. Ther. 24, 369–377.

Bronfort, G., Haas, M., Evans, R., Kawchuk, G., Dagenais, S., 2008. Evidence-informed management of chronic low back pain with spinal manipulation and mobilization. Spine J. 8, 213–225.

Cherkin, D.C., MacCornack, F.A., 1989. Patient evaluations of low back pain care from family physicians and chiropractors. West. J. Med. 150, 351–355.

Christensen, M., Kollasch, M., Ward, R., Webb, K., Day, A., ZumBrunnen, J., 2005. Job Analysis of Chiropractic. NBCE, Greeley, CO.

Coulehan, J.L., 1985. Chiropractic and the clinical art. Soc. Sci. Med. 21, 383–390.

Coulter, I.D., 1990. The chiropractic paradigm. J. Manipulative Physiol. Ther. 13, 279–287.

Cramer, G., Budgell, B., Henderson, C., Khalsa, P., Pickar, J., 2006. Basic science research related to chiropractic spinal adjusting: the state of the art and recommendations revisited. J. Manipulative Physiol. Ther. 29, 726–761.

Fichera, A.P., Celander, D.R., 1969. Effect of osteopathic manipulative therapy on autonomic tone as evidenced by blood pressure changes and activity of the fibrinolytic system. J. Am. Osteopath. Assoc. 68, 1036–1038.

Fuhr, A.W., 2005. Low-force and instrument technique. In: Haldeman, S. (Ed.), Principles and Practice of Chiropractic. McGraw-Hill, York, PA, pp. 787–804.

Galm, R., Rittmeister, M., Schmitt, E., 1998. Vertigo in patients with cervical spine dysfunction. Eur. Spine J. 7, 55–58.

Gatterman, M.I., 2004. Chiropractic Management of Spine Related Disorders, second ed. Lippincott Williams & Wilkins, Baltimore, MD.

Glazener, C.M., Evans, J.H., Cheuk, D.K., 2005. Complementary and miscellaneous intervention for nocturnal enuresis in children. Cochrane Database Syst. Rev. 2.

Goertz, C.H., Grimm, R.H., Svendsen, K., Grandits, G., 2002. Treatment of Hypertension with Alternative Therapies (THAT) Study: a randomized clinical trial. J. Hypertens. 20, 2063–2068.

Grod, J., Diakow, P., 2002. Effect of neck pain on verticality perception: a cohort study. Arch. Phys. Med. Rehabil. 83, 412–415.

Guiney, P.A., Chou, R., Vianna, A., Lovenheim, J., 2005. Effects of osteopathic manipulative treatment on pediatric patients with asthma: a randomized controlled trial. J. Am. Osteopath. Assoc. 105, 7–12.

Hawk, C., 2007. Are we asking the right questions? Chiropractic Journal of Australia 37, 15–18.

Hawk, C., Long, C.R., Boulanger, K.T., 2001. Prevalence of nonmusculoskeletal complaints in chiropractic practice: report from a practice-based research program. J. Manipulative Physiol. Ther. 24, 157–169.

Hawk, C., Long, C.R., Rowell, R.M., Gudavalli, M.R., Jedlicka, J., 2005. A randomized trial investigating a chiropractic manual placebo: a novel design using standardized forces in the delivery of active and control treatments. J. Altern. Complement. Med. 11, 109–117.

Hawk, C., Khorsan, R., Lisi, A.J., Ferrance, R.J., Evans, M.W., 2007. Chiropractic care for nonmusculoskeletal conditions: a systematic review with implications for whole systems research. J. Altern. Complement. Med. 13, 491–512.

Heikkila, H., Johansson, M., Wenngren, B.I., 2000. Effects of acupuncture, cervical manipulation and NSAID therapy on dizziness and impaired head repositioning of suspected cervical origin: a pilot study. Man. Ther. 5, 151–157.

Hondras, M.A., Long, C.R., Brennan, P.C., 1999. Spinal manipulative therapy versus a low force mimic maneuver for women with primary dysmenorrhea: a randomized, observer-blinded, clinical trial. Pain 81, 105–114.

Hughes, S., Bolton, J., 2002. Is chiropractic an effective treatment in infantile colic? Archives of Diseases of Children 86, 382–384.

Hurwitz, E.L., Carragee, E.J., van der Velde, G., et al., 2008. Treatment of neck pain: noninvasive interventions. Spine 33, S123–S152.

Institute of Medicine. 2005. Complementary and Alternative Medicine in the United States. In: National Academies Press.

Karlberg, M., Magnusson, M., Malmstrom, E.M., Melander, A., Moritz, U., 1996. Postural and symptomatic improvement after physiotherapy in patients with dizziness of suspected cervical origin. Archives of Physical Medicine and Rehabilitation 77, 874–882.

Khalsa, P.S., Eberhart, A., Cotler, A., Nahin, R., 2006. The 2005 conference on the biology of manual therapies. J. Manipulative Physiol. Ther. 29, 341–346.

Kokjohn, K., Schmid, D.M., Triano, J.J., Brennan, P.C., 1992. The effect of spinal manipulation on pain and prostaglandin levels in women with primary dysmenorrhea. J. Manipulative Physiol. Ther. 15, 279–285.

Leboeuf, C., Brown, P., Herman, A., Leembruggen, K., Walton, D., Crisp, T.C., 1991. Chiropractic care of children with nocturnal enuresis: a prospective outcome study. J. Manipulative Physiol. Ther. 14, 110–115.

Leboeuf-Yde, C., Pedersen, E.N., Bryner, P., et al., 2005. Self-reported nonmusculoskeletal responses to chiropractic intervention: a multination survey. J. Manipulative. Physiol. Ther. 28, 294–302; discussion 365–366.

Marincola, F.M., 2003. Translational medicine: A two-way road. Journal of Translational Medicine 1, 1.

Masarsky, C.S., Todres-Masarsky, M., 2001. Somatovisceral Aspects of Chiropractic: An Evidence-Based Approach. Churchill Livingstone, Philadelphia, PA.

Meeker, W.C., Haldeman, S., 2002. Chiropractic: a profession at the crossroads of mainstream and alternative medicine. Ann. Intern. Med. 136, 216–227.

Miller, F.G., Kaptchuk, T.J., 2008. The power of context: reconceptualizing the placebo effect. J. R. Soc. Med. 101, 222–225.

Morgan, J.P., Dickey, J.L., Hunt, H.H., Hudgins, P.M., 1985. A controlled trial of spinal manipulation in the management of hypertension. J. Am. Osteopath. Assoc. 85, 308–313.

Nielsen, N.H., Bronfort, G., Bendix, T., Madsen, F., Weeke, B., 1995. Chronic asthma and chiropractic spinal manipulation: a randomized clinical trial. Clin. Exp. Allergy 25, 80–88.

Olafsdottir, E., Forshei, S., Fluge, G., Markestad, T., 2001. Randomised controlled trial of infantile colic treated with chiropractic spinal manipulation. Archives of Diseases of Children 84, 138–141.

Oths, K., 1994. Communication in a chiropractic clinic: how a D.C. treats his patients. Cult. Med. Psychiatry 18, 83–113.

Pickar, J.G., Sung, P.S., Kang, Y.M., Ge, W., 2007. Response of lumbar paraspinal muscles spindles is greater to spinal manipulative loading compared with slower loading under length control. Spine J. 7, 583–595.

Proctor, M., Hing, W., Johnson, T., Murphy, P., 2004. Cochrane Menstrual Disorders and Subfertility Group/Spinal manipulation for primary and secondary dysmenorrhoea. Cochrane Database Syst. Rev. 3.

Reed, W.R., Beavers, S., Reddy, S.K., Kern, G., 1994. Chiropractic management of primary nocturnal enuresis. J. Manipulative Physiol. Ther. 17, 596–600.

Reid, S.A., Rivett, D.A., 2005. Manual therapy treatment of cervicogenic dizziness: a systematic review. Manual Therapeutics 10, 4–13.

Rogers, R., 1997. The effects of spinal manipulation on cervical kinesthesia in patients with chronic neck pain: a pilot study. J. Manipulative Physiol. Ther. 20, 80–85.

Snyder, B.J., Sanders, G.E., 1996. Evaluation of the Toftness system of chiropractic adjusting for subjects with chronic back pain, chronic tension headaches, or primary dysmenorrheal. Chiropractic Technique 8, 3–9.

So, P.S., Jiang, Y., Qin, Y., 2008. Touch therapies for pain relief in adults. Cochrane Database Syst. Rev. CD006535.

Thomason, P., Fisher, B.L., Carpenter, P.A., Fike, G.L., 1979. Effectiveness of spinal manipulative therapy in treatment of primary dysmenorrhea: A pilot study. J. Manipulative Physiol. Ther. 2, 140–145.

Triano, J., 2005. The theoretical basis for spinal manipulation. In: Haldeman, S. (Ed.), Principles and Practices of Chiropractic. McGraw-Hill, New York, pp. 361–381.

Verhoef, M.J., Lewith, G., Ritenbaugh, C., Boon, H., Fleishman, S., Leis, A., 2005. Complementary and alternative medicine whole systems research: beyond identification of inadequacies of the RCT. Complement. Ther. Med. 13, 206–212.

Wagnon, R., Sandefur, R.M., Ratliff, C.R., 1988. Serum aldosterone changes after specific chiropractic manipulation. American Journal of Chiropropractic Medicine 1, 66–70.

Wiberg, J.M., Nordsteen, J., Nilsson, N., 1999. The short-term effect of spinal manipulation in the treatment of infantile colic: a randomized controlled clinical trial with a blinded observer. J. Manipulative Physiol. Ther. 22, 517–522.

Woolf, S.H., 2008. The meaning of translational research and why it matters. J. Am. Med. Assoc. 299, 211–213.

Yates, R.G., Lamping, D.L., Abram, N.L., Wright, C., 1988. Effects of chiropractic treatment on blood pressure and anxiety: a randomized, controlled trial. J. Manipulative Physiol. Ther. 11, 484–488.

A physical therapist's perspective on manual therapy: clinical effectiveness and selected mechanism

Steven Z George

Introduction

Physical therapists have historically used manual therapy to treat musculoskeletal pain. Manual therapy was introduced to the profession by physical therapists who trained with osteopathic, chiropractic, and orthopedic physicians. James Cyriax (United Kingdom) seems to be the most commonly mentioned name associated with early mentoring of physical therapists in the practice of manual therapy.

Physical therapists such as Gregory Greive (United Kingdom), Freddy Kaltenborn (Norway), and Geoffrey Maitland (Australia) would eventually adopt their own manual therapy techniques and philosophies and begin widespread teaching to other therapists. Grieve, Kaltenborn, and Maitland also worked to develop a governing body for physical therapists practicing manual therapy, and in the late 1960s each was involved in the creation of the International Federation of Orthopaedic Manipulative Therapy (IFOMT). Stanley Paris (New Zealand) was the founding chairman of IFOMT and is credited with accelerating the use of manual therapy in the United States, through his participation in the Orthopedic Section of the American Physical Therapy Association (APTA), the founding of a physical therapy school, and continuing education programs.

As is typical in manual medicine, the use of manual therapy by physical therapists is linked to specific philosophies and approaches. For example, therapists trained in Maitland techniques would be expected to commonly utilize oscillatory joint mobilization techniques, and much less frequently to use high-velocity, low-amplitude thrust techniques. Although this culture of trainer-specific approaches still exists in physical therapy, recent trends indicate a shift away from this emphasis in the use of manual therapy.

Standardization of manual therapy instruction

The standardization of manual therapy teaching is one example of a move away from trainer-specific approaches. Historically in the United States, there was considerable variation in whether manual therapy was taught in entry-level physical therapy programs and, if taught, what philosophies and techniques were included. One model of standardization is evidenced in the *Guide to Physical Therapist Practice* (2001), which outlines broad utilization parameters for manual therapy. For example, the guide describes the use of mobilization and manipulation and outlines practice patterns which are appropriate for treatment with manual therapy. Another source of standardization provided by the APTA is the *Manipulation Education Manual*. This provides information on specific examination skills and manual therapy techniques in which physical therapists should be proficient.

It is appropriate to note that a majority of the language provided by the APTA describes physical therapists' use of manual therapy as focused to 'joint and soft tissue' structures. The application of manual therapy to visceral targets is not explicitly addressed, although the language related to 'soft tissue' is vague enough to allow for alternate interpretations. Anecdotally, visceral manipulation is rarely taught in entry-level education programs, but can be accessed by physical therapists through continuing education formats. Visceral manipulation techniques attempt to effect visceral structures through external body contact and are more common in massage and osteopathic practice (Barral & Mercier 1998). When visceral approaches are used by physical therapists the focus remains on the treatment of chronic pain, instead of directly affecting visceral function.

Clinical implementation of manual therapy

Clinical decision making is another recent trend affecting the use of manual therapy by physical therapists. Clinical decision making has undergone a paradigm shift over the past 10 years, and much of the supporting research for this has been led by physical therapists. Traditionally, appropriateness for manual therapy hinged on the identification of key structural or movement faults believed to be pathological or abnormal. After the pathology or abnormality was identified, manual therapy was utilized to 'correct' the fault, resulting in less pain and improved function for the patient. It is beyond the purpose of this chapter to exhaustively review all manual therapy approaches to demonstrate this common link; instead, a specific example will be provided.

In 1995, a treatment-based classification (TBC) system was proposed for low back pain (Delitto et al. 1995). Within this system there were two treatment categories appropriate for manual therapy. One hinged on the identification of static or dynamic pelvic asymmetry through palpation of key bony landmarks such as the anterior and posterior superior iliac spine (ASIS and PSIS, respectively). Palpation of these landmarks and positional tests served to determine whether asymmetry or pain existed, and whether the patient was appropriate for manual therapy. For example, an anterior innominate could be detected by comparing bilateral ASIS and PSIS positions. In the original article, either a pelvic manipulation technique applied through the ASIS or a pelvic muscle energy technique was suggested to correct the rotation (Delitto et al. 1995). Another treatment category hinged on the identification of lumbar movement faults consistent with 'blocked' facet joints. These movement faults were identified by recognizing opening and closing movement patterns during lumbar movement testing, as well as complementary findings when passive intervertebral mobility of the lumbar spine was tested. In this treatment category an appropriately directed lumbar manipulation technique (posterior/inferior for closing restriction and anterior/superior for opening restriction) was recommended to correct the movement fault (Delitto et al. 1995).

These 'correction' approaches, and others like them, have been widely taught to physical therapy students and are commonly implemented in physical therapy clinical settings. However, research reported in the peer-reviewed literature questions the validity of treatment approaches based solely on the identification of structural pathology as normally performed by manual therapists (i.e., through palpation, pain provocation, movement testing, and observation). Again, it is beyond the purposes of this chapter to exhaustively review this literature. Instead, the focus will be on examples that represent general trends in the literature suggesting that correction-focused application of manual therapy is a questionable treatment strategy.

One apparent trend in the literature is that the reliability of identification of structural pathology by palpation is poor. Two studies (Levangie 1999a, Riddle & Freburger 2002) have reported that the inter-rater reliability of the identification of pelvic asymmetry, with either a static or a dynamic approach,

is too low for use in most clinical settings. Furthermore, there is no strong association between pelvic asymmetry and low back pain, which also questions the use of these techniques in clinical settings (Levangie 1999b). Another trend noted in the literature is that manual therapy is applied with forces that are variable (Herzog et al. 2001, Hessell et al. 1990), nonspecific (Herzog et al. 2001 Ross et al. 2004), and does not result in measurable positional changes in targeted joints (Tullberg et al. 1998). Specifically, in a study of 10 consecutive patients identified with sacroiliac joint dysfunction and treated with an appropriate spinal manipulation technique, clinicians noted an improvement in sacroiliac joint dysfunction on clinical examination, although the reference standard (roentgen stereophotogrammetric analysis) did not detect any change in joint motion that exceeded measurement error (Tullberg et al. 1998).

These trends de-emphasizing the importance of identifying structural pathology continue in studies with a clinical focus. A study of 140 subjects with low back pain suggested that although pain relief was an expected outcome, there was no difference in outcomes if a specific lumbar manual therapy technique was selected by experienced clinicians, or whether the technique was randomly determined (Chiradejnant et al. 2003). In another study, subjects underwent an extensive physical examination including static, dynamic, and provocation tests for commonly utilized pelvic assessment (Flynn et al. 2002). Patients were then treated with a specific manipulation technique and range of motion exercises, regardless of whether the examination results indicated that treatment was indicated. This study design may seem counterintuitive at first; however, it must be stressed that this is an appropriate methodology to determine which baseline examination characteristics predict a favorable response to a selected intervention. Essentially, this design allows determination of how variability in patient baseline status affects variability in outcome. The results of the study indicated something very interesting: namely, that the presence of pelvic asymmetry (dynamic or static) was not predictive of a successful outcome from the manipulation (Flynn et al. 2002).

These studies highlight a shift in philosophy that de-emphasizes the importance of identifying specific structural pathology before the application of manual therapy. Instead, the identification of clinical factors that indicate a favorable response has been emphasized (Fig. 14.1). Essentially, the identification of responder subgroups is now a treatment priority, because it appears that larger treatment effects are observed if focused manual therapy is applied to those likely to respond (Brennan et al. 2006, Childs et al. 2004, Fritz et al. 2003). In the case of lumbar spinal manipulation, a clinical prediction rule consisting of five factors (duration of symptoms, location of symptoms, lower score on psychological distress questionnaire, presence of lumbar hypomobility at any segment, and hip internal range of motion >35°) has been identified and validated (Childs et al. 2004). Derivation clinical prediction rules for a variety of other musculoskeletal pain conditions have been reported by physical therapy researchers (Table 14.1). This philosophical shift is still in its professional infancy, but it is quite clear that is has an immediate impact on physical therapy practice, and it is highly likely that the profession will de-emphasize the application of manual therapy based solely on biomechanical theory and continue to develop and validate clinical prediction rules.

Table 14.1 Clinical prediction rule studies for utilization of manual therapy by physical therapists that have been reported in the peer-review literature

Clinical prediction rule Reference	Target condition
Muscle trigger point therapy Fernandez-de-las-Penas et al. (2008)	Chronic tension headache
Lack of improvement following lumbar spinal manipulation Fritz et al. (2004)	Low back pain
Improvement following thoracic spine manipulation Cleland et al. (2007)	Cervical pain
Improvement following cervical spine manipulation Tseng et al. (2006)	Cervical pain
Improvement following lumbopelvic manipulation Iverson et al. (2008)	Patellofemoral pain
Improvement following hip mobilization Currier et al. (2007)	Knee pain/ osteoarthritis

Selected mechanism of pain inhibition for manual therapy

From the previously cited examples it appears that manual therapy has great potential to be effective for musculoskeletal pain. However, many questions remain regarding the mechanisms of manual therapy for pain relief. Neurophysiological effects have always been associated with manual therapy, but over the last 15–20 years mechanistic studies have emphasized the importance of reflex mechanisms, as reviewed by Pickar (2002). It is beyond the scope of this chapter to review neurophysiological mechanisms involving muscle spindles, Golgi tendon organ, paraspinal muscle reflexes and/or motor neuron excitability. This is not meant to diminish these topics, but rather to allow for focus on a reflex that directly involves the processing of pain.

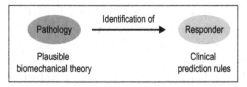

Figure 14.1 Shift in clinical decision making of utilization of manual therapy.

Surprisingly, manual therapy's direct effect on pain has not been extensively covered in the literature, as indicated in a qualitative review (Vernon 2000). Prior studies consistently reported hypoalgesia, or a lessening of pain, reports in response to a standard stimulus. Therefore, hypoalgesia following manual therapy is commonly reported in the literature. However, previous methodologies have only studied general aspects of hypoalgesia and have not been able to discern specific mechanisms.

Manual therapy's effect has been hypothesized as a 'counterirritant' stimulus to nociceptive input received by dorsal horn cells (Boal & Gillette 2004). Specifically, manual therapy activates joint and muscle spindle mechanoreceptors, with the potential of activating low (Aβ) and high (Aδ, C) threshold afferents. This afferent input converges on the spinal cord, where inhibition of dorsal horn cells is physiologically plausible (Boal & Gillette 2004).

In the author's opinion a likely explanation for the effectiveness of manual therapy could be that it has an inhibition effect that is specific to C-fiber-mediated pain perception. Numerous animal studies have suggested that central sensitization of nociceptive systems leading to pain is a specific neurophysiological mechanism associated with the development and maintenance of chronic pain syndromes (Dickenson & Sullivan 1987, 1990, Price et al. 1978, 1994, Vierck et al. 1997, Woolf & Thompson 1991). 'Wind-up' is a specific example of central sensitization within dorsal horn cells which results from tonic, peripheral nociceptive C-fiber input. The tonic, nociceptive input activates N-methyl-D-aspartate (NMDA) and substance P receptors in a wide dynamic range and nociceptive-specific dorsal horn cells. The activation of these cells induces a central hyperalgesia mediated at the spinal cord level, such that subsequent evoked pain stimuli are relayed from dorsal horn cells as increasing in intensity, despite their being of standard amplitude. In animal models,

the temporal parameter (frequency of nociceptive input) is a primary factor in eliciting wind-up (Price et al. 1978).

Direct measurement of wind-up is not feasible in humans, but temporal summation of thermal stimuli is an accepted behavioral measure of wind-up (Price 1999). The use of temporal summation as a proxy measure of wind-up is supported by human studies, which consistently demonstrate that an increase in the frequency of standard nociceptive input is associated with an increase in pain perception (Price et al. 2002, Robinson et al. 2004, Staud et al. 2001). Specifically, thermal input at 0.33 Hz or higher frequencies tends to induce temporal summation in humans, whereas input at 0.20 Hz or slower frequencies does not (Price 1999). It should be noted that this explanation is currently speculative, as only one study directly links temporal summation with disability from chronic LBP (George et al. 2006b).

If manual therapy has the potential to inhibit pain directly, it would have a measurable hypoalgesic effect on pain perception. As was previously mentioned, manual therapy hypoalgesia has been observed by decreased cutaneous receptive field from pin-prick (Glover et al. 1974), tolerance from electrical current (Terrett & Vernon 1984), and mechanical pressure (Vernon et al. 1990). Collectively, these results demonstrate manual therapy's potential for general dorsal horn-mediated pain inhibition. There are, however, several important, unresolved issues regarding manual therapy hypoalgesia, and these provided the impetus for a novel line of research that will be highlighted in this chapter.

The previously cited studies reported a hypoalgesic response in anatomical areas with the same or overlapping dermatomes as those treated with manual therapy (Glover et al. 1974, Terrett & Vernon 1984, Vernon et al. 1990), for example assessing hypoalgesic response to cervical manipulation only in anatomical areas innervated by cervical nerve roots, such as the upper extremity

(Vernon et al. 1990). As a result, these studies were unable to determine whether the observed hypoalgesia was a general effect or a specific effect local to the spinal levels involved with the manipulation (Vernon, 2000). Previous studies utilized pain induction protocols assessing general peripheral pain perception, instead of distinguishing manual therapy's separate effect on Aδ- and C-fiber-mediated pain perception (Price 1999).

Manual therapy's potential for specific inhibition of C-fiber-mediated pain perception has not been widely tested in human studies. Previously cited data support the relevance of investigating manual therapy's effect on wind-up (or temporal summation) in commonly encountered chronic pain states such as fibromyalgia and low back pain. However, it is also important to note that we do not know whether this mechanism of acute central sensitization generated by stimulation of nociceptors and the mechanisms of central sensitization underlying chronic pain conditions are the same.

In our proposed line of research we hypothesized that the effectiveness of manual therapy was through inhibition of dorsal horn wind-up. This would be detectable in experimental settings by measuring decreased temporal summation following the application of manual therapy. If this hypothesis was confirmed, manual therapy could be viewed as a treatment with the potential to reduce the development of chronic pain syndromes, at least those associated with dorsal horn wind-up. This hypothesis was further supported by a previous cross-sectional study in which increased temporal summation was associated with increased self-reporting of disability in patients with chronic low back pain (George et al. 2006b). Therefore, the overriding purpose of this line of research was to determine whether:

1. manual therapy suppressed temporal summation;
2. the hypoalgesia associated with manual therapy was specific to anatomical location (i.e. does lumbar manual therapy only affect temporal summation in lumbar innervated structures); and,
3. hypoalgesia from manual therapy could be influenced by subject expectation of pain relief.

Common experimental methods

The studies reviewed in this chapter used a common methodology for assessing pain perception. Subjects underwent quantitative sensory testing according to previously established protocols involving thermal stimuli (Price et al. 2002, Robinson et al. 2004, Staud et al. 2001, 2003). We selected this protocol because thermal stimuli are sensitive enough to differentiate Aδ- and C-fiber-mediated pain perception.

Thermal stimuli were delivered via contact thermode and a computer-controlled Medoc Neurosensory Analyzer (TSA-2001, Ramat Yishai, Israel) with a handheld, peltier element-based stimulator. Stimuli were applied to the subjects' non-dominant sides, and stimulus sites included areas innervated by lumbar dermatomes (the plantar surface of the foot, the posterior calf, and proximal to posterior superior iliac spine). Control sites included areas innervated by cervical dermatomes (the palmar surface of the hand and forearm). The order of stimulation sites was counterbalanced to prevent ordering effects, and exact stimulation sites were varied to prevent carryover effects due to spatial summation, local sensitization, or suppression of nociceptors. The interval between stimuli was at least 60 seconds to avoid carryover effects for the preceding thermal stimulus. Subject response to thermal stimuli was determined by a numerical rating scale (NRS) for evoked pain intensity, which ranged from 0 (no pain) to 100 (worst pain imaginable).

Subjects were familiarized with the thermal stimuli by a practice session in which a continuous heat stimulus was delivered to their dominant arm. The stimulus started at 35°C and was increased at a rate of 0.5°C/s, with subjects terminating the stimulus when the temperature reached pain threshold. This was repeated three times and the average threshold was calculated. In addition to familiarizing the subjects with thermal stimuli, the pain threshold data allowed us to investigate whether the intervention groups were confounded by general pain sensitivity. We then assessed specific components of thermal pain sensitivity used in previously reported studies (Price et al. 2002, Robinson et al. 2004, Staud et al. 2001).

First pain response

Heat stimuli of 3 seconds' duration were applied to the subjects' skin. The temperature rose rapidly (10°C/s) from a baseline of 35°C to a randomly determined peak of 45, 47, 49, or 50°C. The research assistant recorded NRS ratings of pain intensity. Subjects were asked to rate their first pain intensity felt. These ratings are believed to be primarily mediated by input from Aδ fibers (Price 1999, Price et al. 2002).

Temporal summation

A train of 10 consecutive heat pulses of <1 s duration at an inter-stimulus interval of 0.33 Hz was delivered to the subjects. This frequency was selected to ensure the development of temporal summation (Price 1999). The temperature of the heat pulses rapidly fluctuated (10°C/s) from a low of 35°C to a peak of 47°C. Temperature levels were monitored by a contactor-contained thermistor, and returned to a preset baseline of 35°C by active cooling. The research assistant recorded NRS ratings of pain intensity. Subjects were asked to rate their delayed (second) pain intensity associated with the first, third, and fifth heat pulses.

These ratings are believed to be primarily mediated by C-fiber input (Price 1999, Price et al. 2002).

Healthy subjects' immediate response to spinal manipulation

This study has been previously published and readers interested in a detailed summary are encouraged to investigate the original source (George et al. 2006a). Sixty healthy subjects with no current pain conditions were recruited and gave informed consent for study participation. They were randomly assigned to receive stationary bicycle riding, prone lumbar extension exercises, or a specific spinal manipulation technique for treatment. The subjects were instructed that each treatment is commonly used to treat low back pain. The purpose of the study was to determine the immediate effect of treatment on first pain and temporal summation, and to determine whether this effect differed for pain perception in lumbar and cervical innervated areas.

Each treatment was performed under the supervision of a physical therapist and limited to 5 minutes. Pain perception was tested before random assignment and then 5 minutes after the treatment. Data were analyzed with repeated-measures ANOVA that investigated for group × time interactions in pain perception in lumbar and cervical innervated areas.

The results suggested that there was an inhibition of first pain (Aδ fiber-mediated pain perception) that was statistically significant from pre to post treatment time (p < 0.05). However, the group × time interaction was not statistically significant, indicating that the pain inhibition was similar for all subjects (p > 0.05). These effects were only observed in the lumbar innervated areas, not the cervical areas.

There was also an inhibition of temporal summation (C-fiber-mediated pain

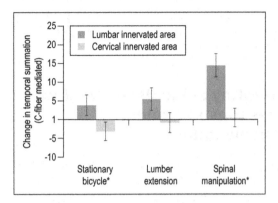

Figure 14.2 Lumbar spinal manipulation specifically inhibits temporal summation in lumbar innervated areas.

perception) that was statistically significant from pre to post treatment time (p < 0.05). In this instance the group × time interaction was statistically significant (p < 0.05). Post-hoc analysis of the interaction indicated that the pain inhibition was greater in those receiving spinal manipulation than in those receiving bicycle (p < 0.05) and lumbar exercise (p < 0.10). These effects were only observed in the lumbar innervated areas, not the cervical areas (Fig. 14.2).

Subjects with low back pain: immediate response to spinal manipulation

This study used parallel methods to investigate a cohort of subjects with chronic low back pain. Thirty subjects were recruited and gave informed consent for study participation. They were asked to withhold pain medication for the 3 hours prior to testing. Subjects were randomly assigned to stationary bicycle riding, prone lumbar extension exercises, or a specific spinal manipulation technique for treatment. The subjects were instructed that each treatment is commonly used to treat low back pain. The purpose of the study was to determine the immediate effect of treatment on temporal summation (C-fiber-mediated pain perception).

Each treatment was performed under the supervision of a physical therapist and

limited to 5 minutes. Pain perception was tested before random assignment and then 5 minutes after treatment. Data were analyzed with paired *t*-tests that assessed pre and post differences in the three treatment groups.

The results suggested that there was an inhibition of temporal summation (C-fiber-mediated pain perception) that was statistically significant from pre to post treatment time for those receiving spinal manipulation (p < 0.05), but no inhibition of temporal summation was observed for those randomly assigned to stationary bicycle (p > 0.05) and lumbar exercise (p > 0.05).

These data were completed in a patient sample, so the results had more ecological validity than the data generated involving healthy subjects. Therefore, the data can be viewed as additional evidence to support the notion that the clinical effectiveness of spinal manipulation is related to inhibition of central sensitization at the dorsal horn.

Influence of pain expectation on healthy subjects' immediate response to spinal manipulation

This study has been previously published and readers interested in a detailed summary are encouraged to investigate the original source (Bialosky et al. 2008b). Sixty healthy subjects with no current pain conditions were recruited and gave informed consent for study participation. All received the same manipulation technique, but were randomly assigned to receive a positive, neutral, or negative expectation of the technique's effect on perception of thermal pain. The purpose of the study was to determine whether subject expectation, a proxy measure of descending inhibition, influenced temporal summation following lumbar spinal manipulation.

Each treatment was performed under the supervision of a physical therapist and limited to 5 minutes. Pain perception was tested before random assignment and then 5 minutes after treatment. Data were analyzed with repeated-measures ANOVA that investigated for group × time interactions in pain perception based on the expectation received.

The results suggested that there was a statistically significant shift in subject expectation consistent with the randomly assigned instructional set ($p < 0.05$). For example, the subjects receiving the positive instructional set reported a larger expected decrease in pain than those receiving the neutral or negative instructional sets. When the actual pain perception testing was performed there was no effect of the instructional set for the lower extremity, as all groups reported decreased temporal summation. However, for pain perception testing in the trunk, a significant group × time interaction ($p > 0.05$) was detected. The nature of this interaction was that those receiving the negative instructional set reported *increased temporal summation* following the lumbar manipulation, whereas those receiving the positive and neutral instructional set reported *decreased temporal summation*. These expectation-specific effects were only observed in the back, not the lower extremity. Expectation is one factor believed to be an 'active agent' for placebo effects associated with manual therapy. Readers interested in more information on placebo effects should refer to Chapter 11.

Summary of studies and limitations to consider

These studies provide preliminary evidence to support our hypotheses that spinal manipulation specifically inhibits temporal summation, a proxy measure of dorsal horn wind-up. The results indicate that these effects were observed in healthy subjects and those with low back pain, and were local to areas innervated by the

lumbar spine, as similar changes were not observed in areas innervated by the cervical spine. Furthermore, the results indicate that the inhibition of temporal summation could be altered by an instructional set for negative expectation of pain relief. Collectively these studies suggest that the clinical effects of spinal manipulation could be due to inhibition of wind-up at the dorsal horn, and that this effect on wind-up is modifiable by descending inhibition related to expectation of pain relief.

A primary limitation of this study was that we used an acute cutaneous thermal stimulus that may not represent the type of pain commonly experienced by patients. Furthermore, we only investigated the immediate effects of manipulation, and cannot comment on the duration of these observed effects. Last, we cannot directly transfer these results to chronic or deep somatic pain because of the differences in neural mechanisms between cutaneous and deeper anatomical structures. Another limitation is that in our thermal stimuli testing protocol we did not consider vertebral alignment or the subsequent effects of manipulation on motor neuron activity. Therefore, we were not able to comment on whether the inhibition of wind-up we observed supports or refutes the concept of a 'facilitated segment' (see Chapters 1 and 12).

Conclusions and future directions

This chapter started with a clinical emphasis by summarizing a current model of manual therapy application that emphasizes the identification of responder characteristics. It then moved to a consideration of a specific mechanism that might explain how manual therapy inhibits pain. Although these topics may seem discordant, there is overlap. Each shifts manual therapy away from biomechanical and structural criteria, and focuses on clinical criteria. In this manner, manual therapy functions as a regulator of the musculoskeletal system by the brain and the somatomotor system (including afferent feedback from Aδ and C-fibers). Our data suggest that inhibition of temporal summation and descending inhibition by expectation may have important implications for pain relief. However, these are only two of the potential nervous system pathways for the therapeutic effect of manual therapy. In our comprehensive model we outline other ways in which manual therapy could induce pain relief, involving peripheral and central nervous system pathways (Bialosky et al. 2008a). Given the wide range of potential effects of manual therapy, there is a unique opportunity for collaborative teams to study both clinical effects and mechanisms of manual therapy using more complex models with advanced assessment techniques.

References

American Physical Therapy Association, 2001. Guide to Physical Therapist Practice, second ed. Physical Therapy vol. 81. 9–746.

Barral, J.P., Mercier, P., 1998. Visceral Manipulation. Eastland Press, Seattle, WA.

Bialosky, J.E., Bishop, M.D., Price, D.D., Robinson, M.E., George, S.Z., 2008a. The mechanisms of manual therapy in the treatment of musculoskeletal pain: A comprehensive model. Man Ther.

Bialosky, J.E., Bishop, M.D., Robinson, M.E., Barabas, J.A., George, S.Z., 2008b. The influence of expectation on spinal manipulation induced hypoalgesia: an experimental study in normal subjects. BMC Musculoskelet. Disord. 9, 19.

Boal, R.W., Gillette, R.G., 2004. Central neuronal plasticity, low back pain and spinal manipulative therapy. J. Manipulative Physiol. Ther. 27, 314–326.

Brennan, G.P., Fritz, J.M., Hunter, S.J., Thackerary, A., Delitto, A., Erhard, R.E., 2006. Identifying subgroups of patients with 'non-specific' low back pain: results of a randomized clinical trial. Spine 31, 623–631.

Childs, J.D., Fritz, J.M., Flynn, T.W., et al., 2004. A clinical prediction rule to identify patients with low back pain most likely to benefit from spinal manipulation: a validation study. Ann. Intern. Med. 141, 920–928.

Chiradejnant, A., Maher, C.G., Latimer, J., Stepkovitch, N., 2003. Efficacy of 'therapist-selected' versus 'randomly selected' mobilisation techniques for the treatment of low back pain: a randomised controlled trial. Aust. J. Physiother. 49, 233–241.

Cleland, J.A., Childs, J.D., Fritz, J.M., Whitman, J.M., Eberhart, S.L., 2007. Development of a clinical prediction rule for guiding treatment of a subgroup of patients with neck pain: use of thoracic spine manipulation, exercise, and patient education. Phys. Ther. 87, 9–23.

Currier, L.L., Froehlich, P.J., Carow, S.D., et al., 2007. Development of a clinical prediction rule to identify patients with knee pain and clinical evidence of knee osteoarthritis who demonstrate a favorable short-term response to hip mobilization. Phys. Ther. 87, 1106–1119.

Delitto, A., Erhard, R.E., Bowling, R.W., 1995. A treatment-based classification approach to low back syndrome: identifying and staging patients for conservative treatment [see comments]. Phys. Ther. 75, 470–485.

Dickenson, A.H., Sullivan, A.F., 1987. Evidence for a role of the NMDA receptor in the frequency dependent potentiation of deep rat dorsal horn nociceptive neurones following C fibre stimulation. Neuropharmacology 26, 1235–1238.

Dickenson, A.H., Sullivan, A.F., 1990. Differential effects of excitatory amino acid antagonists on dorsal horn nociceptive neurones in the rat. Brain Res. 506, 31–39.

Fernandez-de-las-Penas, C., Cleland, J.A., Cuadrado, M.L., Pareja, J.A., 2008. Predictor variables for identifying patients with chronic tension-type headache who are likely to achieve short-term success with muscle trigger point therapy. Cephalalgia 28, 264–275.

Flynn, T., Fritz, J., Whitman, J., et al., 2002. A clinical prediction rule for classifying patients with low back pain who demonstrate short-term improvement with spinal manipulation. Spine 27, 2835–2843.

Fritz, J.M., Delitto, A., Erhard, R.E., 2003. Comparison of classification-based physical therapy with therapy based on clinical practice guidelines for patients with acute low back pain: a randomized clinical trial. Spine 28, 1363–1371.

Fritz, J.M., Whitman, J.M., Flynn, T.W., Wainner, R.S., Childs, J.D., 2004. Factors related to the inability of individuals with low back pain to improve with a spinal manipulation. Phys. Ther. 84, 173–190.

George, S.Z., Bishop, M.D., Bialosky, J.E., Zeppieri Jr., G., Robinson, M.E., 2006a. Immediate effects of spinal manipulation on thermal pain sensitivity: an experimental study. BMC Musculoskelet. Disord. 7, 68.

George, S.Z., Wittmer, V.T., Fillingim, R.B., Robinson, M.E., 2006b. Fear avoidance beliefs and temporal summation of evoked thermal pain influence self-report of disability for patients with chronic low back pain. J. Occup. Rehabil. 16, 95–108.

Glover, J.R., Morris, J.G., Khosla, T., 1974. Back pain: a randomized clinical trial of rotational manipulation of the trunk. Br. J. Ind. Med. 31, 59–64.

Herzog, W., Kats, M., Symons, B., 2001. The effective forces transmitted by high-speed, low-amplitude thoracic manipulation. Spine 26, 2105–2110.

Hessell, B.W., Herzog, W., Conway, P.J., McEwen, M.C., 1990. Experimental measurement of the force exerted during spinal manipulation using the Thompson technique. J. Manipulative Physiol. Ther. 13, 448–453.

Iverson, C.A., Sutlive, T.G., Crowell, M.S., et al., 2008. Lumbopelvic manipulation for the treatment of patients with patellofemoral pain syndrome: development of a clinical prediction rule. J. Orthop. Sports Phys. Ther. 38, 297–309.

Levangie, P.K., 1999a. Four clinical tests of sacroiliac joint dysfunction: the association of test results with innominate torsion among patients with and without low back pain. Phys. Ther. 79, 1043–1057.

Levangie, P.K., 1999b. The association between static pelvic asymmetry and low back pain. Spine 24, 1234–1242.

Pickar, J.G., 2002. Neurophysiological effects of spinal manipulation. Spine J. 2, 357–371.

Price, D.D., 1999. Psychological Mechanisms of Pain and Analgesia. International Association for the Study of Pain Press, Seattle, WA.

Price, D.D., Hayes, R.L., Ruda, M., Dubner, R., 1978. Spatial and temporal transformations of input to spinothalamic tract neurons and their relation to somatic sensations. J. Neurophysiol. 41, 933–947.

Price, D.D., Mao, J., Frenk, H., Mayer, D., 1994. The N-methyl-D-aspartate receptor antagonist dextromethorphan selectively reduces temporal summation of second pain in man. Pain 59, 165–174.

Price, D.D., Staud, R., Robinson, M.E., Mauderli, A.P., Cannon, R., Vierck, C.J., 2002. Enhanced temporal summation of second pain and its central modulation in fibromyalgia patients. Pain 99, 49–59.

Riddle, D.L., Freburger, J.K., 2002. Evaluation of the presence of sacroiliac joint region dysfunction using a combination of tests: a multicenter intertester reliability study. Phys. Ther. 82, 772–781.

Robinson, M.E., Wise, E.A., Gagnon, C., Fillingim, R.B., Price, D.D., 2004. Influences of gender role and anxiety on sex differences in temporal summation of pain. J. Pain 5, 77–82.

Ross, J.K., Bereznick, D.E., McGill, S., 2004. Determining cavitation location during lumbar and thoracic spinal manipulation: is spinal manipulation accurate and specific? Spine 29, 1452–1457.

Staud, R., Vierck, C.J., Cannon, R.L., Mauderli, A.P., Price, D.D., 2001. Abnormal sensitization and temporal summation of second pain (wind-up) in patients with fibromyalgia syndrome. Pain 91, 165–175.

Staud, R., Robinson, M.E., Vierck Jr., C.J., Cannon, R.C., Mauderli, A.P., Price, D.D., 2003. Ratings of experimental pain and pain-related negative affect predict clinical pain in patients with fibromyalgia syndrome. Pain 105, 215–222.

Terrett, A.C., Vernon, H., 1984. Manipulation and pain tolerance. A controlled study of the effect of spinal manipulation on paraspinal cutaneous pain tolerance levels. Am. J. Phys. Med. 63, 217–225.

Tseng, Y.L., Wang, W.T., Chen, W.Y., Hou, T.J., Chen, T.C., Lieu, F.K., 2006. Predictors for the immediate responders to cervical manipulation in patients with neck pain. Man. Ther. 11, 306–315.

Tullberg, T., Blomberg, S., Branth, B., Johnsson, R., 1998. Manipulation does not alter the position of the sacroiliac joint. A roentgen stereophotogrammetric analysis. Spine 23, 1124–1128.

Vernon, H., 2000. Qualitative review of studies of manipulation-induced hypoalgesia. J. Manipulative Physiol. Ther. 23, 134–138.

Vernon, H.T., Aker, P., Burns, S., Viljakaanen, S., Short, L., 1990. Pressure pain threshold evaluation of the effect of spinal manipulation in the treatment of chronic neck pain: a pilot study. J. Manipulative Physiol. Ther. 13, 13–16.

Vierck Jr., C.J., Cannon, R.L., Fry, G., Maixner, W., Whitsel, B.L., 1997. Characteristics of temporal summation of second pain sensations elicited by brief contact of glabrous skin by a preheated thermode. J. Neurophysiol. 78, 992–1002.

Woolf, C.J., Thompson, S.W., 1991. The induction and maintenance of central sensitization is dependent on N-methyl-D-aspartic acid receptor activation implications for the treatment of post-injury pain hypersensitivity states. Pain 44, 293–299.

CHAPTER

15

Therapeutic massage and bodywork: overview of the practice and evidence of a developing health profession

Janet R Kahn

Introduction

Although therapeutic massage is an ancient healing art, its development as a healthcare profession is quite recent. In seeking to understand therapeutic massage in its current North American incarnation, it is helpful to keep the simultaneously ancient and newborn aspects in mind. Although massage has been an aspect of every form of medicine around the world and through the ages, its development as a profession began late in the 20th century, with great strides having been made in the last few decades (Moyer et al. 2009). It is definitely still 'under construction' as a profession, and this reflects real ambivalence among massage therapists about whether the advantages of joining the health professions fold outweigh the costs.

The choice, however, may not be up to the current practitioners of therapeutic massage. Professionalization is happening, due in no small part to the popularity of massage with the public, with the increased scrutiny that inevitably – and responsibly – follows. One aspect of the increased interest is reflected in the growing body of research on massage. A Medline search using massage as a single keyword, limited to clinical trials, randomized controlled trials (RCTs), and meta-analyses published in the last 10 years yielded 680 citations. Although this may not seem like much compared to other manual therapies, a search using the same limits for the previous 10 years yielded only 152 citations, and for the 10 years prior to that, only 26. From this perspective the field of massage research is burgeoning.

There are a number of challenges to research on massage, and many have written about this. Moyer et al. (2009) convened a working group to address these issues at the 2009 North American Research Conference on Complementary and Integrative Medicine. Among other things, the authors suggest looking to the field of psychotherapy, as they feel that profession and therapeutic massage share some key qualities, including that '...both forms of treatment (a) have existed for a considerable time; (b) have scientifically documented effects, but (c) no clear scientific consensus on the mechanisms that underlie their effects; (d) have numerous schools and approaches in which therapists are trained, and which guide their assumptions and selection of specific techniques; and (e) have numerous structural similarities, including typical session length, number of sessions that make up a course of treatment, and the likelihood of repeated, private interpersonal contact between therapist and patient.'

The diversity of the field poses a real challenge to the outsider. To understand the whole of contemporary therapeutic massage it helps to recognize that it has lineages that address somewhat distinct and overlapping 'problems' through repertoires of treatment that are similarly overlapping. Specifically, contemporary massage has roots in medicine (both Eastern and Western), sports and fitness (from the original Olympians onward), the natural health movements in Europe and the US, and the human potential movement, which brought particular attention to the interactions between mind and body. This chapter presents an overview of the contemporary practice of therapeutic massage, the state of the profession, and the current evidence base.

Overview of the profession

Massage is a fast-growing form of complementary and alternative medicine (CAM) in the US, whether measured in number of clients, practitioners, educational institutions, or dollars spent on it. Between 1990 and 1997 the annual percentage of American adults using massage in a 12-month period increased from 6.9% to 11.1% (Eisenberg et al. 1998). A 2007 survey sponsored by the American Massage Therapy Association (AMTA) estimated that 24% of Americans had received a massage in the previous year. Eisenberg et al. estimated that in 1997 13.5 million Americans visited massage therapists, collectively making 114 million visits, which the AMTA estimated cost between $4 and $6 billion. Recent surveys have suggested the current expenditure to be between $6 and $15 billion. The number of hospitals offering massage increased by 30% between 2003 and 2005 alone (American Hospital Association, 2006).

The AMTA has been a major driver of the professionalization of massage. It is responsible for the first council of massage schools (1982), the creation of the Commission of Massage Therapy Accreditation (1989), initiation of the National Certification Board for Therapeutic Massage and Bodywork (1992), and the founding and ongoing financial support of the Massage Therapy Foundation (1993), which funds research, outreach, and scholarship grants. The Massage Therapy Foundation has also advanced massage research through the creation of a massage research database, the creation of the first research agenda for massage (Kahn 2001) and the creation of a curriculum to bring research education into massage schools (Dryden & Achilles 2003). The AMTA and the Association of Bodywork and Massage Professionals (ABMP) have been the organizations promoting state licensure for massage therapists.

Massage is currently licensed in 42 states and the District of Columbia. Standards for licensure vary somewhat, but typically require a minimum of 500 hours of training from an accredited institution, and passage of one of two certification exams. The AMTA estimates that there are currently 265 000–300 000 massage therapists and massage school students in the United States.

There is wide variety in the education of massage therapists, with over 300 accredited massage schools in the US and an estimated 1200 massage training programs that are not accredited. Many of these programs are quite small. Only 93 schools in the US are accredited by the Commission on Massage Therapy Accreditation (COMTA), the sole accrediting agency in the field recognized by the US Department of Education and authorized to accredit at both institutional and programmatic level. A study of licensed massage therapists in Connecticut and Washington found that they had on average 625 hours of initial training (Cherkin et al. 2002). A recent AMTA survey concurred, reporting that massage therapists have an average of 633 hours of initial training and complete an average 25 hours per year of continuing education, most of this used to acquire new techniques. A small minority of massage schools require a BA for admission.

What is massage?

The term massage is used to refer to a wide array of ways to touch the human body. In this chapter the term therapeutic massage and bodywork will refer to purposeful manipulation of the soft tissue (with or without active or passive movements and verbal cuing), performed with the intention of alleviating pain and/or resolving structural imbalances or other abnormalities in the tissue to restore health, wellbeing, and/or ease. Only Western forms of massage will be included in the research reviewed here. Similarly, research involving massage and aromatherapy is not included. The breadth of this definition is driven by what massage therapists do in their practices. The overlap

with other manual therapies discussed in this book is inevitable, as there has been give and take between them over the decades. In recent years, massage therapists have studied methods originated in osteopathy or physical therapy. Craniosacral therapy, a method developed in osteopathy, may currently be practiced by more massage therapists than osteopaths.

There are many elements in a massage treatment, and distinguishing their individual contributions to the effect of a treatment is one challenge in the research. In fact, it may be impossible. At the very least we recognize that therapeutic massage includes the impact of compassionate human touch (see Chapter 9) with or without manipulation, the manual therapy or specific manipulation itself, the relationship of therapist and client, the effects of the healing environment, the client's expectations of the treatment, and the therapist's intention (see Chapter 11).

There is no definitive taxonomy of therapeutic massage, but there are three projects under way which may take us nearer that goal. One is the Massage Body of Knowledge project, a joint effort of the AMTA and ABMP. The second is an effort of the Best Practices Committee of the Massage Therapy Foundation, which has recently put forth a proposal for a process to create massage therapy guidelines (Grant et al. 2008). The third is a taxonomy drafted by the Massage Therapy Research Consortium, a consortium of massage schools in the US and Canada working to build research capacity within their schools and to create aids for all massage therapy researchers.

Here we offer two approaches to thinking about massage technique. For descriptive purposes, the primary techniques are:

- Light hand contact with no force using energetic and/or mental intention to obtain changes (e.g., craniosacral techniques)
- Light rhythmic strokes (e.g., manual lymph drainage techniques)

- Gliding and kneading strokes done with various degrees of pressure (e.g. Swedish massage techniques)
- Friction strokes done with sustained pressure (cross-fiber, transverse, circular, and longitudinal)
- Rocking, jostling, gentle shaking (included in trager and other applications)
- Sustained stretch moving toward or away from a barrier (e.g., myofascial techniques)
- Sustained compression without friction (e.g., trigger point technique)
- Passive movement (e.g., positional release techniques).

Andrade and Clifford offer a taxonomy organized by the intended effect (Andrade & Clifford 2008), and include:

- Superficial reflex techniques
  - Engage only the skin and may produce reflex effects but no mechanical effects
- Superficial fluid techniques
  - Engage the skin, superficial fascia, and subcutaneous fat down to the investing layer of the deep fascia
  - Produce mechanical effects on superficial lymphatics and possibly the venous circulation
- Neuromuscular techniques
  - Engage muscle and the tissues it contains
  - Affect the function of the contractile element, connective tissue hydration, and lymphatic return
  - May also produce complex reflex effects
- Percussive techniques
  - Deform and release tissues quickly
  - Engage different tissues depending on the force with which therapists apply them
  - May also produce useful reflex neuromuscular effects
- Connective tissue techniques
  - Engage superficial and deep layers of connective tissue
  - Mechanically affect the hydration, extensibility, and modeling of connective tissue; may also produce complex reflex effects
- Passive movement techniques
  - Produce substantial tissue or joint motion without effort on the part of the client
  - Engage multiple tissues and structures and have wide-ranging effects on fluid flow, connective tissue, and the neural control of muscle tone.

Presence

No matter what technique is used, Andrade and Clifford (2008) stress the role of 'intelligent touch,' which they say has three dimensions. The first is attention and concentration, or the therapist's capacity to focus on the 'sensory information that they receive primarily, but not exclusively, through their hands.' The second is the capacity of discrimination, which is described as the therapist's 'ability to distinguish fine gradations of sensory information.' Finally there is identification, which they describe as the therapist's ability to distinguish between healthy and dysfunctional tissue states and to identify structures and their response to applied forces. These or similar concepts are a part of most massage therapy training programs, and massage trainees receive instructor feedback on their palpatory skill in identifying these tissue states, as well as their skill in applying appropriate levels of pressure and sensing the client's/body's response.

In addition to these skills, most massage therapists put much weight on the therapist's compassionate intention and holistic view of the client as aspects of the treatment – the view that a client's physical, spiritual, cognitive, and emotional aspects are essentially inseparable from one another, and that all are in some real sense 'touched' by the treatment. Whereas to the researcher working within a reductionist framework the results of such care may be a placebo or non-specific effect (see Chapter 11), to the massage therapist they are often central to treatment. Walton (1999) described it this way: 'By touching a body, we touch every event it has experienced. For a few brief moments we hold all of a client's stories in our hands. We witness someone's experience of their own flesh, through some of the most powerful means possible: the contact of our hands, the acceptance of the body without judgment, and the occasional listening ear. With these gestures, we reach across the isolation of the human experience and hold another person's legend. In massage therapy, we show up and ask, in so many ways, what it is like to be another human being. In doing so, we build a bridge that may heal us both.'

Albeit more eloquent than most, Walton is nonetheless within an accepted massage tradition of speaking poetically or metaphorically rather than clinically. I would not be surprised to hear from a patient that the poetic description meets their experience well. The psychiatric concept of 'somatization,' wherein psychological stress is manifested in some physical or 'somatic' way (e.g., tight neck or GERD) speaks to the 'pathological' states that can arise through the mind–body interface. Walton's language is larger than pathology, as implied in the notion of accepting the body without judgment, as well as in the prohibition of diagnosis by massage therapists. To the extent that science has a description of the experience Walton describes, it may be the concept of a resonant field being created between the therapist and patient or within which they meet one another. Within such a field, the physical contact of the massage therapist may not have any 'otherness,' and benefit may be derived that affects both parties and which involves more for the patient than simply the application of manual forces.

Walton's view, shared by many massage therapists, probably reflects the influence of the human potential movement on the development of therapeutic massage in the US. At the Esalen Institute, among other places, the intermingling of bodyworkers and psychotherapists led to an exploration of the links between mental and bodily ease and distress, notions of wellness were expanded, and new modalities such as Rolfing, bioenergetics, and Aston Patterning were developed. This deepened exploration of the relationship between human structure and consciousness, which had begun earlier in Europe and which is probably the greatest American contribution to the field (Johnson 1995). It brought attention to the relationship between practitioner and client in creating and maximizing therapeutic effects, an aspect of healing still in need of systematic investigation.

What clients seek

Clients come to massage therapists because of illness and injury, and a desire for wellbeing (Cherkin et al. 2002). In their 1999 survey of licensed massage therapists in Washington and Connecticut, Cherkin et al. examined data from over 2000 visits to massage therapists and found that 19% were for wellness or relaxation, 5% for anxiety or stress, and roughly 63% for musculoskeletal complaints. The musculoskeletal visits were three to one chronic over acute, and within that 63% were 20% back, 17% neck, 8% shoulder, and the remainder were small percentages of varied complaints. This is the most systematic available review of what clients seek from massage treatment.

Review of the literature

Massage for musculoskeletal pain

Given the finding that 63% of visits to massage therapists are primarily for a musculoskeletal complaint (Cherkin et al. 2002), the body of research in this area is strikingly small. Back pain, the most rigorously investigated area, illustrates some of the challenges in massage research. A 2002 review of studies on massage for back pain, for instance, found only eight trials that included a massage arm (Furlan et al. 2002), and in half of these massage was included as a control arm in a study of something else. One of the other studies compared two German forms of 'massage' not typically practiced in the United States (Teil massage, and acupressure using a metal roller). Of the remaining three studies, one utilized a combination of massage and selected exercise (Preyde 2000), and the two that used massage alone as the intervention utilized somewhat different protocols (Cherkin et al. 2001, Hernandez-Reif et al. 2001). The lack of comparable and consistent techniques across studies makes reviews challenging and meta-analyses virtually impossible.

With these caveats, the preponderance of evidence is that massage appears effective in reducing pain and restoring function in patients with subacute and chronic nonspecific low back pain, especially when combined with exercises and education (Cherkin et al. 2009, 2001, Furlan et al. 2009, Hernandez-Reif et al. 2001, Preyde 2000). A relatively large (n = 232) and rigorous study (Cherkin et al. 2001) found massage to offer modest cost savings compared to acupuncture or self-help education via book and video, when accounting for a patient's use of health services for back pain during the year following treatment.

The massage protocol in the Cherkin study was not a strict protocol, but rather gave the therapists parameters within which they could use their clinical judgment to design a treatment for each patient encounter. In this way it closely replicated massage as it is practiced. Viewed in one light this is a strength, as many early massage studies offered as an intervention either a length of session or a type of massage that was not regularly practiced in the 'real' world, leaving many wondering what the implications were for clinical practice. A shortcoming of the approach in Cherkin's study,

however, is that as most of the treatments given in the study involved myofascial techniques, neuromuscular techniques, or both, it was unclear whether similar results could be expected from other kinds of massage. In particular, from a public health standpoint the study did not answer the question of whether 'most massage therapists' who have graduated from a 500-hour program (which many state licensure laws set as the bar) would be likely to produce similar results.

Recent progress in research on massage for musculoskeletal pain

To address this question we conducted a study comparing two distinct massage protocols. Each was designed by leading massage educators to utilize different techniques and presumably different mechanisms of action (Cherkin et al. 2009).

This most recent Cherkin study on massage for back pain was an RCT which randomized 402 subjects with chronic low back pain to one of three arms: usual care; relaxation massage, which was a full-body protocol of entirely Swedish massage techniques in which the therapist was told to hold the intention of encouraging a generalized relaxation response; and focused structural massage, which was a protocol consisting largely of myofascial and neuromuscular techniques in which the therapist was told to identify the musculoskeletal contributors to each patient's back pain and treat those. The study asked two questions. Is relaxation massage (Swedish techniques) an effective treatment for chronic low back pain? Is focused structural massage (neuromuscular, myofascial techniques) more effective than relaxation massage? The primary outcomes were back-related dysfunction assessed via the Roland Scale, and a visual analog scale of the patients' assessment of the troublesomeness of their back pain symptoms.

Subjects received a maximum of 10 1-hour massages over a 10-week period. Data were collected at baseline, 10 weeks (end of treatment), 26 weeks, and 52 weeks, just as in the earlier study. As Figures 15.1 and 15.2 show, subjects receiving either form of massage fared significantly better than those in usual care by the end of the treatment period (p < 0.001 for each of the two primary vari-ables), and at that time there was no significant difference between the effects of the two forms of massage. At 26 weeks post baseline (4 weeks after the end of the treatment period) both forms of massage were still showing significantly greater effect than usual care in relation to the Roland Scale of disability (p = 0.003), but there were no significant differences at that point in relation to

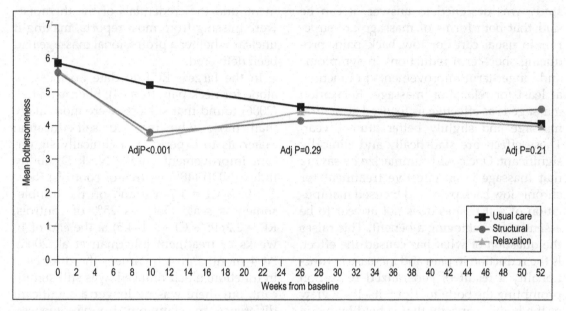

Figure 15.1 **Mean Bothersomeness Scores.** Cherkin 2009 – Symptom Bothersomeness Scores (0–10). (Courtesy of Dan Cherkin; unpublished.)

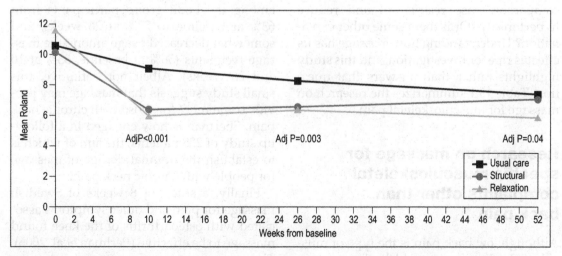

Figure 15.2 **Mean Roland Disability Scores.** Cherkin 2009 – Roland Disability Scale Scores (0–23). (Courtesy of Dan Cherkin; unpublished.)

symptom troublesomeness (p = 0.29). Finally, at the 1-year point the two forms of massage had diverged and, surprisingly – at least to those who value 'advanced' technique – the relaxation massage appeared to be more effective than the focused structural massage: significantly better on the Roland Scale (p = 0.04) and slightly, but not significantly, better on the symptom troublesomeness (p = 0.21).

In short, in terms of the questions the study was designed to answer, it can be said that both forms of massage are superior to usual care for low back pain, producing short-term reductions in symptoms and longer-term improvements in function, at least for relaxation massage. Relaxation massage is as effective as focused structural massage and slightly better after 1 year. These effects are statistically and clinically significant. One could summarize by saying that massage is an effective treatment for chronic low back pain, and focused manipulation of soft tissues does not appear to be essential for achieving a benefit. This raises the question of what has caused the effect. Is the reduction in pain and increase in functionality a result of generalized relaxation prompting the body to 'right' itself – a view of the body's capacity that is held by many CAM therapists? Or do both Swedish and myofascial and neuromuscular techniques comparably ease restrictions and reduce hypertonicity? Or is there some other explanation? Understanding how massage has its effect is ripe for investigation, and this study highlights rather than answers that question. Table 15.1 summarizes the research on massage for musculoskeletal pain.

Research on massage for specific musculoskeletal complaints other than back pain

Although low back pain is the type of musculoskeletal pain for which the greatest research literature on massage exists, a few other forms of musculoskeletal pain have been studied. Reviews of massage for neck pain have found they were unable to make conclusive recommendations for practice (Ezzo et al. 2007). Among other things, most studies were quite small and aggregation of data was impossible because the treatment protocols were often unclear, and, when clear, differed from one another; massage was often part of a multimodal treatment; and the credentials of the therapists were missing from most reports, making it unclear whether a professional massage had been delivered.

In the largest RCT to date on massage alone for neck pain (n = 64), Sherman et al. (2006) found that subjects were more likely than those who received self-education materials to experience a clinically significant improvement on the Neck Disability Index (NDI) (48% vs 18% of controls; RR = 2.7; 95% CI = 1.2–6.5) and on the troublesomeness scale (55% vs 25% of controls; RR = 2.2; 95% CI = 1.1–4.5) at the end of 10 weeks of treatment (Sherman et al. 2006). At 4 months post treatment the difference in function, albeit reduced, was still significant, but there was no longer a significant difference in symptom troublesomeness. There was a difference between the groups in medication usage, with increased usage among the book group participants from 63% at baseline to 77% at 26 weeks, and somewhat decreased usage among the massage recipients (56% at baseline, 53% at 10 and 26 weeks). Albeit not definitive, this small study suggests that massage may provide some relief for those with chronic neck pain. Sherman is now engaged in a follow-up study of 228 patients, the aim of which is to establish the optimal dosage of massage for people with chronic neck pain.

Finally, a study of 8 weeks of Swedish massage for pain and other symptoms associated with osteoarthritis of the knee found massage to be effective (Perlman et al. 2006). The primary outcomes were scores on the Western Ontario and McMaster Universities

Table 15.1 Massage for musculoskeletal pain

Citation	Study design	Sample size	Experimental intervention	Comparison group intervention	Study duration or endpoint(s)	Outcomes
Back pain						
Cherkin et al. 2009	3-armed RCT	402	10 sessions of either RMT or FSMT	UC	10 wks, 26 wks, 52 wks	At 10 wks both RMT & FSMT superior to UC on RDQ & symptom bothersomeness (p < 0.001); at 26 wks RMT & FSMT superior to UC on RDQ (p = 0.003); at 52 wks RMT superior to FSMT on RDQ (p = 0.04) and symptom scale (p = 0.21)
Cherkin et al. 2001	3-armed RCT	262	MT or Acu ≤ 10x/10 wks	Self-care educational materials (SCE)	Weeks 4, 10 & 52 post baseline	10 wks – MT superior to SCE on symptom scale (p = 0.01); on dysfunction scale, MT superior to SCE (p < 0.001) & Acu (p = 0.01). 52 wks – MT superior to Acu on symptom scale (p = 0.002) & dysfunction scale (p = 0.05) MT groups used least medication (p < 0.05) and had lowest costs of subsequent back pain care
Hernandez-Reif et al. 2001	RCT	24	MT 30 min 2x week for 5 weeks	PMR 30 min 2x week for 5 weeks	5 weeks	MT group reported less pain (p < 0.05), less depression (p = 0.05), improved sleep (p = 0.03), improved flexion (p < 0.003), higher serotonin & dopamine (both p = 0.04)
Preyde 2000	4-armed RCT	98	6 sessions of CMT, STM, or REPE w/in 1 month	Sham laser therapy	End of tx & 1 month post end of tx	CMT improvement superior to other 3 arms on function (mean RDQ score 1.54 v. 2.86–6.5, p < 0.001), pain intensity (mean PPI score 0.42 v. 1.18–1.75, p < 0.001) and decrease in the quality of pain (mean PRI score 2.29 v. 4.55–7.71, p = 0.006). CMT & STM both showed clinically significant improvement on function. At 1 mo f/up no pain reported by 63% CMT, 27% STM, 14% REPE & 0% sham laser

(Continued)

Table 15.1 Massage for musculoskeletal pain—Cont'd

Citation	Study design	Sample size	Experimental intervention	Comparison group intervention	Study duration or endpoint(s)	Outcomes
Neck pain						
Sherman et al. 2006	RCT	64	MT, ≤ 10 sessions in ≤ 10 wks	SCE	10 wks; 26 wks	At 10 wks, more MT Ss improved on NDI (48% vs. 18% of SCE; RR = 2.7; 95% CI = 1.2–6.5) & on the bothersomeness scale (55% vs. 25% of SCE; RR = 2.2; 95% CI = 1.1–4.5). At 26 wks dif in NDI reduced but still significant. Med usage decreased for MT (56% at baseline, 53% at 26 wks) but increased for SCE (63% at baseline to 77% at 26 weeks)
Osteoarthritis						
Perlman et al. 2006	RCT	68	MT 2x/wk for 4 wks + 1x/wk for 4 wks	Delayed intervention of same protocol	End of tx (8 weeks)	MT group showed significant improvements in the mean WOMAC global scores (p < 001), pain (p < 0.001), stiffness (p < 0.001), and physical function domains (p < 0.001), and pain VAS (p < 0.001), range of motion in degrees (p = 0.03), and time to walk 50 ft (15 m) in seconds (p < 0.01).

Acu, acupuncture; CMT, comprehensive massage therapy (soft-tissue manipulation, remedial exercise and posture education); FSMT, focused structural massage using largely neuromuscular & myofascial techniques; LBP, lower back pain; LROM, lumbar range of motion as assessed by the Modified Schober test; MT, massage therapy; NDI, Neck Disability Index; PMR, progressive muscle relaxation; RDQ, Roland Disability Questionnaire; REPE, remedial exercise w/postural education; RMT, Relaxation massage of Swedish strokes; SCE, self-care educational materials; STM, soft tissue manipulation alone; UC, usual care; VAS, visual analog scale; WOMAC (Western Ontario and McMaster Universities Osteoarthritis Index) pain and functionality scale.

Osteoarthritis Index (WOMAC) and pain visual analog scale (0 = no pain, 10 = worst pain ever). The 68 subjects were randomized to massage or to a delayed intervention control. In contrast to most studies on massage for pain, which have administered weekly treatments, this study administered full-body Swedish massage twice weekly in the first 4 weeks to build a loading dose, and then once weekly for the next 4 weeks. The massage therapy group demonstrated significant improvements in their WOMAC global score (-21.15 ± 2.46 mm; $p < 0.0001$), stiffness (-21.60 ± 26.99 mm; $p < 0.0001$), physical function domains (-20.50 ± 22.50 mm; $p < 0.0001$) and pain (-17.62 ± 310.06 mm; $p = 0.0023$) at 8 weeks (end of treatment) as well as decreased pain (VAS) and time to walk 50 feet ($p < 0.05$). At 16 weeks (8 weeks post treatment) improvements seen in the massage therapy group generally persisted. The authors conclude that massage seems to be an effective treatment for osteoarthritis of the knee.

Massage and somatovisceral interactions

As stated earlier, the view of the body held by massage therapists emphasizes its intrinsic wholeness. In this view, massage to one area may have impact on the whole body, including internal structures, and at least affects nearby body areas. Juhan, in his classic text *Job's Body*, speaks of the skin being 'no more separated from the brain than the surface of a lake is separate from its depths.' 'The brain,' he goes on, 'is a single functional unit, from cortex to fingertips to toes. To touch the surface is to stir the depths' (Juhan 1987). Indeed, some of the literature on massage seems to support such a 'unified field theory' of the body – or perhaps it is simply that the specific mechanisms of action have not yet been identified. The remainder of this chapter will explore the evidence for massage and somatovisceral interactions.

Massage and stress

In the survey mentioned above (Cherkin et al. 2002), relaxation, stress relief, and anxiety reduction accounted for roughly 24% of visits to massage therapists. A number of small investigations have shown that massage may offer immediate reductions in stress and anxiety in a variety of situations. These include people undergoing short-term stressful medical procedures, such as debridement (Field et al. 1998b) and autologous bone marrow transplant (Ahles et al. 1999), as well as people in more long-term stressful situations such as depressed adolescent mothers (Field et al. 1996a). Although all three of these studies indicate reductions in state anxiety, the latter study, which compared massage with a combination of yoga and progressive muscle relaxation, also showed reductions for the massage group in behavioral ('fidgettiness,' $p < 0.01$) and physiological (pulse and heart rate) signs of anxiety, as well as a reduction in depression ($p < 0.05$). Staff observational reports of behavior indicated that the massage group had improved affect ($p < 0.001$) and cooperation ($p < 0.005$).

Many of the studies by the Touch Research Institute team measured general indicators of relaxation/stress reduction, such as self-reports on the State Trait Anxiety Inventory (Spielberger et al. 1970) or salivary cortisol levels, as well as some measure particular to the condition under study, such as peak air flow for children with cystic fibrosis (Hernandez-Reif et al. 1999), or blood glucose levels in diabetics. Although the value of this Hernandez-Reif study and other early work by this team is diminished by small sample size (n = 20) and lack of blinding, it still offers a line of investigation that could be pursued. In this study the treatment was a 20-minute massage administered by parents to their children for 30 evenings, and the comparison condition was 20 minutes of reading by the parents to the children for the same period. The results indicated a significant reduction in anxiety for parents and children from day

1 to day 30 in the massage group (p < 0.05) and, importantly, an increase in peak air flow for children in the massage group from day 1 to day 30 (p < 0.05).

Perhaps the most common and controversial outcome assessed in a number of studies was salivary cortisol levels. Field and colleagues, in over a dozen early studies, had found significant post-massage increases in serotonin levels and reductions in epinephrine, norepinephrine, and cortisol. However, Moyer and colleagues conducted a meta-analysis of 37 studies measuring nine dependent variables and found that a single massage treatment produced reductions in state anxiety, blood pressure, and heart rate, but not in cortisol levels, and that multiple treatments produced reductions in pain and depression comparable to those with psychotherapy (Moyer et al. 2004). These authors criticized the early work of Field et al. for having reported within-group findings for studies whose design demanded between-group analysis. A more recent study of neurohormonal responses to massage in a sample of healthy men confirms the findings of Moyer and colleagues concerning lack of significant effect upon cortisol levels (Bello et al. 2008). These investigators found no significant differences between the control and the massage conditions for plasma arginine vasopressin (AVP) or plasma cortisol.

Two studies on massage for people experiencing workplace stress included a measure of cognition in addition to some of the more common stress-related outcome measures (Field et al. 1996b, Hodge et al. 2002). Hodge and colleagues investigated seated massage as a workplace stress reduction intervention and randomized 100 employees working in a large teaching hospital to receive either a 20-minute massage twice weekly for 8 weeks (the protocol was a blend of light- to medium-pressure circular motions to the upper body, acupressure to the face and chest, and foot reflexology), or a quiet room in which to take a 20-minute break. Findings indicate that, compared to the control group, the massage group had

significant improvement in cognition scores (p = 0.000), as assessed by the Symbol Digit Modalities Test, a 90-second timed instrument providing indices of normal capacities in adults as well as improvement resulting from specific therapeutic interventions. The massage subjects also showed lower anxiety (state p = 0.009, trait p = 0.04), improved emotional control (p = 0.05), and a reduction in sleep disturbance for massage subjects on 12-hour shifts (p = 0.02).

The Field study also utilized seated massage compared with a rest break. They included EEG readings as an outcome, which indicated that, although subjects receiving both massage and the rest break experienced increased frontal δ power (indicative of increased relaxation), only the massage group also showed the decreased frontal α and β powers that are indicative of enhanced alertness. This interpretation was supported by the finding that the massage subjects were able to complete a set of mathematical computations more quickly and with half the error rate of the control group. The data from these two studies run counter to the expectation of some that subjects would emerge from massage in a relaxed, but somewhat vegetative state – perhaps 'too relaxed' to return to work effectively. It suggests instead that massage induces something like the state of meditation – relaxed and alert. This finding will not surprise those who have come to massage via the human potential movement.

One other effect of massage should be noted, namely enhanced sleep quality. Massage has been shown to improve sleep quality and/or duration for elderly volunteers (Field et al. 1998a), critically ill hospitalized patients (Richards 1998), youths institutionalized for depression or adjustment disorder (Field et al. 1992), hospital workers (Hodge et al. 2002), and cancer patients (Smith et al. 2002). Outcome measures employed included wrist actometer, time-lapse video, and polysomnography in addition to self-reports and report by hospital staff. Table 15.2 summarizes the research on massage for stress-related conditions.

Table 15.2 Massage for stress-related conditions

Citation	Study design	Sample size	Experimental intervention	Comparison group intervention	Study duration or endpoint(s)	Outcomes
Diego & Field 2009	RCT	20 Healthy adults	MT moderate pressure 15 min	MT light pressure 15 min	1 session; EKG* readings at baseline, during and post-MT	Moderate pressure group had increase HF, decreased LF/HF ratio; Light pressure group had decreased HF and increased LF/HF
Bello et al. 2008	RCT	14 Healthy men	MT 20 min/day x 2 days	Reading period 20 min/day x 2 days	Multiple measures during each session	Plasma OT levels increased in both groups (p < 0.05), no sig. dif. between groups
Lawler & Cameron 2006	RCT	47 Migraine patients	MT 45 min 1/wk during wks 5–10 + diary-keeping of sleep & migraine wks 1–13	Diary keeping of sleep & migraine wks 1–13	Baseline to 13 weeks	MT group had decreases in migraine frequency over course of study (p < 0.01), no decrease for controls; MT group, but not controls, had enhanced sleep quality (p < 0.01). Neither had change in sleep quantity
Field et al. 1998b	RCT	28 Burn patients	MT predebridement	UC	Pre & postdebridement	State anxiety and cortisol levels decreased in MT group**
Field et al. 1996a	RCT	32 Adol. mothers	MT 30-min x 10 sessions over 5 weeks	RT 30-min x 10 sessions over 5 weeks	5 weeks	Both groups lower anxiety self-report; MT group only lowered salivary and urine cortisol levels and lowered pulse**
Workplace stress						
Hodge et al. 2002	RCT	100	20 min seated MT 2x/wk x 8 weeks	20 min break in quiet room 2x/wk x 8 weeks	8 weeks	MT group had greater improvement in cognition (SDMT) than controls (p = 0.000), and in emotional control (p = 0.04); as well as less fatigue (p = 0.000), lower anxiety (state p = 0.009, Trait p = 0.04), decreased sleep disturbance for those working 12-hour shifts (p = 0.02)

(Continued)

Table 15.2 Massage for stress-related conditions—Cont'd

Citation	Study design	Sample size	Experimental intervention	Comparison group intervention	Study duration or endpoint(s)	Outcomes
Field et al. 1996b	RCT	50	15 min seated MT 2x/wk for 5 wks	15 min period of relaxation in chair 2x/wk for 5 wks	5 weeks	**EEG** – MT group had increased frontal delta power (relaxation) + decreased frontal alpha and beta (alertness), while controls had increased frontal delta, alpha & beta **POMS** – MT group only had lower anxiety levels post-MT **Computations** – MT group showed increased speed and accuracy on math computations while the control group did not change **Salivary cortisol** – MT group had lowered salivary cortisol levels on Day 1 only, controls not at all

BMT, autologous bone marrow transplant; OT, plasma oxytocin; POMS, Profile of Mood States; RT, relaxation therapy of unknown non-touch description; SDMT, Symbol Digit Modalities Test – a cognition measure.

*EKG data were used to derive the high-frequency (HF), low-frequency (LF) components of heart rate variability and the low to high frequency ratio (LF/HF) as noninvasive markers of autonomic nervous system activity.

**Note that little information was available. This is among the Touch Research Institute studies using cortisol levels as an outcome measure that was criticized by Moyer (2004).

Premature infant studies

One of the larger bodies of massage research concerns effects on premature infants of a protocol involving 15-minute massages given three times a day, each of which involves both moderate pressure massage and a kinesthetic component of flexion and extension of the limbs (Vickers et al. 2004). The duration of the treatment period varied across studies from 5 to 10 days. The first of the studies, and many subsequent ones, were conducted by Field's team at the Touch Research Institute, University of Miami. These studies represent perhaps the most concerted effort to elucidate a chain of not only correlation, but causal effect of massage per se.

Although at least one of the later neonate studies included an arm of sham massage, which will be discussed later, the early studies compared neonates who received the massage and kinesthetic activity intervention described above with control neonates who received usual care and nothing more. Outcomes across roughly a dozen studies have been relatively consistent, and included:

- Significantly greater weight gain by massage than control infants, ranging from 28% to 47% greater across studies (Field et al. 1986, Field 1995);
- Significantly fewer postnatal complications and stress behaviors than control infants;
- More mature motor behaviors on the Brazelton scale;
- Discharge from hospital an average of 3–6 days earlier than non-massaged babies, at a hospital cost saving of $3,000+ per infant in 1986 dollars;
- Eight months post discharge, the massaged infants were still showing an advantage on weight, mental and motor development.

The findings were striking but the causal chain was not immediately apparent. Some hypothesized that the weight gain could be due to greater caloric intake, but this was shown not to be the case (Field 2001). The notion that it was a result of increased sleep or decreased activity brought on by massage was pursued, and investigations of that hypothesis found that the massaged neonates were more alert and spent more time in active awake states than control neonates, suggesting that enhanced weight gain was not achieved by decreased activity (Dieter et al. 2003, Lee 2005).

The next hypothesis pursued was that moderate-pressure massage stimulates vagally mediated parasympathetic activity, leading to more efficient food absorption through increased gastric motility and the release of food absorption hormones, such as insulin (Diego et al. 2005). The specification of moderate-pressure massage arose from earlier findings by Field that light touch was responded to as an irritant by neonates, whereas a moderate pressure prompted a favorable response (Field 1995), reiterated in a later study on adults (Diego et al. 2004). Thus the investigation of the increased vagal activity hypothesis was a fully blinded RCT in which 48 premature infants were randomly assigned to either moderate-pressure massage, light-touch massage deemed the sham, or a control condition in which they received neither form of touch. Electrocardiogram (ECG) readings were used to derive measures of heart rate and autonomic nervous system (ANS) function, including Cardiac Vagal Index (CVI) and vagal tone, and electrogastrogram (EGG) readings assessed gastric motility. The results from that study were as follows:

- Neonates in the massage group gained significantly more weight than those in the control or sham massage groups ($F_{(2, 15)} = 6.93$; $p < 0.01$; $h2 = 0.21$), but did not consume any more calories ($F_{(2, 15)} = 0.10$; p = not significant; $h2 = 0.01$).
- The moderate-pressure massage group alone experienced:
  - A significant increase in CVI (linear trend; $F_{(1, 15)} = 8.42$; $p < 0.01$; $h2 = 0.36$) that peaked marginally

during the massage (quadratic trend; $F_{(1, 15)} = 3.13$; $p < 0.1$; $h2 = 0.17$);

- A significant increase in vagal tone (linear trend; $F_{(1, 15)} = 5.62$; $p < 0.05$; $h2 = 0.27$) that peaked during the massage (quadratic trend; $F_{(1, 15)} = 4.54$; $p < 0.05$; $h2 = 0.23$);
- A significant increase in gastric motility (linear trend; $F_{(1, 15)} = 10.66$; $p < 0.01$, $h2 = 0.42$); and
- A significant decrease in tachygastria (linear trend; $F_{(1, 15)} = 9.87$; $p < 0.01$; $h2 = 0.39$).

The authors regarded these findings as partial support for their hypothesized model indicating that moderate-pressure massage leads to greater weight gain through its effects on vagal activity and gastric motility.

Their next effort was an investigation of the effects of vagal activity and gastric motility on food absorption and digestive hormones during massage therapy while controlling for other potential mediating factors (Field et al. 2008). A Swedish team (Uvnas-Moberg et al. 1997) had already found that tactile stimulation led to increased release of gastrin. Field and colleagues examined the potential for massage to increase serum insulin and insulin-like growth factor-1 (IGF-1) in preterm neonates. Forty-five preterm neonates were randomly assigned to either usual care with the massage and kinesthetic activity intervention, or to usual care alone. Treatment period was 5 days. Results indicated that although the groups did not differ on caloric consumption (kcal/kg) during the study period, the massage group showed:

- A greater increase in weight gain ($F = 6.07$; $p < 0.02$)
- A greater increase in insulin ($F = 4.75$; $p < 0.001$)
- A greater increase in IGF-1 ($F = 4/93$; $p < 0.05$)

Correlation analyses suggested significant relations between these growth variables for the massage group but not for the control group, as follows: (1) weight gain was related to increased insulin, $r = 0.60$, $p = 0.05$; and (2) weight gain was related to increased IGF-1, $r = 0.46$, $p = 0.02$. Calorie consumption was not related to any of these variables.

Guzzetta and colleagues (2009) had also identified increased IGF-1 as a result of massage. In a very different line of inquiry, they investigated the effects of massage on both human infants and rat pups and found higher levels of blood IGF-1 in both populations than in the counterpart controls for each. In the human infants they also found accelerated maturation of electroencephalographic activity and of visual function, in particular visual acuity. In the rat pups they found that massage accelerated the maturation of visual function and increased the level of IGF-1 in the cortex. These findings, they assert, demonstrate that massage can have an influence on brain development, and in particular on visual development, with an indication that its effects are mediated by specific endogenous factors such as IGF-1.

Relating these studies of premature infant weight gain to the work on massage as a stress reducer, Field et al. hypothesize that one mechanism through which massage therapy could contribute to weight gain is by increasing insulin and IGF-1, as insulin promotes the conversion of glucose to both short-term and long-term storage, and IGF-1 stimulates cell growth and multiplication. Stress is known to be common among preterm neonates and can contribute to dysregulation of glucose metabolism, including hyperglycemia and insulin resistance (Mericq 2006, Mitanchez 2007). It has been shown that massage has reduced stress behaviors and increased calmer states in preterm neonates (Hernandez-Reif et al. 2007). Field et al. hypothesize that this is '…likely associated with both the decreased cortisol levels (Acolet et al. 1993) and increased vagal parasympathetic activity (Diego et al. 2005) noted in preterm infants following moderate pressure massage. Increased vagal activity may lead to greater weight gain by both increasing gastric activity and promoting the release of insulin. Further, massage therapy may lead to greater weight gain by reducing the inhibitory effects of cortisol on insulin secretion. In addition, massage therapy may lead to greater weight gain by decreasing cortisol and, in turn, increasing IGF-1, as chronically high levels of cortisol inhibit growth hormone secretion (Duclos et al. 2007, Tsigos & Chrousos 2002), and growth hormone stimulates the production of IGF-1' (Field et al. 2008, p. 4). Table 15.3 summarizes the research on massage in infants and children.

Thoughts on mechanism of action

Given the diverse benefits of massage for people with a wide range of conditions, it is tempting to look for a single underlying mechanism of action. This tendency is reinforced by the recent finding from Cherkin et al. (2009) that even musculoskeletal pain may ease in response to generalized relaxation, rather than to specific local manipulation.

Diego and Field suggest this underlying mechanism may be a parasympathetic nervous system response set in motion by the stimulation of pressure receptors in the skin responding to a moderate level of pressure. Their hypothesis regarding the role of enhanced vagal tone in premature infants is presented above.

Kerr and colleagues present a different view concerning the route of massage's varied effects. They suggest that what they call touch healing therapies (TH) may be effective in chronic pain treatment through four features that jointly encourage neural plasticity, particularly the reformation of the somatosensory cortical map (Kerr et al. 2007). These four features, any and all of which can be present in a massage treatment, are light tactile stimulation, a behaviorally relevant and relaxed context, repeated sessions, and directed somatosensory attention. It is known that chronic pain is sometimes

centrally maintained, meaning that it can persist even when there is no remaining damage to the tissue and hence no current nociception to account for the pain sensation. Cortical dysregulation has been associated with centrally maintained pain (Flor 2003, Price 2002). Studies have indicated that remodeling is possible in the somatosensory maps of adults (Pascual-Leone & Torres 1993). Body maps of chronic pain patients have shown enlargement in the areas related to the painful body regions (Flor et al. 1995, 1997, Maihofner et al. 2003). Taking all this into account, Kerr et al. hypothesize that touch healing 'modalities work to renormalize somatotopic maps via a therapeutic plasticity mechanism.'

As Juhan has told us, 'The skin is no more separated from the brain than the surface of a lake is separate from its depths.' There is a mystery to human unity, human integrity. Although reductionist science can show this mystery's existence and effects exquisitely, it may not be the best approach when we seek to 'explain' or 'reveal' it. The Kerr hypothesis points to the synergistic effect of four factors which may, individually or in various combinations, prompt self-healing. For what is renormalization of somatotopic maps via a therapeutic plasticity mechanism other than a statement of our great potential for self-healing, for remaking ourselves well when we have become unwell? Massage and other touch healing therapies point out the wonder of another human being aiding in this self-healing process.

However, although the four factors identified all appear to aid in activating this normalization, it has not yet been shown whether there is one among them that must always be present. If Field et al. are correct that this healing is prompted by engagement of pressure receptors, then the light tactile touch of Kerr's formula would be required. Yet, research on the effects of progressive muscle relaxation (PMR) and other meditative approaches would indicate that touch may not be necessary, or that minds

Table 15.3 Massage in infants and children

Citation	Study design	Sample size	Experimental intervention	Comparison group intervention	Study duration or endpoint(s)	Outcomes
Preterm infants						
Guzzetta et al. 2009	Matched case control	20	15 min MT 3× day × 10 days w/classical music	Classical music only	12 days	MT group had more rapid visual maturation; higher levels of blood IGF-1
Field et al. 2008	RCT	42	MTKS 15 min 3×/day	Standard NICU care	5 days	MTKS group showed greater increases during the 5-day period in (1) weight gain; (2) serum levels of insulin; and (3) IGF-1. Increased weight gain was significantly correlated with insulin and IGF-1
Diego et al. 2005	RCT	48	MPMT 15 minute massage 3× day	LPMT 15 min 3×/day OR no tx control (unspecified)	5 days	MPMT group gained sig. more weight with same calorie intake as other 2 groups ($p < 0.01$); had increased CVI ($p < 0.01$); Vagal ton ($p < 0.05$); an increase in gastric motility and decrease in tachygastria
Dieter et al. 2003	RCT	32	MT 15 min 3×/day	UC in NICU	5 days	Massage group had 53% greater avg daily weight gain, reduction time sleeping

Study	Type	N	Treatment	Control	Duration	Results
Field et al. 1986	RCT	40	MTKS 15 min 3x/day	UC in NICU	10 days	MTKS group had avg 47% greater weight gain, were more active and alert during sleep/wake behavior observations, and showed more mature habituation, orientation, motor, and range of state behavior on Brazelton scale, hospitalization 6 days shorter, avg savings of $3,00
Children						
Escalona et al. 2001	RCT	20	MT by parent 15 min/night before bed	Parent read Dr Seuss 15 min/night before bed	1 month	MT group had improved on-task behavior in school, improved sleep at home, decrease in salivary and urine cortisol levels*
Hernandez-Reif et al. 1999	RCT	20 w/cystic fibrosis 5-15 years of age	MT by parent 20 min/night	Parental reading 20 min/night	30 days	MT group had greater reduction in anxiety than control ($p < 0.01$); Group by days interaction effect showed MT had increased peak air flow after 1 month ($p < 0.05$) but not controls

CVI, cardiac vagal index; LPMT, light pressure massage; MPMT, moderate pressure massage; MTKS, massage therapy for 10 min + tactile stimulation of limb movement for 5 min.
*Little information available, e.g., no p values.

are capable of 'touching,' and that directed somatosensory attention may be key. If we begin with Kerr's hypothesis and explore the four factors in a variety of permutations to see what can be left out without destroying effect, we may learn something.

Alternatively, we could turn our attention away from the therapist and towards the client, away from the changer towards the changee. For this changee may also be the changer. Investigations of mean changes in response to massage therapy wash out the range of change that occurs in these experiments. I suggest that we begin to look at the base states and talents of the clients to understand what readiness for self-healing looks like; what might indicate or reflect great versus limited capacities for self-healing. Any manual therapist can tell of clients who transformed beyond all expectation in response to a modest intervention, or of the ones who were so tight/resistant/out of body, whatever, that 'nothing 'would have 'worked.' Where the ready client meets the potentially effective treatment may turn out to be where the rubber meets the road.

Summary

There is a growing and increasingly rigorous body of research literature concerning a host of somatoemotional and somatovisceral effects of massage. Despite this, there are major lacunae in the literature. Relatively little investigation has addressed hypotheses regarding the causal route of the effects seen from massage. The term massage still too often remains a black hole, with investigators failing to describe their research protocols in sufficient detail for replication, and virtually always failing to provide any rationale for the protocol chosen. Best practices need to be further developed by the profession and tested by the research community. Related to best practices, to date there has been no focused attention on the issue of massage dosing, either in terms of the duration of an individual massage session or the number and/or frequency of total sessions in a treatment period.

From a public health standpoint, we should focus on establishing the range of situations for which a massage intervention would be safe and effective, and ultimately what would be the 'best' intervention, where best is understood to include comparisons of efficacy, cost, ease of access, and the like. For those engaged in the mystery of the human mind/body, there is plenty of room for exploration.

References

Acolet, D., Modi, N., Giannakoulopoulos, X., et al., 1993. Changes in plasma cortisol and catecholamine concentrations in response to massage in preterm infants. Archives of Diseases in Children 68, 29–31.

Ahles, T.A., Tope, D.M., Pinkson, B., et al., 1999. Massage therapy for patients undergoing autologous bone marrow transplantation. J. Pain Symptom Manage. 18 (3), 157–163.

American Hospital Association, 2006. Massage Therapy Industry Fact Sheet. Online. Available http://www.amtamassage.org/news/MTIndustryFactSheet.html#6.

Andrade, C., Clifford, P., 2008. Outcome-based massage, second ed. Lippincott Williams & Wilkins.

Bello, D., White-Traut, R., Schwertz, D., et al., 2008. An exploratory study of neurohormonal responses of healthy men to massage. J. Altern. Complement. Med. 14 (3), 387–394.

Cherkin, D.C., Eisenberg, D., Sherman, K.J., et al., 2001. A randomized trial comparing traditional Chinese medical acupuncture, therapeutic massage and self-care education for chronic low back pain. Arch. Inter. Med. 161, 8.

Cherkin, D.C., Deyo, R.A., Sherman, K.J., et al., 2002. Characteristics of licensed acupuncturists, chiropractors, massage therapists, and naturopathic physicians. J. Am. Board Fam. Med. 15 (5), 378–390.

Cherkin, D.C., Sherman, K., Cook, A., et al., 2009. A randomized trial comparing relaxation massage, focused structural massage, and usual care for chronic low back pain. Altern. Ther. Health Med. 15 (3), S99–S100.

Diego, M.A., Field, T., 2009. Moderate pressure massage elicits a parasympathetic nervous system response. Int. J. Neurosci. 119 (5), 630–638.

Diego, M.A., Field, T., Sanders, C., et al., 2004. Massage therapy of moderate and light pressure and vibrator effects on EEG and heart rate. Int. J. Neurosci. 114 (1), 31–44.

Diego, M.A., Field, T., Hernandez-Reif, M., 2005. Vagal activity, gastric motility and weight gain in massaged preterm neonates. J. Pediatr. 147 (1), 50–55.

Dieter, J.N., Field, T., Hernandez-Reif, M., et al., 2003. Stable preterm infants gain more weight and sleep less after five days of massage therapy. J. Pediatr. Psychol. 28, 403–411.

Dryden, T., Achilles, R., 2003. Massage therapy research curriculum kit. Massage Therapy Foundation, Evanston, IL.

Duclos, M., Guinot, M., Le Bouc, Y., 2007. Cortisol and GH: odd and controversial ideas. Appl. Physiol. Nutr. Metab. 32, 895–903.

Eisenberg, D.M., Davis, R.B., Ettner, S.L., et al., 1998. Trends in alternative medicine use in the United States, 1990–1997. Results of a follow-up national survey. JAMA 280, 1569–1575.

Escalona, A., Field, T., Singer-Strunck, R., et al., 2001. Brief report: improvements in the behavior of children with autism following massage therapy. J. Autism Dev. Disord. 31, 513–516.

Ezzo, J., Haraldsson, B., Gross, A., et al., 2007. Massage for mechanical neck disorders: a systematic review. Spine 32 (3), 353–362.

Field, T., 1995. Massage therapy for infants and children. J. Dev. Behav. Pediatr. 16 (2), 105–111.

Field, T., 2001. Massage therapy facilitates weight gain in preterm infants. Current Directions in Psychological Science 10, 51–54.

Field, T., Schanberg, S.M., Scafidi, F., et al., 1986. Tactile/kinesthetic stimulation effects on preterm neonates. Pediatrics 77 (5), 654–658.

Field, T., Morrow, C., Valdeon, C., et al., 1992. Massage reduces anxiety in child and adolescent psychiatric patients. J. Am. Acad. Child Adolesc. Psychiatry 31, 125–131.

Field, T., Grizzle, N., Scafidi, F., et al., 1996. Massage and relaxation therapies effects on depressed adolescent mothers. Adolescence 31 (124), 903–911.

Field, T., Ironson, G., Scafidi, F., et al., 1996. Massage therapy reduces anxiety and enhances EEG pattern of alertness and math computations. Int. J. Neurosci. 86, 3–4, 197–205.

Field, T., Hernandez-Reif, M., Quintino, O., et al., 1998. Elder retired volunteers benefit from giving massage therapy to infants. J. Appl. Gerontol. 17, 229–239.

Field, T., Peck, M., Krugman, S., et al., 1998. Burn injuries benefit from massage therapy. J. Burn Care Rehabil. 19 (3), 241–244.

Field, T., Diego, M., Hernandez-Reif, M., et al., 2008. Insulin and insulin-like growth factor-1 increased in preterm neonates following massage therapy. J. Dev. Behav. Pediatr. 29 (6), 463–466.

Flor, H., 2003. Cortical reorganization and chronic pain: implications for rehabilitation. J. Rehabil. Med. 41, 66–72.

Flor, H., Elbert, T., Knecht, S., et al., 1995. Phantom-limb pain as a perceptual correlate of cortical reorganization following arm amputation. Nature 375, 482–484.

Flor, H., Braun, C., Elbert, T., et al., 1997. Extensive reorganization of primary somatosensory cortex in chronic back pain patients. Neurosci. Lett. 224, 5–8.

Furlan, A.D., Brosseau, L., Imamura, M., et al., 2002. Massage for low back pain. Cochrane Database Syst. Rev. 2, CD001929.

Furlan, A.D., Imamura, M., Dryden, T., et al., 2009. Massage for low back pain: An updated systematic review within the framework of the Cochrane back review group. Spine Jun 25 Epub ahead of print.

Grant, K., Balletto, J., Gowan-Moody, D., et al., 2008. Steps toward massage therapy guidelines: a first report to the profession. International Journal of Therapeutic Massage and Bodywork 1 (1), 19–36.

Guzzetta, A., Baldini, S., Bancale, A., et al., 2009. Massage accelerates brain development and the maturation of visual function. J. Neurosci. 29 (18), 6042–6051.

Hernandez-Reif, M., Field, T., Krasnegor, J., et al., 1999. Children with cystic fibrosis benefit from massage therapy. J. Pediatr. Psychol. 24 (2), 175–181.

Hernandez-Reif, M., Field, T., Krasnegor, J., et al., 2001. Lower back pain is reduced and range of motion increased after massage therapy. Int. J. Neurosci. 106, 3–4, 131–145.

Hernandez-Reif, M., Diego, M., Field, T., 2007. Preterm infants show reduced stress behaviors and activity after 5 days of massage therapy. Infant Behav. Dev. 30 (4), 557–561.

Hodge, M., Robinson, C., Boehmer, J., et al., 2002. Employee outcomes following work-site acupressure and massage. In: Rich, G.J. (Ed.), Massage Therapy: The Evidence for Practice. Mosby, St. Louis.

Johnson, D.H., 1995. Bone. Practices of Embodiment. North Atlantic Books, Berkeley, Breath and Gesture.

Juhan, D., 1987. Job's Body: A Handbook for Bodywork. Station Hill Press, New York.

Kerr, C., Wasserman, R., Moore, C., 2007. Cortical plasticity as a therapeutic mechanism for touch healing. J. Altern. Complement. Med. 13 (1), 59–66.

Lawler, S., Cameron, L., 2006. A randomized, controlled trial of massage therapy as a treatment for migraine. Ann. Behav. Med. 32 (1), 50–59.

Lee, H., 2005. The effect of infant massage on weight gain, physiological and behavioral responses in premature infants. Taehan Kanho Hakhoe Chi 35, 1451–1460.

Maihofner, C., Handwerker, H.O., Neundorfer, B., et al., 2003. Patterns of cortical complex regional pain syndrome. Neurology 61, 1707–1715.

Mericq, V., 2006. Prematurity and insulin sensitivity. Horm. Res. 65, 131–136.

Mitanchez, D., 2007. Glucose regulation in preterm newborn infants. Horm. Res. 68, 265–271.

Moyer, C.A., Rounds, J., Hannum, J.W., 2004. A meta-analysis of massage therapy research. Psychol. Bull. 130 (1), 3–18.

Moyer, C.A., Dryden, T., Shipwright, S., 2009. Directions and dilemmas in massage therapy research: a workshop report from the 2009 North American research conference on complementary and integrative medicine. International Journal of Therapeutic Massage and Body Work 2 (2), 15–27.

Pascual-Leone, A., Torres, F., 1993. Plasticity of the sensorimotor cortex representation of the reading finger in Braille readers. Brain 116, 39–52.

Perlman, A., Sabina, A., Williams, A., Njike, V., Katz, D., 2006. Massage therapy for osteoarthritis of the knee: a randomized controlled trial. Arch. Intern. Med. 166.

Preyde, M., 2000. Effectiveness of massage therapy for subacute low-back pain: a randomized controlled trial. Can. Med. Assoc. J. 162, 13.

Price, D., 2002. Central neural mechanisms that interrelate sensory and affective dimensions of pain. Mol. Interv. 2, 392–403.

Richards, K.C., 1998. Effects of a back massage and relaxation intervention on sleep in critically ill patients. Am. J. Crit. Care 7, 288–299.

Sherman, K.J., Cherkin, D.C., Hawkes, R.J., et al., 2006. Randomized trial of therapeutic massage vs. self-care book for chronic neck pain. Altern. Ther. Health Med. 12 (3), 63.

Smith, M.C., Kemp, J., Hemphill, L., et al., 2002. Outcomes of massage therapy for cancer patients. J. Nurs. Scholarsh. 34, 257–262.

Spielberger, C.D., Gorsuch, R.L., Lushene, R.D., 1970. STAI Manual. Consulting Psychologist, Palo Alto.

Tsigos, C., Chrousos, G.P., 2002. Hypothalamic-pituitary-adrenal axis, neuroendocrine factors and stress. J. Psychosom. Res. 53, 865–871.

Uvnas-Moberg, K., Widstrom, A.M., Marchini, G., et al., 1997. Release of GI hormones in mother and infant by sensory stimulation. Acta Paediatr. Scand. 76, 851–860.

Vickers, A., Ohlsson, A., Lacy, J.B., et al., 2004. Massage for promoting growth and development of preterm and/or low birth-weight infants. Cochrane Database Syst. Rev. (2) CD000390.

Walton, T., 1999. Contraindiations to massage part II: taking a health history. Massage Therapy Journal Winter 37 (4), 70–79.

Section Four
Consensus statements

CHAPTER 16

Basic science on somatovisceral interactions: peripheral and central evidence base and implications for research

Wilfrid Jänig

Acknowledgements

The experimental work was supported by the German Research Foundation.

Introduction

The basic philosophy of osteopathic medicine is a 'whole-person' approach to care and to the understanding of the integrative functioning of the body. This approach is also the basis of so-called 'holistic' or 'integrative' medicine (see Chapter 1). It is included both implicitly and explicitly in all manual therapy or other physical interventions directed at the body in the treatment of dysfunctional states (as practiced by chiropractors, physical therapists, massage therapists, and others). This approach uses the biological mechanisms of the body and brain to correct the pathophysiological regulations of the body tissues (see Chapter 1). Beal (1985) described this focus in a more practical and direct way: 'The concept of viscerosomatic reflexes reflects the strong interest of the osteopathic profession in the relationship of the musculoskeletal system in health and disease. It was apparent to early practitioners in the profession that somatic dysfunction was the result of multiple factors – somatic, visceral, and psychologic.... [Thus] The osteopathic profession has held certain basic tenets to be true – that altered or impaired function frequently occurs in the somatic system, that these somatic components may be manifest as presymptomatic signs of disease, and that they may be expressed as local or remote effects of dysfunction as somatovisceral or viscerosomatic reflexes. ... [Therefore] osteopathic manipulative treatment of viscerosomatic reflexes has been advocated on the basis that it is designed to reduce somatic dysfunction, to interrupt the viscerosomatic reflex arcs, to influence the viscus through stimulation of somatovisceral effects, and to reduce the potential preconditioning effect of somatic dysfunctions to body stressors'.

The physiological and hence also the pathophysiological regulation of body tissues involves the brain and its reciprocal communications with the body. The efferent pathways from the brain are the somatomotor, autonomic, and neuroendocrine systems. The afferent pathways from the body tissues to the brain are the large groups of small-diameter (Aδ- and C-) afferents, which monitor the mechanical, thermal, metabolic, and inflammatory states of the tissues (see Chapter 2 and Fig. 2.1).

Manual and other physical interventions at the somatic body tissues do affect the target tissues locally, independent of their innervation on one side (see Chapter 6) and the somatic afferent innervation of these tissues on the other. The consequences of these therapeutic interventions are complex, as stimulation of the afferent neurons activates (1) reflex circuits in the spinal cord, brain stem, and hypothalamus involved in regulation of somatomotor, autonomic, and endocrine systems; (2) neural pathways and centers related to interoceptive body sensations, which include pain, heat, and other sensations from the skin, and pain and other sensations from deep somatic tissues and viscera; and (3) neural circuits related to affective (emotional) feelings.

How do we bring these levels of neural integration together to understand the mechanisms underlying the potentially curative effects of manual interventions on functional disorders in the deep somatic and visceral body domains? Some mechanisms underlying the neural processes potentially operating during manual therapy are discussed in the chapters of this book. Here I will critically discuss the experimental measurements and clinical observations on which the concepts of *somatic dysfunction* and the *dysfunctional spinal segment* are based. This includes the concept of *somatovisceral interactions*. I will concentrate particularly on the spinal autonomic (largely sympathetic) systems. Then I will summarize some aspects of the integrative functions of the spinal cord and potential mechanisms underlying chronic deep somatic and visceral pain. Finally, I will discuss the role of positive feedback mechanisms involving the somatomotor and spinal autonomic systems. I will not address the philosophical superstructure of osteopathic medicine that is related to 'spirit, mind, brain and body' (but see Introduction and Figure 2.1 in Chapter 2).

Systems and mechanisms involved in manual therapy

Various systems believed to be important in understanding the effectiveness of manual therapy in osteopathic medicine (but also in other medical fields independent of osteopathic medicine) and various underlying mechanisms have been discussed in this book. The common theme in all chapters (with the exception of Chapter 6) is that the integrative action of the central nervous system (which includes the spinal cord!) stands in the center to provide the mechanisms operating in manual therapy. Here I highlight the main topics that have been discussed:

1. Use of the body's recuperative power and the promotion of self-healing in the therapeutic approach of manual medicine (Chapters 1, 9, 10, 12, 13, 15).

2. Integration of brain, body, and mind in the holistic (integrative) approach of manual medicine. Manual medicine as part of complementary and alternative medicine (Chapters 1, 11, 12, 15).

3. The role of the musculoskeletal system, including joints, fascia, and other deep somatic tissues of the spine in the generation of dysfunctional states of deep somatic tissues and viscera, and in the curative effects of manual therapy (Chapters 1, 3, 7, 12, 13, 14).

4. Close interaction between the somatic body domain (in particular deep somatic) and the visceral body domain (somatovisceral interaction) (Chapters 2, 3, 4, 7, 8, 12, 13).

5. Regulation of autonomic targets in the viscera, deep somatic tissues, and skin by the sympathetic nervous system (Chapters 2, 3, 4, 5, 7).

6. Integration of afferent information from deep somatic tissues (in particular skeletal muscle, fascia, and joints of the spine) and its control by supraspinal centers. This integration is believed to be essential in the curative effects of manual therapy to induce changes in the motor systems (skeletal muscle, targets of the sympathetic nervous system) and in the ascending systems related to body sensations, including pain (Chapters 2, 3, 4, 7).

7. Chronic pain in deep somatic tissues (in particular skeletal muscle, fascia, and joints) and viscera. This pain is related to the activation of small-diameter spinal (and trigeminal) afferents from deep somatic tissues (in particular the spine) and viscera, and integrative mechanisms of the central nervous system (Chapters 2, 6, 7, 13, 14).

8. Systemic effects of manual therapy based on central integration of neural regulation of skeletal muscle by the somatomotor system, neural regulation of viscera, blood vessels, and other targets by the autonomic nervous system, neuroendocrine regulation in stress and antistress, and neural regulation of pain behavior (Chapters 7, 8, 9, 10).

Somatic dysfunction and the spinal segmental dysfunction

The scientific basis of osteopathic medicine is related to pathobiological[1] processes in deep somatic tissues, in particular of the spine, and in the viscera; to the role of the afferent and efferent (somatomotor and autonomic) innervation of the diseased tissues; to the integrative neural processes in the spinal cord; and to supraspinal control. This is reflected in the osteopathic practice that consists – to put it simply – of the diagnosis and treatment of (1) structural changes in deep somatic tissues of the spine; (2) restricted mobility of skeletal muscle, joints, and fascia; and (3) changes in soft tissue consisting of alterations of local circulation, muscle tone, deep tissue sensitivity (discomfort and pain); and texture of deep tissues ('trophic changes') (Johnston 1992, Patriquin 2003; see Chapter 12). Interactions occur between the neural and non-neural components, between different deep somatic compartments, between deep somatic and visceral tissues, and between spinal and supraspinal neural circuits. Improvements in the diagnosis and treatment of functional diseases depend greatly on our understanding of the mechanisms of these interactions. In the center of both stands the concept of somatic dysfunction (previously called osteopathic lesion) and the concept of spinal segmental dysfunction (also called lesioned segment, or dysfunctional segment or facilitated segment).

The scientific basis of the 'philosophy of osteopathy' as it is propagated today (Chila 2010; Chapter 1 in this book) was first formulated in its full extent by Korr in 1947 and 1948, and has remained practically unchanged up to the present (Korr 1947, 1948, 1955a,b, 1978, 1979). For example, his keynote article published in 1948

---

[1]Pathobiology includes pathological, functional, structural, biochemical, and psychobiological processes.

in the *Journal of the American Osteopathic Association* was reprinted in the same journal in 2000 without further comments or interpretations in the light of modern research.[2] Korr himself has directed and conducted research in this field, in particular related to spinal sympathetic outflow, in order to give support to his concept (Korr et al. 1958, 1962, 1964, Wright et al. 1960). Korr's scientific ideas and research are mainly rooted in the experimental work of Denslow on the somatomotor system (Denslow 1944; Denslow & Clough 1941; Denslow & Hassett 1942; Denslow et al. 1947) and in the experimental work of Kellgren and Lewis on referred pain and hyperalgesia in the deep somatic tissues and viscera (Kellgren 1938, 1939, 1940, Lewis & Kellgren 1939, Lewis 1942).

The neural concept underlying osteopathic medicine

In the paper 'The neural basis of the osteopathic lesion', Korr (1947) states (I quote this because it makes clear what Korr foreshadowed in his future research and in his overall concept [bold and explanations in squared brackets are from me]):

Four of the main principles in osteopathy appear to be:

1. *Joints and their supports are subject to anatomic and functional derangements.*
2. *These derangements have distant as well as local effects.*

3. *They are related, directly or indirectly, to other pathological influences.*
4. *They may be recognized, and their local and distant effect influenced favorably by manipulation.*

Accepting the existence of joint derangements (osteopathic lesions), it is our purpose in this paper to examine not the mechanical and etiological factors involved, but rather the fundamental basis for principle 2 and 3 [i.e. the neural basis of these principles] and to a small extent principle 4,…

The osteopathic lesion has many aspects which are partly revealed in the local and distant effects referred to as principle 2. Included among these are:

1. *Hyperesthesia, especially of the muscle and the vertebrae [i.e., pain and hyperalgesia].*
2. *Hyperexcitability, reflected in altered muscular activity and in altered states of muscle contraction.*
3. *Changes in tissue texture of muscle, connective tissue, and skin [trophic changes].*
4. *Changes in local circulation and in the exchange between blood vessels and tissues.*
5. *Altered visceral and other autonomic functions.*

How are these effects produced? What are the central factors [factors depending on the central nervous system] responsible for these manifestations of structural and postural abnormalities? What in the intrinsic nature of the osteopathic lesion is the basis for the peripheral, palpable, and clinical effects? What fundamental [neural] changes take place as a result of effective manipulative therapy? [To date, none of these questions have been answered].

---

[2]Lederman (2000) was entirely right in the introductory sentence to his paper 'Facilitated segment: a critical review': *The concept of spinal facilitated segments has dominated osteopathic neurophysiology for over half this century. This concept has been at the heart of osteopathic teachings and is often used both in clinical diagnosis and as part of the rationale of treating different musculoskeletal and visceral conditions. Surprisingly, such an important subject has never been criticized: the existence of facilitated segments and their relevance to manual therapy or osteopathic medicine has never been questioned.*

After an extensive discussion Korr concludes:

*An **osteopathic lesion** represents a **facilitated segment** of the spinal cord maintained in that state by impulses [in primary afferent neurons] of endogenous origin entering the corresponding dorsal root. All structures receiving efferent nerve fibers from that segment are, therefore, potentially exposed to excessive excitation or inhibition.*

Under the heading **Manipulative Therapy** at the end of the paper, Korr states:

*…Since the excessive tendinous and muscular tension produced around a joint, let us say, by some bony displacement tends reflexly to produce more tension, **the manipulative easing of tension breaks a vicious cycle** [involving skeletal muscle, its afferent and efferent innervation, and the spinal cord; see pages 289–291].*

*Still another type of vicious cycle may be in operation and be broken by manipulative therapy… Through **overexcitation of sympathetic fibers** in the segment of lesion, **visceral pathology may be established**. The anterior horn cells may then be subjected to additional bombardment with impulses conveyed by visceral afferents, thus causing exaggeration of the somatic lesion … **Manipulative relaxation of the muscles may break this cycle, too,** [involving the sympathetic outflow to targets in skeletal muscle, e.g. blood vessels or other targets, or visceral targets and feedback via small-diameter afferents and spinal cord] through diminution of proprioceptor discharge into the cord….*

What is stated here in one of the first papers by Korr was repeatedly formulated by him in the subsequent 30 years (see, for example,

Korr 1978). Korr and co-workers developed their own methods to record the electrical skin response (dependent on the activity in sudomotor neurons [Thomas & Korr 1951, 1957, Thomas et al. 1958]), and the blood flow through skin (dependent on activity in cutaneous vasomotor neurons [Wright et al. 1960, Wright & Korr 1965]). Korr (1951) endeavored to develop methods to measure:

1. Blood flow through deep somatic tissues (which is dependent on activity in muscle vasoconstrictor neurons [and local changes]) using special thermocouples inserted into skeletal muscle, tendon, or ligaments;
2. Abnormalities in texture (hardness, resilience) in skeletal muscle and skin (trophic changes);
3. Chemical and metabolic changes in skeletal muscle;
4. Sensory changes such as spontaneous pain, hyperalgesia, and hyperexcitability in the tissues (skeletal muscle, skin, viscera); and
5. Changes in viscera using roentgenologic and other techniques.

Korr's idea was to measure both systematically and quantitatively in humans (healthy subjects and patients) changes in the output channels of the spinal cord (to skeletal muscle, to autonomic targets in somatic tissues and viscera, to supraspinal centers [responsible for generating the sensations, including pain]) under controlled conditions in order to learn about the mechanisms underlying the osteopathic lesion and the facilitated segment. For Korr it was clear that both animals and more direct methods, such as electrophysiology, have to be used in research.

Korr hoped to work out why manual therapeutic interventions can be successful and how these interventions can be optimized to generate better and mechanism-based manual treatments. This was a modern research concept. Korr was fully aware that the main problems to be solved are (1) to work out the mechanism of the lesion process (preferentially in the skeletomotor system of the spine); (2) to learn about as to how this lesion process develops over time, i.e. to study its development under chronic conditions; and (3) how this lesion process is modulated (enhanced or attenuated) by supraspinal centers, in particular the telencephalon (Korr 1951).

Korr's conclusions

Korr concluded from his research, using the measurements of the electrical skin response and cutaneous vasomotor response, that:

1. The activity in the sympathetic neurons to skin increased in patients with an osteopathic lesion;
2. This increase in activity in sympathetic neurons is restricted to a spinal segment and its neighboring segments;
3. This increased activity is a sign of increase of activity in *all* sympathetic outflow channels of these segments (i.e., also to the viscera and to the deep somatic tissues); and
4. This increased activity in sympathetic neurons indicates a general increase of excitability in these spinal segments (hence also of the somatomotor system, and of the systems mediating the afferent information to supraspinal centers) (Fig. 16.1).

Korr believed that the main 'motor' or origin of the increased excitability is located in the (paraspinal) musculoskeletal system, and that it is maintained by multiple positive feedback circles (vicious circles) between skeletal muscle and spinal cord, as well as between viscera and spinal cord. Any neural impulse activity impinging on the facilitated segment was to contribute to this process, whether originating in the musculoskeletal system, the viscera, or supraspinal centers. By the same token he argued that therapeutic interventions at the deep somatic tissues (in particular of the spine), the skin, or the forebrain could interrupt this pathophysiological process.

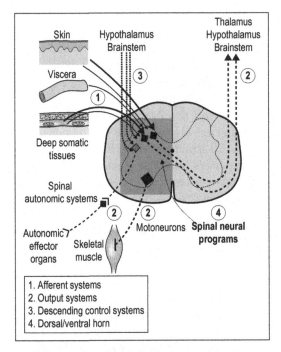

Figure 16.1 The spinal cord as integrative organ.
1, Afferent inputs from skin, deep somatic tissues and viscera; *2*, efferent outputs to skeletal muscles, autonomic effector cells (organs), supraspinal brain centers and other spinal segments; *3*, descending systems from supraspinal centers (in brain stem and hypothalamus) to modulate processing of information from body tissues by neurons in the spinal gray; *4 (shaded box)*, ensemble of spinal neuronal programs ('spinal reflex circuits') processing transmission of activity in afferent neurons and systems projecting from supraspinal centers to the output systems of the spinal cord (see 2). After Jänig (2005).

Korr's concept in the light of modern neurobiological research

Is Korr's concept, which is at the heart of teaching, diagnosis, and treatment in osteopathic medicine (Lederman 2000), supported by modern neurobiological research? Here I will raise some critical questions in the light of such research conducted in the fields of pain and the autonomic nervous system. These critical remarks do not belittle what Korr has tried to achieve: Korr was modern in his time, as he tried to formulate testable scientific questions.

1. The research strategy recommended by Korr to explore the neural mechanisms

of the osteopathic lesion and of the facilitated segment was absolutely correct. However, the actual design of the investigations was too much guided to justify the concept of the facilitated segment. Furthermore, the investigations conducted so far lack sound quantification and statistical comparisons, thereby weakening the conclusions drawn. This is of course also related to the technical limitations of the 1950s and 1960s that Korr was struggling with.

2. The mechanisms of the facilitated segment are explained by a general increase in the excitability of all systems in the spinal cord. I question whether these conclusions are sufficiently supported by the data that have been published.

3. In Chapter 2 of this book I stated that the sympathetic nervous system consists of many functional subsystems which are defined by the targets they innervate and regulate. In the periphery these systems consist of separate pre- and postganglionic channels that transmit the centrally generated impulse activity to the target cells. Every peripheral sympathetic pathway is connected to distinct neural circuits in the spinal cord, brain, and hypothalamus. Thus, I am skeptical that generalizations about the activity in sympathetic systems occurring under pathophysiological conditions such as Korr has made can be substantiated. From the increase in electrodermal skin responses generated during quasi-experimental interventions in humans, it cannot be inferred that the activity of sympathetic systems innervating skeletal muscle or viscera has also increased.

4. Korr's generalization about sympathetic activity and his connecting this increase in sympathetic activity with the generation of diseases (e.g., in the viscera or deep somatic structures) and its decrease with the curative effects of manual therapy is questionable and unjustified, at least when based on the human or animal studies conducted so far. How important this concept was in Korr's view can be seen from the title of his article 'Sustained sympathicotonia as a factor of disease' (Korr 1978).

5. The idea of vicious circles (positive feedback loops) involving skeletal muscle, viscera, and spinal cord is fascinating (see Chapter 7). However, this idea was not supported by the experimental data. It is still very much debated and remains an enigma, as we lack convincing experimental investigations on animal models and humans to support this concept (see below).

6. The integration between spinal circuits connected to the efferent motor systems (somatomotor system, sympathetic systems), the ascending tract neurons, and supraspinal control centers (see Fig. 16.1) is important in order to understand the mechanisms underlying the changes in the myotomes, viscera, and dermatomes. Korr knew this. He nonetheless assumed that the neural processes in the spinal cord (which include inhibitory and excitatory interneurons and output neurons) dictate the pathophysiological processes.

7. What is the experimental and clinical evidence (quantitative data) for osteopathic medicine to focus in teaching, clinical diagnosis, and treatment, primarily on the paraspinal skeletomotor system? In other words, why is the paraspinal skeletomotor system at the center of osteopathic medicine? What is functionally special with this system in relation to health and disease?

8. Korr showed that individual healthy subjects have specific (spatially relative invariant) patterns of electrodermal skin responses. He inferred that these patterns are enhanced during visceral diseases or myofascial diseases of the paraspinal apparatus (Korr et al. 1958, 1962). What is the quantitative evidence to support this conclusion? It has never been systematically studied in individual subjects that patterns of electrodermal skin responses present in healthy conditions remain invariant, but become stronger in intensity during disease. This does not question the findings of Beal and others that visceral diseases (e.g., of the heart, respiratory tract, different sections of the gastrointestinal tract, kidney, pelvic organs) are manifested in somatic tissues (deep somatic [myotomes, sklerotomes], skin [dermatomes]) in typical segmental patterns (Beal 1983, 1985, Beal & Dvorak 1984, Beal & Kleiber 1985, Beal & Morlock 1984, Hansen & Schliack 1962, Johnston et al. 1987, Schliack & Schiffter 1976).

9. The concept of the 'facilitated segment' and the 'osteopathic lesion' is interesting and fascinating. However, it needs better support based on quantitative measurements conducted in patients, healthy subjects, and animal models.

10. Research on human subjects (healthy controls, patients) is needed in which the sensory changes (including pain and discomfort) are compared quantitatively with the changes in skin (in the referred zones, dermatomes), in skeletal muscle (paraspinal and other; in the referred myotomes), and in the viscera (if possible).

Conclusion

Based on clinical observations and measurements in humans, Korr formulated the concept of the 'osteopathic lesion' (now somatic dysfunction) and the 'facilitated segment' (now spinal segmental dysfunction). He formulated testable scientific questions or hypotheses and tried to test them in human subjects, measuring changes in skin resistance and cutaneous blood flow. The attraction of Korr's concept was that it included the somatic and autonomic motor components in explaining the mechanisms of functional deep somatic and visceral diseases. Thus, it was an integrative concept. Unfortunately, this concept was not developed further, and Korr's investigations were not systematically followed. Thus, his ideas and conclusions were never challenged. Today we have the tools to do so.

The spinal cord as integrative organ

Organization of the spinal cord and its output systems

In Chapters 2 and 7 it was emphasized that the spinal cord is an integrative organ in its own right in the regulation of activity in spinal preganglionic neurons, and hence in the neural regulation of autonomic effector organs by spinal autonomic systems. The same principle applies to the regulation of activity in somatomotor neurons and hence of skeletal muscles. Thus the spinal cord contains a wealth of excitatory and inhibitory interneurons (segmental, propriospinal) which are involved in the following functions (Fig. 16.1):

1. Transmission and processing of afferent activity from the peripheral tissues (skin deep somatic tissues, viscera) to the output systems (somatomotor neurons, preganglionic neurons, ascending tract neurons projecting to brain stem, hypothalamus, and thalamus; 2 in Fig. 16.1).

2. Modulation of transmission of activity from premotor neurons located in the brain stem, hypothalamus, or cortex (for somatomotor neurons) to somatomotor neurons and to preganglionic neurons

involved in the regulation of autonomic targets in somatic tissues or in the regulation of viscera (3 in Fig. 16.1). In this important function, activity in premotor neurons projecting to the spinal cord and activity in spinal circuits involving different groups of spinal excitatory and inhibitory interneurons are integrated (see pp. 28–35 [Spinal Cord] and Figs. 2.10 and 2.11 in Chapter 2).

3. Control of synaptic transmission from primary afferent neurons to second-order neurons in the dorsal horn by systems in the brain stem (this probably applies not only to transmission of nociceptive impulse activity, but most likely also to transmission of activity in all functional types of small-diameter afferent neurons [Aδ- and C-fibers] which monitor the mechanical, thermal, and metabolic states of the body tissues) (3 in Fig. 16.1).

4. Coordination of somatomotor systems, spinal autonomic systems, and systems controlling the synaptic transmission of afferent activity to second-order neurons.

The number of spinal interneurons (segmental and propriospinal) outnumber the number of spinal output neurons (motor neurons, preganglionic neurons, neurons projecting to supraspinal centers in brain stem, hypothalamus, and thalamus [ascending tract neurons]) by one order of magnitude (Polgar et al. 2004, Spike et al. 2003), indicating how important these interneurons are in the integrative activity of the spinal cord. Furthermore, in primates (and probably other mammalian species as well) the number of supraspinal neurons projecting to the spinal cord is probably much higher than the number of ascending tract neurons projecting to supraspinal centers, indicating how powerful the supraspinal control of spinal circuits is. This is also reflected in the fact that the volume of the spinal cord is about 2% of the volume of the brain in primates, but 35% in the rat (Swanson 1995).

This argues that top-down control by the telencephalon is becoming quantitatively more important with the encephalization in evolution. It does not argue that the results we obtained in research on rodents do not apply to humans.

The dorsal horn of the spinal cord (and the trigeminal nucleus) can be divided functionally into three parts (Craig 2003a, 2008a, Dostrovsky & Craig 2006). This subdivision is somewhat speculative and not generally accepted. However, it helps to distinguish integrative aspects of interoception[3] (pain in the three body domains, thermal sensations, other sensations of the skin [e.g., itch, sensual touch], sensations of the deep somatic tissues, visceral sensations, etc.), of exteroception (pressure, touch, vibration), and of regulation of somatomotor neurons and spinal preganglionic neurons:

1. The neurons in the superficial laminae I and II of the dorsal horn preferentially serve interoception of the body, and probably are also involved in autonomic reflexes. The ascending tract neurons in lamina I transmit impulse activity in afferent neurons with small-diameter (Aδ- and C-) fibers (from nociceptors, thermoreceptors, chemoreceptors in the skin; from mechanoreceptors and chemoreceptors in deep somatic tissues [skeletal muscle, joints, fascia] or viscera). These ascending tract neurons are specialized or relatively specialized with respect to the different types of afferent input (at least for the skin). Some of these lamina 1 tract neurons are convergent (wide dynamic range) neurons. Lamina I tract neurons project mainly to the posterior part of the ventromedial nucleus of the thalamus (VMpo), which in turn projects to the dorsal posterior insular cortex (dpINS). They also project to various nuclei in the brain stem and hypothalamus, and to the medial

[3]See Craig (2002, 2003c, 2008b) and pages 16–18 in Chapter 2 for the definition of interoception.

thalamus. The VMpo is developed in primates, particularly in humans, and appears to be either absent or rudimentary in other species, such as rats (Craig 2003a, 2004, Craig & Blomquist 2002). In the VMpo and the dpINS the body tissues are topographically represented. The dpINS is the interoceptive cortex (sometimes also called 'limbic sensory cortex') according to Craig (Craig 2002, 2003b,c, 2008b).

2. Lamina II (substantia gelatinosa Rolandi) contains only interneurons and propriospinal neurons, but no ascending tract neurons. This lamina is preferentially specialized for processing information in small-diameter afferents from the skin.

3. Laminae III and IV of the dorsal horn, together with the dorsal column–medial lemniscal system, serve exteroception and proprioception.

4. Most ascending tract neurons (and interneurons) in the deep dorsal horn (lamina V, VI, VII, X) can be activated by afferent neurons with Aβ-fibers as well as afferent neurons with small-diameter (Aδ- and C-) fibers (which include nociceptive afferents). They are convergent ('wide dynamic range') neurons which have large receptive fields and receive convergent afferent inputs from the three body domains. Their synaptic activation by stimulation of afferent neurons is mostly not monosynaptic and not modality specific. Ascending tract neurons in these laminae project to special nuclei in the thalamus that project to the somatomotor cortex. These tract neurons (and therefore also the interneurons in the spinal laminae of the deep dorsal horn) serve motor control (somatomotor and probably autonomic motor control); they are probably not involved in pain sensations or other interoceptive sensations (Craig 2006, 2008a, Craig & Zhang 2006). However,

this subject is controversially discussed (Craig & Blomqvist 2002, Willis et al 2002, Willis & Coggeshall 2004).

These data and neurophysiological studies of spinal autonomic systems (see Chapter 2 in this book and Chapters 4 and 9 in Jänig 2006) strongly argue that the spinal cord contains the neural machineries that could explain the reciprocal relations between the three body domains (skin, deep somatic tissues, viscera). Thus they could explain:

1. Why functional diseases or dysfunctional states of viscera or deep somatic structures are expressed in changes to the corresponding dermatomes and myotomes;

2. Why manual and other interventions in one body domain (e.g., skin or paraspinal musculoskeletal system) could have beneficial effects on the corresponding diseased body tissues; and

3. Why supraspinal centers controlling the spinal circuits are important in interactions between the different body tissues.

Functional plastic changes of dorsal horn neurons in the spinal cord

Inflammation of peripheral tissues leads to sensitization of nociceptive primary afferent neurons (Fig. 16.2). This is reflected in the following changes of the nociceptive afferent neurons: development of ongoing (spontaneous) activity; decreased activation threshold and larger responses upon mechanical or thermal stimulation; and recruitment of mechanoinsensitive (silent) afferent neurons with unmyelinated axons. The cellular and subcellular (molecular) mechanisms of this sensitization are partially known, at least for the acute phase of sensitization (Hucho & Levine 2007, Julius & McCleskey 2006, Meyer et al. 2006, Ringkamp & Meyer 2009, Woolf & Ma 2007). However, it is debated whether the mechanisms of sensitization are the same in the chronic stage.

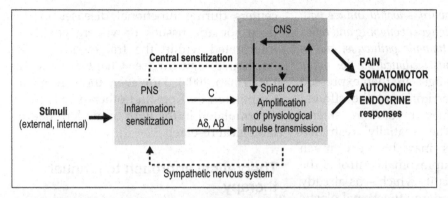

Figure 16.2 Concept of generation of peripheral and central hyperexcitability during stimulation of nociceptors (e.g., by inflammation) leading to pain. The pain is always associated with motor, autonomic, and endocrine responses. The upper interrupted arrow indicates that the central changes are generated (and possibly maintained) by persistent activity of nociceptors with unmyelinated (C-) fibers (e.g., during chronic inflammation) called here 'central sensitization'. The lower interrupted arrow indicates the potential efferent feedback via the sympathetic nervous system (including the sympathoadrenal system) (see Fig. 16.4). The transmission of nociceptive impulses is under multiple control of the brain (arrows upper right). The sensitization of nociceptors entails sensitization of central neurons (e.g., in the dorsal horn) and changes of the central representations (of the somatosensory system) which may become irreversible. The central changes, induced by persistent activity in afferent nociceptive neurons, are also reflected in the activity of sympathetic systems and somatomotor systems that may establish positive feedback loops to the primary afferent neurons. CNS, central nervous system; PNS, peripheral nervous system.

The sensitization of nociceptive primary afferent neurons generates a sensitization of second-order neurons (interneurons, tract neurons) in the spinal (or trigeminal) dorsal horn, called *central sensitization*. It is expressed as an amplification of transmission of nociceptive impulses in the dorsal horn, and is a short-term functional plastic change of dorsal horn neurons (Fig. 16.2). Phenomenologically, this sensitization consists of the development or increase of ongoing activity, decrease of threshold and increase of activation to peripheral mechanical or thermal stimulation, enlargement and development of new receptive fields in the peripheral tissues, and the development of responses to novel stimuli. The underlying mechanisms are related to the local inhibitory and excitatory interneurons and to changes in the descending control systems. The molecular translational and transcriptional changes, including the changes in the glial cells, occur over minutes, hours, and days. Many of these changes have been explored and can be described (Julius & McCleskey 2006, Latremoliere & Woolf 2009, McMahon

et al. 2006, Sandkühler 2009, Woolf & Salter 2006). Whether the mechanisms of sensitization in the spinal cord are the same in acute and chronic conditions is debated.

The plastic functional changes in the dorsal horn may be followed or paralleled by functional plastic changes in supraspinal centers such as the brain stem, hypothalamus, thalamus, and telencephalon. This in turn will change the supraspinal control of the spinal circuits (3 in Fig. 16.1; Fields et al. 2006, Heinricher & Ingram 2009, Ren & Dubner 2009).

Whatever the detailed mechanisms of chronic sensitization of dorsal horn neurons under pathophysiological conditions and the subsequent changes in supraspinal centers (including telencephalon) are, it is not far-fetched to assume that these changes occur in *all* second-order neurons receiving nociceptive synaptic afferent input and transmitting and processing afferent activity to ascending tract neurons, preganglionic neurons or somatic motor neurons. *Thus, during disease of a visceral organ or a deep somatic structure, persistent activity in nociceptive afferent neurons would induce pain and discomfort and changes of ongoing and reflex activity in spinal autonomic pathways, and in somatic motor neurons mediated by the spinal cord.* The neural changes are then expressed in the projection territories of the efferent neurons (dermatomes, myotomes, sclerotomes, viscera). The spatially restricted functional changes may be very much dependent on the supraspinal control of the spinal neuronal circuits which – as already mentioned – also undergo functional plastic changes. Whether these changes are maintained by a very low rate of ongoing activity in peripheral nociceptive afferent neurons or whether they may become independent of this activity in chronic conditions needs to be explored.

One component addressed below is feedback via the spinal autonomic systems and the somatomotor system to the peripheral body tissues (Fig. 16.2; see also Fig. 16.4). Under physiological conditions the activity in the efferent neurons to the effectors and the activity in the spinal and vagal afferent neurons innervating the effectors are entirely in balance (see Chapter 7). However, in pathophysiological conditions both may form feedback loops and contribute a further component (see below). One disorder showing this is complex regional pain syndrome (CRPS).[4] CRPS is probably a disorder of the central nervous system involving the somatosensory systems, the sympathetic systems, and the somatomotor system (Jänig & Baron 2002, 2003, Jänig & Levine 2006). In this disorder the efferent sympathetic feedback to the affected extremity may contribute to the changes related to the somatosensory stem (including the nociceptive systems), the sympathetic nervous system, and the somatomotor system.

These multiple mechanisms operating in the spinal dorsal horn and supraspinal centers during functional diseases in the deep somatic tissues or viscera could be interpreted within the framework of the 'facilitated segment' (see Chapters 1 and 12; Lederman 2000). However, the concept as formulated by Korr and others needs to be reformulated in the light of modern neurobiological research.

Theoretical approach to manual therapy

Any therapy for functional disorders in the somatic deep tissues or viscera should be anchored in the peripheral and central nervous system mechanisms that underlie those disorders. In view of the lack of detailed knowledge about these mechanisms, it is not surprising that most suggested treatments are based purely on practical experience, i.e., they are empirical. However, as discussed in this book, it can clearly be concluded that the consequences of such therapeutic interventions should occur both at the periphery of the body (i.e., at the deep somatic tissues or skin) and centrally. This applies to manual, physical, occupational, and 'psychological' therapies. Taking the example of complex regional pain syndrome (CRPS),[4] some of these therapies are indeed to a certain degree mechanism based. This applies to the mirror image therapy and mirror image program (McCabe et al. 2003, 2008, Moseley 2004, 2005, 2006), to sympathetic blocks, and to various types of physical therapy (Baron 2006, 2009).

Manual and related therapies acting on deep somatic body tissues or skin areas related to them or viscera 'manipulate' the different integration centers in the brain (spinal cord, brain stem, hypothalamus, telencephalon) by stimulating the populations of small-diameter afferents innervating skin or deep somatic tissues that monitor the mechanical, thermal, and metabolic states of these tissues (Jänig 2009b). Thus these therapies may affect the diseased

---

[4]See footnote 8.

tissues via the spinal reflex circuits and via the supraspinal centers and – as has been shown in patients with CRPS – may contribute to the correction of the mismatch between the afferent inflow from the body tissues (and this includes the nociceptive as well as the non-nociceptive afferent feedback) and the neural programs that regulate the somatomotor and the autonomic motor outflow to the affected tissues. The correction of the mismatch potentially occurs on all central integration levels, starting in the spinal cord, leading to normal somatic sensations (including a reduction in pain), normal perception of the affected extremity, normal motor behavior, and normal regulation of autonomic parameters by the sympathetic nervous system (i.e., blood flow, sweating and texture of skin; edema and consistency of subcutaneous tissue; tone, irritability, consistency, viscoelastic properties and fluid content of skeletal muscle; texture changes in deep fascial layers and joint capsules; secretion and motility of visceral organs; and blood flow through visceral organs).[5] In fact, a very promising and exciting development is the mirror image therapy and mirror image program as propagated by McCabe and co-workers (2003, 2008) and Moseley (2004, 2005, and 2006) for patients with CRPS.

---

[5]It is commonly assumed that the texture of the skin, subcutaneous edema, and consistency, fluid content and consistency of skeletal muscle, and texture changes in deep fascial layers and joint capsules are dependent on the sympathetic innervation. However, this assumption is based solely on the segmental innervation of the tissues by sympathetic postganglionic neurons, and not on functional studies. Furthermore, peptidergic primary afferent neurons with unmyelinated fibers may also be involved, e.g., by activity-dependent release of substance P and CGRP (calcitonin gene-related peptide), leading acutely to neurogenic inflammation, and chronically probably to other changes related to the trophic changes (see Jänig 2006, Chapter 2; Jänig 1993; Schaible et al 2005). In essence, the neural mechanisms underlying these tissue changes and developing remotely from the diseased visceral or deep somatic tissues are unknown. See page 35 in Chapter 2.

Conclusion

The spinal cord (and the trigeminal region) is an active neural interface between body tissues and brain in the regulation of skeletal muscle, autonomic targets, and tissue sensations. It is the main input and output gate from and to the body tissues, the other gate to and from the visceral organs being the nucleus of the solitary tract together with the dorsal motor nucleus of the vagus and the nucleus ambiguus. The spinal cord contains the neural circuits to process incoming information from the body tissues and relay it to supraspinal centers. It contains the circuits that shape the patterns of signals in the efferent, somatomotor, and autonomic output systems to the body tissues. Supraspinal centers (in brain stem, hypothalamus, and cerebral hemispheres) use these spinal circuits in their control and coordination of the spinal motor output systems, and in their control of the incoming afferent information from the three body domains. The spinal circuits, together with their supraspinal control, are important for the interaction between the three body domains in health and disease (somatic dysfunction). During disease of deep somatic tissues or viscera the neural regulation of these tissues becomes deficient. The beneficial effect of manual and other physical interventions in the deep somatic tissues of the spine and other somatic body tissues may be mainly mediated by these spinal neural circuits, always in coordination with the supraspinal control independent of their local effects.

Pain behavior and chronic pain as disease

Pain is a complex multidimensional event that cannot be reduced to the nociceptive sensation (sensory-discriminative component) but includes formally the affective component, the cognitive component, and the motor component (somatomotor, autonomic,

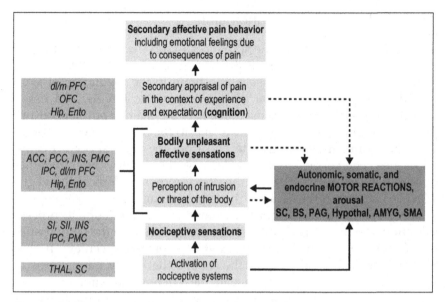

Figure 16.3 The interaction between nociceptive sensations, bodily unpleasant affective sensations, and secondary affective pain behavior and the brain centers possibly involved. Activation of endocrine, somatic, and autonomic motor systems occur on all integrative levels during activation of the centers representing nociception and pain. The mechanisms of activation of these motor systems by higher centers (see interrupted arrows) have been little studied. Simplified scheme. ACC, anterior cingular cortex; AMYG, amygdala; BS, brain stem; Ento, entorhinal cortex; Hip, hippocampus; Hypothal, hypothalamus; INS, insular cortex; IPC, inferior parietal cortex; PAG, periaqueductal gray; PCC, posterior cingulate cortex; PFC, prefrontal cortex (dl, dorsolateral; m, medial); PMC, premotor cortex; SC, spinal cord; SI, SII, primary and secondary somatosensory cortex; SMA, supplementary motor area; THAL, Thalamus. Modified after Casey & Tran (2006) and Price (2000).

neuroendocrine). All dimensions together describe the pain behavior or the secondary affective pain behavior (Fig. 16.3). Using modern imaging and other techniques it has been shown that various centers in spinal cord, brain stem, hypothalamus, and telencephalon are involved in the generation of this pain behavior (Bushnell & Apkarian 2006; Casey & Tran 2006; Lorenz & Tracey 2009; Tracey & Mantyh 2007; Treede & Apkarian 2009) (see left side of Fig. 16.3). They are activated by experimental or natural stimulation of peripheral nociceptive afferent neurons and sometimes globally described as 'neural pain matrix' (Melzack 1999) or 'neural signature of pain' (Tracey & Mantyh 2007). As expected and in accordance with the definition of pain by Price (1999), the higher centers are also activated during imagined painful events without obvious tissue damage, i.e. without an activation of nociceptors. Thus, severe pain can also be experienced without afferent nociceptive or with trivial nociceptive input and this pain is as real as pain emerging during nociceptive afferent input. Neuroimaging studies have emphasized this important point and future investigations probably will show that the mechanisms of this pain are particularly important in chronic pain conditions.

As discussed by Casey and Tran (2006) and Treede and Apkarian (2009), different cortical areas participate in different aspects (components) of pain (sensation, affection, cognition, somatic and autonomic motor responses). We have to keep in mind that:

1. None of these functions can be assigned to only one forebrain structure, i.e., each function is represented in more than one brain structure.

2. Processing of nociceptive information occurs sequentially as well as in parallel. Figure 16.3 does not imply strictly sequential processing. Thus, activation

of ascending nociceptive systems activates cortical systems in parallel as well as sequentially.

3. Cortical systems are activated in overlapping time domains of milliseconds, seconds, hours, and months to years (Casey & Tran 2006). In these time domains early identification and recognition of the nociceptive events, as well as immediate reactions and evaluation of them, and generation of sustained pain behavior occur.

4. Activation of the ascending nociceptive system in the spinal cord or caudal trigeminal nucleus (in particular neurons in the lamina I, see above) and in the thalamus generates nociceptive sensations. These sensations are dependent on the activation of the primary and secondary somatosensory cortices and of the dorsal posterior insular cortex (dpINS) via the posterior ventromedial nucleus of the thalamus (VMpo). The role of the VMpo/dpINS system in the perception of type, localization, duration, and intensity of nociceptive sensations is controversial (Bushnell & Apkarian 2006, Craig 2003a-c, 2004, 2008b, Dostrovsky & Craig 2006).

5. In parallel with the generation of the nociceptive sensation, protective somatic, autonomic, and neuroendocrine processes are activated via the spinal cord, brain stem, hypothalamus, and amygdala and other brain centers in a stereotyped fashion.

6. The generation of nociceptive sensations is followed and paralleled by a perception of bodily unpleasant affective sensations signaling the injury or impending injury. These affective sensations occur during the activation of the insular cortex (presumably also the anterior insular cortex), the anterior and posterior cingulate cortex, the inferior parietal cortex, and the premotor cortex. The activation of the medial thalamus – and probably of the hypothalamus

via a parallel pathway including the parabrachial nucleus (not shown in Fig. 16.3) – is presumably also involved in the generation of this affective pain component.

7. The secondary (cognitive) appraisal of the nociceptive events and attention to them in the context of experience (memory), expectations, and environmental context leads to the secondary affective pain behavior. This behavior is dependent on the activation of the medial and dorsolateral prefrontal cortices, orbitofrontal cortex, the hippocampus, and the entorhinal cortex.

8. During the perception of threat to the body and secondary (cognitive) appraisal, the (somatic, autonomic, neuroendocrine) motor components involving higher brain centers are also activated (see interrupted arrows in Fig. 16.3). These motor components are parts of the secondary affective pain behavior and are orchestrated by the anterior cingulate cortex and the amygdala (Neugebauer et al. 2009).

9. The transmission of nociceptive impulses in the spinal and trigeminal dorsal horn (and probably the transmission of impulses in small-diameter [Aδ-, C-] afferents monitoring the tissue states and associated with non-painful interoceptive sensations) is controlled by supraspinal centers. Activation of these centers, represented in the periaqueductal gray, in the dorsolateral pontine tegmentum and in the ventromedial medulla oblongata (including the caudal raphe nuclei) may generate antinociception or pronociception, depending on the behavioral context. These centers are in turn under the control of the cerebral hemispheres (orbitofrontal cortex, prefrontal cortex, anterior insula, anterior cingulate cortex, etc.; Fields et al. 2006, Heinricher & Ingram 2009, Ren & Dubner 2009).

This sequential and parallel activation of forebrain centers resulting in pain behavior occurs under biological conditions during transient activation of nociceptors or activation of nociceptors in a recuperative (healing) phase, e.g., in inflammatory pain following tissue injury. The imaging studies on which the data are based show forebrain responses in a correlation manner. They do not tell us in which way individual forebrain structures are causally involved in the characteristics of the different components of pain (Apkarian et al. 2005, Treede & Apkarian 2009). It is likely that most brain structures activated during acute pain are also activated during stimulation of other non-nociceptive small-diameter afferent neurons that monitor the metabolic, mechanical, and/or thermal states of the body tissues. As is the case with the nociceptive afferent neurons, activation of which is important for the regulation of protective body processes, the activation of these non-nociceptive afferent neurons is important for many homeostatic regulations. These regulations are paralleled by interoceptive sensations that also have distinct sensory, affective, and cognitive components.

How does this complex neural system behave in chronic pain, i.e., under pathophysiological conditions when pain is no longer a warning sign (Apkarian et al. 2009, Casey & Tran 2006, Mayer & Bushnell 2009)? The example of chronic low back pain may be taken as an example (see Apkarian et al. 2009 and Robinson & Apkarian 2009 for review and literature):

1. Only 5% or less of individuals with acute low back pain develop subacute and then chronic low back pain. The majority (>90%) of individuals with acute low back pain may experience episodes of low back pain, but usually recover in days or weeks.
2. Peripheral physical factors diagnosed radiographical and physical trauma are poorly correlated with the frequency of chronic low back pain.
3. Treatment of low back pain with non-steroidal anti-inflammatory drugs (NSAIDs) or antidepressants is not significantly different in clinical effectiveness from placebo treatment.
4. Psychosocial and psychological factors are poorly correlated with the development of chronic low back pain, i.e. these factors provide poor predictors regarding chronic pain, as is the clinical effectiveness of psychosocial treatment.

This situation of low back pain, as far as the underlying mechanisms, the role of the central nervous system, and current treatment strategies are concerned, may apply to most chronic pain syndromes (Mayer & Bushnell 2009). Imaging studies of chronic low back pain patients show that chronic pain is correlated with plastic changes of cortical brain structures. These are reflected in changes of brain activity, chemistry, and morphology, which are most dramatically expressed in reductions in the volume of gray matter in the prefrontal cortex, reduced activity in cortical structures related to control of sensory processing, and probably leading to loss of control of nociceptive impulse processing. Thus, there may be a change in the balance between or impairments of neural controls of the sensory component, the affective component, and the cognitive component (Apkarian et al. 2009, Robinson & Apkarian 2009, Treede & Apkarian 2009).

What are the consequences for the treatment? Is the body's recuperative power promoting the body's self-healing under these conditions still strong enough to be activated by therapeutic approaches used in manual therapy? A main priority of manual and similar therapies is probably to prevent the development of chronic deep somatic or visceral pain, with its disastrous long-term consequences for the central nervous system, and to prevent the abuse of pharmacological treatments. Are we able to show that manual therapeutic interventions lead to reorganization of cortical centers and repair of maladaptive cortical representations, which are then correlated with attenuation of chronic pain and normal regulation of body functions (Kerr et al. 2007)? This is in accordance with the notion that therapies acting through interventions at somatic body tissues not only influence the spinal and supraspinal reflex centers, but modulate forebrain centers involved in affective (emotional) and cognitive aspects of body sensations, including pain. By the same token, it may be hypothesized that these therapeutic interventions, that act via the forebrain centers, activate the neural motor circuits, resulting in normal coordinated movements. To be more efficient in these manual and related treatments we need a better understanding of the mechanisms underlying deep (somatic and visceral) chronic pain.

Conclusion

The sensory–discriminative, affective, cognitive, and motor (somatic, autonomic, neuroendocrine) components of pain constitute pain behavior. These components are organized in various parts of the telencephalon, diencephalon, and brain stem, forming the 'neural pain matrix' or 'neural signature of pain.' This includes, at the telencephalic level, the primary and secondary somatosensory cortices, the insula, the inferior parietal cortex, the anterior and posterior cingulate cortex, the orbitofrontal cortex, and the medial and lateral prefrontal cortex. At all levels of integration, starting in the spinal cord, the motor components are integrated. How these centers interact, generating the different types of chronic clinical pain, and how they generate chronic pain without obvious tissue damage is poorly understood. By the same token, we do not understand how manual and other physical therapeutic interventions modulate this neural network leading to a reduction in pain.

Are positive feedback mechanisms important?

Can activity in efferent systems enhance the activity in primary afferent nociceptive and non-nociceptive neurons to the spinal cord so as to establish with the spinal reflex circuits positive feedback circles ('vicious circles'; Fig. 16.4)? Such positive feedback mechanisms could maintain the abnormal sensations (e.g., pain and discomfort), the somatomotor activity, and events dependent on the sympathetic outflow

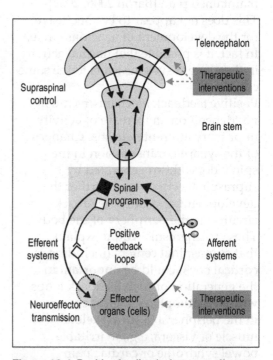

Figure 16.4 Positive feedbacks between efferent systems (motoneurons, autonomic spinal systems), effector cells, spinal afferent systems supplying the body tissues, and spinal cord. The spinal neuronal programs are under supraspinal control. Positive feedback coupling can presumably develop in various ways: by changes of the afferent activity (e.g., sensitization of noziceptive neurons, recruitment of silent [mechoinsensitive] afferents), sensitization of neurons in the spinal cord, changes of neuroeffector transmission, changes of the descending control, etc. The therapeutic interventions may act at the afferent neurons and the effector tissue. Not only peripheral tissues are influenced in this way, but also spinal and supraspinal reflex circuits and processes in the forebrain (hypothalamus, telencephalon).

(e.g., vasoconstrictions with ischemias). They have been postulated by Korr and others (see Chapter 28 in Bonica 1953 and Chapter 15 in Livingston 1943). Whether such efferent feedback mechanisms are important in the generation of pain and associated changes (increase of skeletal muscle tone, vasoconstrictions, etc.) has not been proved beyond doubt.

1. It is tacitly assumed that the activity in the efferent (somatomotor or sympathetic) systems is increased (e.g., in patients with complex regional pain syndrome [CRPS][6] and sympathetically maintained pain [Baron 2006, 2009]). This does not appear to be conclusive for the development of a vicious circle. In fact, it is possible that normal activity in the efferent systems leads to the same changes.

2. Positive feedback mechanisms must not depend on an increase of activity in primary afferent neurons. Changes of the synaptic transmission in the spinal dorsal horn generated by supraspinal centers may further the development of positive feedback circuits via the periphery of the body. These mechanisms would explain that supraspinal centers (including cortical ones) could be important in the generation of such feedback loops, without pathophysiological changes in the peripheral tissues (skeletal muscle or viscera; e.g., in irritable bowel syndrome or cardiac pain [see Chapter 7]).

3. The clinical phenomena suspected to be dependent on positive feedback loops via the peripheral tissues (e.g., pain, changes of somatomotor or autonomic motor activity) can also occur independently of them. Thus, a sympathetically maintained pain (e.g., in patients with CRPS) can clinically only

be diagnosed after blockade of the activity in the sympathetic innervation of the affected extremity.

4. The efferent feedback is mostly only *one* component in the generation of the clinical phenomenology.

5. The concept of positive feedback mechanisms operating via deep somatic tissues or viscera could be important not only to understand the clinical phenomenology in functional disorders of the deep somatic or visceral domains, but also to understand the mechanisms by which manual and other physical therapies applied to the body surface or the deep somatic tissues work. These therapies activate small-diameter myelinated and unmyelinated afferents (by manipulation of the effector tissues) that monitor the state of the body tissues, and may interrupt the positive feedback loops involving the somatomotor and autonomic neuronal programs in spinal cord and supraspinal centers which control somatomotor and autonomic regulation, as well as the transmission of impulse activity in the dorsal horn (Fig. 16.4). However, this interesting idea, which is implicit in the neurobiological concept of osteopathic manual therapy, is hypothetical and not yet supported by experimental data. We need quantitative investigations on patients (and healthy subjects) and from animal experiments in vivo to test this idea.

Role of feedback mechanisms in pain of the skeletomotor system

Pain in skeletal muscle is dependent on the excitation of small-diameter myelinated (Aδ-) and unmyelinated (C-) afferents. Knowledge about spinal mechanisms and their supraspinal control, as well as the thalamocortical mechanism underlying these pains (see Figs. 16.2, 16.3), is still incomplete (Graven-Nielsen et al. 2008, Mense 1993,

---

[6]See footnote 8 for CRPS.

Mense & Simons 2001, Schaible 2006, Schaible & Grubb 1993). The excitation of the nociceptors may also be dependent on the tone of the skeletal musculature that is regulated via the α- and γ-motor neurons. The mechanisms by which activity in the motor neurons can contribute to excitation and/or sensitization of nociceptive muscle and other deep somatic afferents and can lead to form a positive feedback to the spinal cord that maintains the excitation of nociceptors, the central sensitization, the muscle pain, and the increased tone of skeletal muscle are poorly understood (Mense & Simons 2001).

The excitation and/or sensitization of deep somatic nociceptive afferents is presumably generated by ischemia and other metabolic changes, uncoordinated contractions of motor units (resulting in shearing forces between muscle fibers), and tonic contractions. In myofascial pain syndromes myofascial trigger points in skeletal muscle are hypothesized to be important in the persistent excitation of nociceptors, and to be one component in the positive feedback circle.[7] This persistent excitation of nociceptors in skeletal muscle may maintain a sensitization of dorsal horn neurons, which together with the efferent feedback to skeletal muscle forms the vicious circle. This hypothetical feedback mechanism is at various sites under the control of brain stem and cortex. The supraspinal control may act via various pools of spinal interneurons that are synaptically connected to the α- and γ-motor

neurons and integral components of the spinal motor reflexes. The supraspinal control can principally maintain or attenuate the positive feedback circle. Cortically induced protective motor behavior during chronic pain could perhaps promote such a positive feedback mechanism. Manual interventions at somatic tissues could interrupt this mechanism via the cerebral centers.

The positive feedback mechanisms that are possibly active in the generation of deep somatic pain (including its reference into other deep somatic structures, viscera or possibly skin) appear to be dependent on too many peripheral and central neural variables to be proven. Thus, the concept of the role of a positive feedback mechanism in the maintenance of deep somatic pain and associated changes is difficult to prove experimentally and very much debated (see Johansson et al. and Graven-Nielsen et al. in Johansson et al. 2003, and Chapter 5 in Mense & Simons 2001).

The working model of a positive feedback mechanism of skeletal muscle and spinal cord could explain the therapeutic effects of manual and other physical interventions. These interventions could act via stimulation of spinal afferent neurons (of the deep somatic tissues and skin) and influence integrative neuronal processes in spinal cord and supraspinal centers. This would lead to changes of activity in the efferent neurons (somato-motor neurons, sympathetic neurons), a reduction of activity in nociceptive afferent neurons, and a reduction of pain and discomfort. The therapeutic interventions would also influence the tissues directly, with improvements in the nutritive situation of the tissues in the micromilieu of the nociceptors with decrease of activity in the nociceptors. Interventions at the primary myofascial trigger points in myofascial pain syndromes (manually, by cooling, by needling, by local anesthetic) could also interrupt a positive feedback mechanism (but see footnote 7).

---

[7]The mechanisms underlying the myofascial trigger points and the connected sensitization and excitation of nociceptors with Aδ- and C-fibers are still an enigma. Most cellular mechanisms discussed on the basis of Simon's 'integrated myofascial trigger point hypothesis' are not based on experimental evidence and measurements (see Mense & Simons 2001, Simons 2004). Clinical studies to objectively reproduce the identification of myofascial trigger points, as well as quantitative investigations of the success of therapeutic interventions at the myofascial trigger points, remain incomplete (Lucas et al 2009, Myburgh et al 2008, Tough et al 2009).

Sympathetic nervous system and pain

Patients with complex regional pain syndrome (CRPS)[8] and patients with neuropathic pain may have pain that is dependent on activity in sympathetic neurons innervating the affected extremity. This is called sympathetically maintained pain (SMP) (Baron 2006, 2009). A positive feedback loop via the sympathetic innervation of the affected extremity was postulated under pathophysiological conditions. Efferent sympathetic neurons are directly or indirectly coupled back to primary afferent neurons and contribute to their excitation and/or sensitization (see Fig. 16.2). This concept is based on experimental investigations of patients with SMP and on experimental investigations using animal models (Baron et al. 2002a, Jänig 2002, 2009a, Price et al. 1998, Torebjörk et al. 1995).

Spinal autonomic systems and visceral pain

Visceral pain is dependent on the activation of spinal thoracolumbar or sacral visceral afferent neurons, the synaptic transmission of this afferent impulse activity in the spinal dorsal horn, and its control by supraspinal centers, transmission to supraspinal centers in brain stem and thalamus (probably mainly the posterior ventromedial nucleus in the thalamus [VMpo] of primates [Craig 2004, Craig & Blomquist 2002]), and central cortical representations, one primary representation being probably the interoceptive cortex of the dorsal posterior insula (see Fig. 16.3) (Bielefeld & Gebhart 2006, Craig 2002, 2003b,c, 2008b, Foreman 1999, Gebhart & Bielefelt 2009). Vagal afferents are not involved in visceral pain except for the proximal part of the esophagus and trachea. They are, however, involved in central inhibitory control of transmission of impulses in spinal visceral afferents to second-order neurons in the spinal dorsal horn (see Chapter 7; Jänig 2005, 2006, 2009c).

Here it is hypothesized that spinal autonomic non-vasoconstrictor pathways to visceral organs (see Chapter 2) are probably important in the generation of pain and other sensations in visceral organs. The neurons of these autonomic pathways are integrated in the regulation of the visceral organs. Reflex activity in these spinal autonomic neurons may change when the spinal visceral afferents are continuously active or sensitized, or when normally silent visceral afferent neurons are recruited (Cervero 1994, Jänig 2006, Jänig & Häbler 1995). This process could lead to sensitization of second-order neurons in the spinal dorsal horn. By activating spinal autonomic systems, positive feedback loops might be established between visceral afferent neurons, spinal cord, spinal autonomic systems, and visceral effector organs (e.g., smooth musculature of gastrointestinal tract or urinary bladder; heart). Supraspinal centers, which normally control transmission of synaptic impulses from visceral afferents to second-order neurons in the spinal cord, could promote (or inhibit) these positive feedback loops. Furthermore, changes in supraspinal centers occurring without peripheral visceral trauma and

---

[8]CRPS syndromes were originally known under the terms reflex sympathetic dystrophy or causalgia (or several other terms depending on medical specialty and country; Wilson & Bogduk 2005). However, these terms were thought to be inappropriate as a clinical designation. They were sloppily used to describe an extensive range of clinical presentations, and the pathophysiological mechanisms underlying these syndromes were poorly understood. The new terminology is descriptive and based entirely on elements of history, symptoms, and findings on clinical examination, with no implied pathophysiological mechanism avoiding any mechanistic implications (Stanton-Hicks et al 1995). According to the International Association for the Study of Pain "Classification of Chronic Pain", reflex sympathetic dystrophy and causalgia are now called complex regional pain syndromes (CRPS). In CRPS type I (reflex sympathetic dystrophy) minor injuries at the limb or lesions in remote body areas precede the onset of symptoms. CRPS type II (causalgia) may develop after injury of a major peripheral nerve (Merskey & Bogduk 1994).

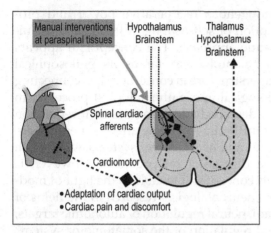

Figure 16.5 Positive feedback between spinal cardiac afferents and sympathetic pathways to the heart involving the spinal cord. A hypothesis. Under physiological conditions afferent feedback from the heart enhances the activity in sympathetic premotor neurons in the rostral ventrolateral medulla and presumably the ventromedial medulla and cardiomotor neurons (CM) directly or indirectly via spinal interneurons. This afferent feedback contributes to the adaptation of cardiac output during exercise. In pathophysiological conditions (e.g., ischemia or stress) activity in the sympathetic cardiomotor neurons may enhance the activity in the spinal cardiac afferents. This leads to cardiac pain and further enhancement of activity in the cardiomotor neurons via the positive feedback loop. The neurons in the dorsal horn of the upper thoracic segments are now sensitized. Manual interventions at paraspinal tissues may lead to activation of deep somatic afferents which may interrupt the positive feedback loop by interfering with the spinal circuits connected to the cardiomotor neurons, cardiac afferents, and supraspinal control systems (see Chapter 7).

without sensitization of visceral spinal afferents could establish feedback loops between visceral organs and spinal cord and lead to visceral pain. These positive feedback loops may turn out to be important mechanisms of cardiac pain without ischemia, non-cardiac chest pain, pain in non-ulcer dyspepsia, pain in irritable bowel disease, and pain in other functional visceral diseases (Bradesi et al. 2009, Cohn et al. 2003, Henningsen 2007, Mayer & Bushnell 2009).

A hypothetical example is demonstrated in Figure 16.5. Resting activity and physiological stimulation of spinal visceral afferents innervating the heart or the large blood vessels elicit no sensations under healthy conditions. This activity is integrated in the neural regulation of the heart (contractility, heart rate). During physical exercise, activity in spinal cardiac afferents synaptically enhances the activation of sympathetic preganglionic cardiomotor neurons (and of interneurons associated with them) generated by sympathetic premotor neurons in the lower brain stem. In this way, cardiac output is adapted and maintained in relation to the level of exercise.

In pathophysiological conditions (e.g., atherosclerotic changes of the coronary arteries, resulting in ischemia), positive feedback coupling may have serious consequences. Cardiac spinal afferent neurons are excited and sensitized by ischemia, which leads to sensitization of neurons in the thoracic spinal dorsal horn, causing cardiac pain with referral to the dermatomes, myotomes, and sklerotomes that correspond to the thoracic spinal segments T2–T6 and C2–C4 (Foreman 1999; see Chapter 7 for details). Whether the spinal cardiac afferents that are excited by ischemia are the same as those that are excited during exercise and increase of cardiac output, or whether a special group of cardiac afferents is excited that has nociceptive functions, we do not know. The latter is tacitly assumed (Coleridge & Coleridge 1980), but this may not be the case at all (Malliani 1982, Malliani et al. 1986). Stimulation of spinal cardiac afferent neurons excites the sympathetic cardiomotor neurons via the cardiocardiac spinal reflex pathway. This activation in turn enhances the excitation of spinal cardiac afferents via an enhanced contraction of the ventricles and an increased heart rate. A positive feedback reflex loop, which adapts the work of the heart under physiological conditions of exercise, may now have fatal consequences under pathophysiological conditions. This idea is discussed in more detail in Chapter 7 (Foreman et al.). It has furthermore been described (1) that the cardiocardiac spinal reflex pathway involving the sympathetic cardiomotor neurons is integrated with a positive feedback circuit between the paraspinal skeletomotor system and the spinal cord, and (2) that this integrated neural feedforward system is under supraspinal excitatory and inhibitory control involving vagal afferents from thoracic organs, the spinoreticular system, the nucleus of the solitary tract, the gigantocellular tegmental field in the lower brain stem, and the spinal segments C1–C2 (see Fig. 7.10 in Chapter 7).

Manual interventions applied to the upper thoracic and cervical paraspinal tissues could lead to a reduction in heart rate and contractility of the heart, as well as in cardiac pain. It is hypothesized that this somatovisceral intervention interferes with the spinal and supraspinal neural circuits involved in the regulation of cardiac output and its adaptation during muscular exercise (see Chapter 7). The mechanisms mediating these therapeutically positive effects have yet to be worked out.

Conclusion

It has long been debated whether positive feedback loops between peripheral body tissues and the spinal cord can operate to maintain pain, discomfort, and dysfunctional tissue states. Such feedback loops would include the motor neurons to skeletal muscle, spinal autonomic neurons to autonomic effector organs, the effector tissues, the feedback from the tissues in afferent neurons with small-diameter fibers, the spinal neural circuits, and their supraspinal control (Fig. 16.5). With the exception of complex regional pain syndromes, the existence of these positive feedback mechanisms remains hypothetical and unproven. Research on patients is needed to test this hypothesis.

Synopsis and outlook

Korr's concept of the 'osteopathic lesion' and the 'facilitated segment' has dominated osteopathic medicine for more than 50 years. The core of this concept is to use the body's

endogenous recuperative power and promotion of self-healing in the manual therapeutic approach. The concept still appears to be modern as far as its philosophical superstructure is concerned, i.e., connecting biological and pathobiological processes in the deep body domains and their regulation by the brain, involving afferent, neuroendocrine, and neural motor systems, with health and disease of the organism. However, is this concept still tenable in the light of modern neurobiological research in the fields of pain, neural regulation of autonomic targets, and regulation of the somatomotor system? Does it reflect mechanistically the neurobiological complexities on which the functioning of the body in health and disease and the curative manual interventions in disease are based? Will this concept lead to answers explaining why manual therapeutic interventions can be successful in the treatment of dysfunctional body states? Does the concept supply us with ideas as to how functional disorders of the body are anchored and can be explained in the frame of modern neurobiology? I think that we have to reformulate the concept on the basis of modern research in neurobiology. We must reformulate the research questions and restructure the research approach. Clinical investigations on patients, research on the human subject as model (healthy subjects and patients), and research on animal models must be more closely integrated. The way to achieve this aim resembles the situation regarding unraveling the mechanisms at the base of complex regional pain syndrome, with the aim of developing new treatment strategies (Baron et al. 2002b, Jänig & Baron 2004, 2009).

References

Apkarian, A.V., Bushnell, M.C., Treede, R.D., Zubieta, J.K., 2005. Human brain mechanisms of pain perception and regulation in health and disease. Euro. J. Pain 9, 463–484.

Apkarian, A.V., Baliki, M.N., Geha, P.Y., 2009. Towards a theory of chronic pain. Prog. Neurobiol. 87, 81–97.

Baron, R., 2006. Complex regional pain syndromes. In: McMahon, S.B., Koltzenburg, M. (Eds.), Wall & Melzack's Textbook of Pain, fifth ed. Elsevier Churchill Livingstone, Amsterdam, Edinburgh, pp. 1011–1027.

Baron, R., 2009. Complex regional pain syndromes. In: Basbaum, A.L., Bushnell, M.C. (Eds.), Science of Pain. Academic Press, San Diego, pp. 909–918.

Baron, R., Schattschneider, J., Binder, A., Siebrecht, D., Wasner, G., 2002a. Relation between sympathetic vasoconstrictor activity and pain and hyperalgesia in complex regional pain syndromes: a case-control study. Lancet 359, 1655–1660.

Baron, R., Fields, H.L., Jänig, W., Kitt, C., Levine, J.D., 2002b. National Institutes of Health Workshop: reflex sympathetic dystrophy/complex regional pain syndromes–state-of-the-science. Anesth. Analg. 95, 1812–1816.

Beal, M.C., 1983. Palpatory testing for somatic dysfunction in patients with cardiovascular disease. J. Am. Osteopath. Assoc. 82, 822–831.

Beal, M.C., 1985. Viscerosomatic reflexes: a review. J. Am. Osteopath. Assoc. 85, 786–801.

Beal, M.C., Dvorak, J., 1984. Palpatory examination of the spine. A comparison of the results of two methods and their relationship to visceral disease. Manual Medicine 1, 25–32.

Beal, M.C., Kleiber, G.E., 1985. Somatic dysfunction as a predictor of coronary artery disease. J. Am. Osteopath. Assoc. 85, 302–307.

Beal, M.C., Morlock, J.W., 1984. Somatic dysfunction associated with pulmonary disease. J. Am. Osteopath. Assoc. 84, 179–183.

Bielefeld, T.K., Gebhart, G.F., 2006. Visceral pain: basic mechanisms. In: McMahon, S.B., Koltzenburg, M. (Eds.), Wall and Melzack's Textbook of Pain, fifth ed. Churchill Livingstone, Amsterdam Edinburgh, pp. 721–736.

Bonica, J.J., 1953. Causalgia and other reflex sympathetic dystrophies. In: Bonica, J.J. (Ed.), Management of Pain. Lea and Febiger, pp. 913–978.

Bradesi, S., Mayer, E.A., Schwetz, I., 2009. Irritable bowel syndrome. In: Basbaum, A.L., Bushnell, M.C. (Eds.), Science of Pain. Academic Press, San Diego, pp. 571–578.

Bushnell, M.C., Apkarian, A.V., 2006. Representation of pain in the brain. In: McMahon, S.B., Koltzenburg, M. (Eds.), Wall and Melzack's Textbook of Pain, fifth ed. Livingstone Churchill, Amsterdam Edinburgh, pp. 107–124.

Casey, K.L., Tran, T.D., 2006. Cortical mechanisms mediating acute and chronic pain in humans. In: Cervero, F., Jensen, T.S. (Eds.), Pain, vol. 81. Handbook of Clinical Neurology, Aminoff MJ, Boller F, Swaab DF (series eds), Elsevier, Edinburgh, pp. 159–177.

Cervero, F., 1994. Sensory innervation of the viscera: peripheral basis of visceral pain. Physiol. Rev. 74, 95–138.

Chila, A.G. (Ed.), 2010. Foundations for Osteopathic Medicine, third ed. Lippincott Williams & Wilkins, Philadelphia.

Cohn, P.F., Fox, K.M., Daly, C., 2003. Silent myocardial ischemia. Circulation 108, 1263–1277.

Coleridge, H.M., Coleridge, J.C., 1980. Cardiovascular afferents involved in regulation of peripheral vessels. Annu. Rev. Physiol. 42, 413–427.

Craig, A.D., 2002. How do you feel? Interoception: the sense of the physiological condition of the body. Nat. Rev. Neurosci. 3, 655–666.

Craig, A.D., 2003a. Pain mechanisms: labeled lines versus convergence in central processing. Annu. Rev. Neurosci. 26, 1–30.

Craig, A.D., 2003b. A new view of pain as a homeostatic emotion. Trends Neurosci. 26, 303–307.

Craig, A.D., 2003c. Interoception: the sense of the physiological condition of the body. Curr. Opin. Neurobiol. 13, 500–505.

Craig, A.D., 2004. Distribution of trigeminothalamic and spinothalamic lamina I terminations in the macaque monkey. J. Comp. Neurol. 477, 119–148.

Craig, A.D., 2006. Retrograde analyses of spinothalamic projections in the macaque monkey: input to ventral posterior nuclei. J. Comp. Neurol. 499, 965–978.

Craig, A.D., 2008a. Retrograde analyses of spinothalamic projections in the macaque monkey: input to the ventral lateral nucleus. J. Comp. Neurol. 508, 315–328.

Craig, A.D., 2008b. Interoception and emotion. A neuroanatomical perspective. In: Lewis, M., Haviland-Jones, J.M., Barrett Feldman, L. (Eds.), Handbook of Emotions, third ed. The Guilford Press, New York, pp. 272–288.

Craig, A.D., Blomqvist, A., 2002. Is there a specific lamina I spinothalamocortical pathway for pain and temperature sensations in primates? J. Pain 3, 95–101.

Craig, A.D., Zhang, E.T., 2006. Retrograde analyses of spinothalamic projections in the macaque monkey: input to posterolateral thalamus. J. Comp. Neurol. 499, 953–964.

Denslow, J.S., 1944. An analysis of the variability of spinal reflex thresholds. J. Neurophysiol. 207–215.

Denslow, J.S., Clough, G.H., 1941. Reflex activity in the spinal extensors. J. Neurophysiol. 4, 430–434.

Denslow, J.S., Hassett, C.C., 1942. The central excitatory state associated with postural abnormalities. J. Neurophysiol. 5, 393–402.

Denslow, J.S., Korr, I.M., Krems, A.D., 1947. Quantitative studies of chronic facilitation in human moto neuron pools. Am. J. Physiol. 105, 229–238.

Dostrovsky, J.O., Craig, A.D., 2006. Ascending projection systems. In: McMahon, S.B., Koltzenburg, M. (Eds.), Wall and Melzack's Textbook of Pain, fifth ed. Livingstone Churchill, Amsterdam, Edinburgh, pp. 187–204.

Fields, H.L., Basbaum, A.I., Heinricher, M.M., 2006. Central nervous system mechanisms of pain modulation. In: McMahon, S.B., Koltzenburg, M. (Eds.), Wall and Melzack's Textbook of Pain, fifth ed. Elsevier Churchill Livingstone, Amsterdam, Edinburgh, pp. 125–142.

Foreman, R.D., 1999. Mechanisms of cardiac pain. Annu. Rev. Physiol. 61, 143–167.

Gebhart, G.F., Bielefeldt, T.K., 2009. Visceral pain. In: Basbaum, A.L., Bushnell, M.C. (Eds.), Science of Pain. Academic Press, San Diego, pp. 543–570.

Graven-Nielsen, T., Arendt-Nielsen, L., Mense, S. (Eds.), 2008. Fundamentals of Musculoskeletal Pain. IASP Press, Seattle.

Hansen, K., Schliack, H., 1962. Segmentale Innervation [Segmental Innervation]. Thieme-Verlag, Stuttgart.

Heinricher, M.M., Ingram, S.L., 2009. The brain stem and nociceptive modulation. In: Basbaum, A.L., Bushnell, M.C. (Eds.), Science of Pain. Academic Press, San Diego, pp. 593–626.

Henningsen, P., Zipfel, S., Herzog, W., 2007. Management of functional somatic syndromes. Lancet 369, 946–955.

Hucho, T., Levine, J.D., 2007. Signaling pathways in sensitization: toward a nociceptor cell biology. Neuron 55, 365–376.

Jänig, W., 1993. Spinal visceral afferents, sympathetic nervous system and referred pain. In: Vecchiet, L., Albe-Fessard, D., Lindblom, U., Giamberardino, M.A. (Eds.), 'New Trends in Referred Pain and Hyperalgesia', Pain Research and Clinical Management, vol. 7. Elsevier Science Publishers, Amsterdam, pp. 83–92.

Jänig, W., 2002. Pain and the sympathetic nervous system: pathophysiological mechanisms. In: Mathias, C.J., Bannister, R. (Eds.), Autonomic Failure, fourth ed. Oxford University Press, Oxford, pp. 99–108.

Jänig, W., 2005. Vagal afferents and visceral pain. In: Undem, B., Weinreich, D. (Eds.), Advances in Vagal Afferent Neurobiology. CRC Press, Boca Raton, pp. 465–493.

Jänig, W., 2006. The Integrative Action of the Autonomic Nervous System. Neurobiology of Homeostasis. Cambridge University Press, Cambridge, New York.

Jänig, W., 2009a. Autonomic nervous system and pain. In: Basbaum, A.L., Bushnell, M.C. (Eds.), Science of Pain. Academic Press, San Diego, pp. 193–225.

Jänig, W., 2009b. Autonomic nervous system dysfunction. In: Mayer, E.A., Bushnell, M.C. (Eds.), Functional Pain Syndromes: Presentation and Pathophysiology. IASP Press, Seattle, pp. 265–300.

Jänig, W., 2009c. Vagal afferent neurons and pain. In: Basbaum, A.I., Bushnell, M.C. (Eds.), Science of Pain. Academic Press, San Diego, pp. 245–251.

Jänig, W., Baron, R., 2002. Complex regional pain syndrome is a disease of the central nervous system. Clin. Auton. Res. 12, 150–164.

Jänig, W., Baron, R., 2003. Complex regional pain syndrome: mystery explained? Lancet Neurol. 2, 687–697.

Jänig, W., Baron, R., 2004. Experimental approach to CRPS. Pain 108, 3–7.

Jänig, W., Baron, R., 2009. Mechanisms and treatment strategy of complex regional pain syndromes. In: Weinman, M.H., Weinblatt, M.E., Louie, J.S., van Vollenhoven, R.F. (Eds.), Targeted Treatment of the Rheumatic Diseases. Elsevier, Amsterdam, pp. 286–401.

Jänig, W., Häbler, H.J., 1995. Visceral-autonomic integration. In: Gebhart, G.F. (Ed.), Visceral Pain; Progress in Pain Research and Management, vol. 5. IASP Press, Seattle, pp. 311–348.

Jänig, W., Levine, J.D., 2006. Autonomic-neuroendocrine-immune responses in acute and chronic pain. In: McMahon, S.B., Koltzenburg, M. (Eds.), Wall & Mezack's Textbook of Pain, fifth ed. Elsevier Churchill Livinstone, Amsterdam, Edinburgh, pp. 205–218.

Johansson, H., Windhorst, U., Djupsjöbacka, M., Passatore, M. (Eds.), 2003. Chronic Work-Related Myalgia. Neuromuscular Mechanisms Behind Work-Related Chronic Muscle Pain Syndromes. University of Gävle Press, Gävle, Sweden.

Johnston, W.L., 1992. Osteopathic clinical aspects of somatovisceral interaction. In: Patterson, M.M., Howell, J.N. (Eds.), The Central Connection: Somatovisceral/Viscerosomatic Interaction. University Classics, Ltd, Athens, OH, pp. 30–46.

Johnston, W.L., Kelso, A.F., Hollandsworth, D.L., Karrat, J.J., 1987. Somatic manifestations in renal disease: a clinical research study. J. Am. Osteopath. Assoc. 87, 61–74.

Julius, D., McCleskey, E.W., 2006. Cellular and molecular properties of primary afferent neurons. In: McMahon, S.B., Koltzenburg, M. (Eds.), Wall and Melzack's Textbook of Pain, fifth ed. Churchill Livingstone, Amsterdam, Edinburgh, pp. 35–48.

Kellgren, J.H., 1938. Observations on referred pain arising from muscle. Clin. Sci. (Lond.) 3, 175–180.

Kellgren, J.H., 1939. On the distribution of pain arising from deep somatic structures with charts of segmental pain areas. Clin. Sci. (Lond.) 4, 35–45.

Kellgren, J.H., 1940. Somatic simulating visceral pain. Clin. Sci. (Lond.) 4, 303–309.

Kerr, C.E., Wasserman, R.H., Moore, C.I., 2007. Cortical dynamics as a therapeutic mechanism for touch healing. J. Altern. Complement. Med. 13, 59–66.

Korr, I.M., 1947. The neural basis of the osteopathic lesion. J. Am. Osteopath. Assoc. 47, 191–198.

Korr, I.M., 1948. The emerging concept of the osteopathic lesion. J. Am. Osteopath. Assoc. 48, 127–138 (reprinted 2000 in J. Am. Osteopath. Assoc. 100: 449–460).

Korr, I.M., 1951. The three fundamental problems in osteopathic research. J. Am. Osteopath. Assoc. 50, 407–416.

Korr, I.M., 1955a. IV. Clinical significance of the facilitated state. J. Am. Osteopath. Assoc. 54, 277–282.

Korr, I.M., 1955b. Symposium on the functional implications of segmental facilitation; a research report. I. The concept of facilitation and its origins. J. Am. Osteopath. Assoc. 54, 265–268.

Korr, I.M., 1978. Sustained sympathicotonia as a factor in disease. In: Korr, I.M. (Ed.), The Neurobiologic Mechanisms in Manipulative Therapy. Plenum Publishing, New York, pp. 229–268.

Korr, I.M., 1979. The spinal cord as organizer of disease processes: II. The peripheral autonomic nervous system. J. Am. Osteopath. Assoc. 79, 82–90.

Korr, I.M., Thomas, P.E., Wright, H.M., 1958. Patterns of electrical skin resistance in man. Acta Neurovege. (Wien) 17, 77–98.

Korr, I.M., Wright, H.M., Thomas, P.E., 1962. Effects of experimental myofascial insults on cutaneous patterns of sympathetic activity in man. Acta Neurovege. (Wien) 23, 329–355.

Korr, I.M., Wright, H.M., Chace, J.A., 1964. Cutaneous patterns of sympathetic activity in clinical abnormalities of the musculoskeletal system. Acta Neurovege. (Wien) 25, 589–606.

Latremoliere, A., Woolf, C.J., 2009. Central sensitization: a generator of pain hypersensitivity by central neural plasticity. J. Pain 10, 895–926.

Lederman, E., 2000. Facilitated segment: a critical review. British Osteopathic Journal 22, 7–20.

Lewis, T., 1942. Pain. Macmillan, New York.

Lewis, T., Kellgren, J.H., 1939. Observations relating to referred pain, visceromotor reflexes and other associated phenomena. Clin. Sci. (Lond.) 4, 47–71.

Livingston, W.K., 1943. Pain Mechanisms. A Physiological Interpretation of Causalgia and Related States. McMillan (reprinted by Plenum Press 1976).

Lorenz, J., Tracey, I., 2009. Brain correlates of pschological amplification of pain. In: Mayer, E.A., Bushnell, M.C. (Eds.), Functional Pain Syndromes: Presentation and Pathophysiology. IASP Press, Seattle, pp. 385–401.

Lucas, N., Macaskill, P., Irwig, L., Moran, R., Bogduk, N., 2009. Reliability of physical examination for diagnosis of myofascial trigger points. Clin. J. Pain 25, 80–89.

Malliani, A., 1982. Cardiovascular sympathetic afferent fibers. Rev. Physiol. Biochem. Pharmacol. 94, 11–74.

Malliani, A., Lombardi, F., Pagani, M., 1986. Sensory innervation of the heart. Prog. Brain Res. 67, 39–48.

Mayer, E.M., Bushnell, M.C. (Eds.), 2009. Functional Pain Syndromes: Presentation and Pathophysiology. IASP Press, Seattle.

McCabe, C.S., Haigh, R.C., Ring, E.F., Halligan, P.W., Wall, P.D., Blake, D.R., 2003. A controlled pilot study of the utility of mirror visual feedback in the treatment of complex regional pain syndrome (type 1). Rheumatology (Oxford) 42, 97–101.

McCabe, C.S., Haigh, R.C., Blake, D.R., 2008. Mirror visual feedback for the treatment of complex regional pain syndrome (type 1). Curr. Pain Headache Rep. 12, 103–107.

McMahon, S.B., Bennett, D.L.H., Bevan, S., 2006. Inflammatory mediators and modulators of pain. In: McMahon, S.B., Koltzenburg, M. (Eds.), Wall and Melzack's Textbook of Pain, fifth ed. Elsevier Churchill Livingstone, Amsterdam, Edinburgh, pp. 49–72.

Melzack, R., 1999. From the gate to the neuromatrix. Pain (Suppl. 6), S121–S126.

Mense, S., 1993. Nociception from skeletal muscle in relation to clinical muscle pain. Pain 54, 241–289.

Mense, S., Simons, D.G., 2001. Muscle Pain. Understanding its Nature, Diagnosis, and Treatment. Lippincott Williams & Wilkins, Philadelphia.

Merskey, H., Bogduk, N., 1994. Classification of Chronic Pain: Descriptions of Chronic Pain Syndromes and Definition of Pain Terms, second ed. IASP Press, Seattle.

Meyer, R.A., Ringkamp, M., Campbell, J.N., Raja, S.N., 2006. Peripheral mechanisms of cutaneous nociception. In: McMahon, S.B., Koltzenburg, M. (Eds.), Wall and Melzack's Textbook of Pain, fifth ed. Elsevier Churchill Livingstone, Amsterdam, Edinburgh, pp. 3–34.

Moseley, G.L., 2004. Graded motor imagery is effective for long-standing complex regional pain syndrome: a randomised controlled trial. Pain 108, 192–198.

Moseley, G.L., 2005. Is successful rehabilitation of complex regional pain syndrome due to sustained attention to the affected limb? A randomised clinical trial. Pain 114, 54–61.

Moseley, G.L., 2006. Graded motor imagery for pathologic pain: a randomized controlled trial. Neurology 67, 2129–2134.

Myburgh, C., Larsen, A.H., Hartvigsen, J., 2008. A systematic, critical review of manual palpation for identifying myofascial trigger points: evidence and clinical significance. Arch. Phys. Med. Rehabil. 89, 1169–1176.

Neugebauer, V., Galhardo, V., Maione, S., Mackey, S.C., 2009. Forebrain pain mechanisms. Brain Res. Rev. 60, 226–242.

Patriquin, D.A., 2003. Chapmans reflexes. In: Ward, R.C. (Ed.), Foundations for Osteopathic Medicine, second ed. Lippincott, Williams & Wilkins, Philadelphia, pp. 1051–1055.

Polgar, E., Gray, S., Riddell, J.S., Todd, A.J., 2004. Lack of evidence for significant neuronal loss in laminae I-III of the spinal dorsal horn of the rat in the chronic constriction injury model. Pain 111, 144–150.

Price, D.D., 1999. Psychological Mechanisms of Pain and Analgesia. IASP Press, Seattle.

Price, D.D., 2000. Psychological and neural mechanisms of the affective dimension of pain. Science 288, 1769–1772.

Price, D.D., Long, S., Wilsey, B., Rafii, A., 1998. Analysis of peak magnitude and duration of analgesia produced by local anesthetics injected into sympathetic ganglia of complex regional pain syndrome patients. Clin. J. Pain 14, 216–226.

Ren, K., Dubner, R., 2009. Descending control mechanisms. In: Basbaum, A.I., Bushnell, M.C. (Eds.), Science of Pain. Academic Press, San Diego, pp. 723–762.

Ringkamp, M., Meyer, R.A., 2009. Physiology of nociceptors. In: Basbaum, A.I., Bushnell, M.C. (Eds.), Science of Pain. Academic Press, San Diego, pp. 97–114.

Robinson, J.P., Apkarian, A.V., 2009. Low back pain. In: Mayer, E.A., Bushnell, M.C. (Eds.), Functional Pain Syndromes: Presentation and Pathophysiology. IASP Press, Seattle, pp. 23–53.

Sandkühler, J., 2009. Models and mechanisms of hyperalgesia and allodynia. Physiol. Rev. 89, 707–758.

Schaible, H.G., 2006. Basic mechanisms of deep somatic pain. In: McMahon, S.B., Koltzenburg, M. (Eds.), Wall and Melzack's Textbook of Pain, fifth ed. Churchill Livingstone, Amsterdam, Edinburgh, pp. 621–634.

Schaible, H.G., Grubb, B.D., 1993. Afferent and spinal mechanisms of joint pain. Pain 55, 5–54.

Schaible, H.G., Del, R.A., Matucci-Cerinic, M., 2005. Neurogenic aspects of inflammation. Rheum. Dis. Clin. North Am. 31, 77–101.

Schliack, H., Schiffter, R., 1976. Klinik der sogenannten vegetativen Schmerzen [Clinic of so-called autonomic pains]. In: Sturm, A., Birkmayer, W. (Eds.), Klinische Pathologie des vegetativen Nervensystems [Clinical Pathology of the Autonomic Nervous System]. Gustav Fischer Verlag, Stuttgart, pp. 498–537.

Simons, D.G., 2004. Review of enigmatic MTrPs as a common cause of enigmatic musculoskeletal pain and dysfunction. J. Electromyogr. Kinesiol. 14, 95–107.

Spike, R.C., Puskar, Z., Andrew, D., Todd, A.J., 2003. A quantitative and morphological study of projection neurons in lamina I of the rat lumbar spinal cord. Euro. J. Neurosci. 18, 2433–2448.

Stanton-Hicks, M., Jänig, W., Hassenbusch, S., Haddox, J.D., Boas, R., Wilson, P., 1995. Reflex sympathetic dystrophy: changing concepts and taxonomy. Pain 63, 127–133.

Swanson, L.W., 1995. Mapping the human brain: past, present, and future. Trends Neurosci. 18, 471–474.

Thomas, P.E., Korr, I.M., 1951. The automatic recording of electrical skin resistance patterns on the human trunk. Electroencephalogr. Clin. Neurophysiol. 3, 361–368.

Thomas, P.E., Korr, I.M., 1957. Relationship between sweat gland activity and electrical resistance of the skin. J. Appl. Physiol. 10, 505–510.

Thomas, P.E., Korr, I.M., Wright, H.M., 1958. A mobile instrument for recording electrical skin resistance patterns of the human trunk. Acta Neurovege. (Wien) 17, 97–106.

Torebjörk, H.E., Wahren, L.K., Wallin, B.G., Hallin, R., Koltzenburg, M., 1995. Noradrenaline-evoked pain in neuralgia. Pain 63, 11–20.

Tough, E.A., White, A.R., Cummings, T.M., Richards, S.H., Campbell, J.L., 2009. Acupuncture and dry needling in the management of myofascial trigger point pain: a systematic review and meta-analysis of randomised controlled trials. Euro. J. Pain 13, 3–10.

Tracey, I., Mantyh, P.W., 2007. The cerebral signature for pain perception and its modulation. Neuron 55, 377–391.

Treede, R.D., Apkarian, A.V., 2009. Nociceptive processing in the cerebral cortex. In: Basbaum, A.I., Bushnell, M.C. (Eds.), Science of Pain. Academic Press, San Diego, pp. 669–698.

Willis, W.D. Jr., Coggelshall, R. E., 2004. Sensory Mechanisms of the Spinal Cord. Ascending Sensory Tracts and Their Descending Control. Vol. 2, third edn. Kluwer Academic Press/Plenum Publishers, New York.

Willis, W.D. Jr., Zhang, X., Honda, C.N., Giesler, G.J. Jr., 2002. A critical review of the role of the proposed VMpo nucleus in pain. J. Pain 3, 79–94.

Wilson, P.R., Bogduk, R.E., 2004. Sensory Mechanisms of the Spinal Cord. Ascending Sensory Tracts and Their Descending Control. In: Wilson, P.R., Stanton-Hicks, M., Harden, R.N. (Eds.), CRPS: Current Diagnosis and Therapy. IASP Press, Seattle, pp. 19–41.

Woolf, C.J., Ma, Q., 2007. Nociceptors–noxious stimulus detectors. Neuron 55, 353–364.

Woolf, C.J., Salter, M.W., 2006. Plasticity and pain. In: McMahon, S.B., Koltzenburg, M. (Eds.), Wall and Melzack's Textbook of Pain, fifth ed. Elsevier Churchill Livingstone, Amsterdam, Edinburgh, pp. 91–105.

Wright, H.M., Korr, I.M., 1965. Neural and supraspinal components of disease: progress in the application of 'thermography'. J. Am. Osteopath. Assoc. 64, 918–921.

Wright, H.M., Korr, I.M., Thomas, P.E., 1960. Local and regional variations in cutaneous vasomotor tone of the human trunk. Acta Neurovege. (Wien) 22, 33–52.

Clinical applications of manual therapy on physiologic functions and systemic disorders: evidence base and implications for research

Hollis H King • Michael M Patterson

Introduction

Manual therapy has not only come of age in the era of evidenced-based medicine for the treatment of musculoskeletal disorders, but also shows intriguing promise of benefit for systemic disorders. Albeit still early in the development of an evidence base compared to other medical and therapeutic practices, progress in manual therapy research is substantial and manual therapy warrants consideration as an appropriate treatment modality in many types of disorders and pain conditions. The 2008 symposium 'Delineating the Evidence Base for Somato-visceral Interactions and Autonomic Mechanisms of Manual Therapy' (Osteopathic Research Center 2008), which was the impetus for this book, was a benchmark event in that it came about in part with NIH-NCCAM grant support and brought together all of the manual therapy professions (see Chapters 12–15) as well as basic scientists whose research pertained to neuromusculoskeletal mechanisms of action (see Chapters 2–10). Manual therapy is a significant portion of the services provided by osteopathic physicians and physical therapists, and is the primary modality of service for chiropractic and therapeutic massage professionals. As discussed in Chapter 12, musculoskeletal pain is the most common reason for a person to seek primary medical care in the US (United States Bone and Joint Decade [USBJD] 2009), and around the world musculoskeletal disorders are the leading cause of disability, accounting for 25% of the total cost of illness (International Bone and Joint Decade 2006).

The intention of the 2008 symposium was to examine the evidence base for the concept of somatovisceral interactions and to examine the role not only of spinal cord but also of cortical and subcortical influences on these interactions, and to examine the possible role of manual therapy on somatovisceral and visceral interactions. A fundamental belief in the practice of manual therapy is that through somatovisceral interactions the treatment of somatic structures can influence visceral function. However, it is becoming more evident not only that spinal pathways are involved in these interactions, but that supraspinal (cortical and subcortical) structures have a strong influence on the interactions between somatic and visceral domains. Basic science evidence related to the nature of somatovisceral/viscerosomatic interactions and higher-center influences is presented in detail in Chapters 2–5, 7, and 10, and discussed in Chapter 16.

Each of the clinical research chapters (Chapters 12–15) has a section on the nature of the profession, whether osteopathic medicine/osteopathy, chiropractic, physical therapy, or therapeutic massage, which is intended to give the reader unfamiliar with a particular profession an overview that places the reported research in some perspective. For the purposes of this book, the umbrella term manual therapy encompasses the services delivered by providers in the professions listed above and represented in this text. Although there are differences in the scope of practice of the manual therapy professions in the US and worldwide, the research pertaining to the effects brought about by manual therapy providers is comparable, as many of the outcome measures and the hypothesized mechanisms of action are the same.

This chapter will review and summarize the evidence base for manual therapy and highlight the most promising areas for further research.

Manual therapy in musculoskeletal disorders – axial skeleton pain

Evidence for the benefit of manual therapy for musculoskeletal pain and its applications in the treatment of musculoskeletal disorders has reached the point where there is little doubt about its efficacy for several common musculoskeletal disorders. As discussed in Chapters 12 and 13, there has been a practice guideline statement from a US federal agency (Bigos et al. 1994) and a number of meta-analyses and systematic reviews (Assendelft et al. 2004, Bronfort et al. 2008, Cherkin et al. 2003, Licciardone et al. 2005) showing the benefit of manual therapy for some types of low back pain. Other research and reviews conclude there is benefit of manual therapy for neck pain from the chiropractic literature (Hurwitz et al. 2002, 2008), the osteopathic literature (McReynolds & Sheridan 2005), and the therapeutic massage literature (Sherman et al. 2009). However, with neck pain and other musculoskeletal conditions, more clinical trials are needed to reach the level of the evidence base for some types of low back pain.

Physical therapists have historically used manual therapy to treat musculoskeletal pain along with a number of other modalities. Research by physical therapists has tended to focus on specific modalities, rather than a general study of the efficacy of physical therapist application of manual therapy. Typical of this perspective is the research reported by George in Chapter 14, which describes the benefit of manual therapy in reducing musculoskeletal pain (George et al. 2006).

From the therapeutic massage perspective, Kahn, in Chapter 15, describes the preponderance of evidence as demonstrating that massage appears effective in reducing pain and restoring function in patients with subacute and chronic nonspecific low back pain, especially when combined with exercises and education (Cherkin et al. 2001, 2009, Furlan et al. 2009, Hernandez-Reif et al. 2001, Preyde et al. 2000). Cherkin et al.'s (2009) study on massage for back pain was a randomized controlled trial (RCT) which randomized 402 subjects with chronic low back pain to one of three arms: (1) usual care; (2) relaxation massage, which was a full-body protocol of entirely Swedish massage techniques in which the therapist was told to hold in mind the intention of encouraging a generalized relaxation response; and (3) focused structural massage, which was a protocol consisting largely of myofascial and neuromuscular techniques in which the therapist was told to identify the musculoskeletal contributors to each patient's back pain and treat those. Both forms of massage were superior to usual care for low back pain, producing short-term reductions in symptoms and longer-term improvements in function. This study is representative of the progress made in clinical research design, which is now typical in manual therapy research.

It is beyond the scope of this chapter to exhaustively review these and other published research reports supportive of the benefit of manual therapy in musculoskeletal pain and musculoskeletal disorders. However, the summary and conclusions offered in this chapter are based on an integrated review of research from all the manual therapy professions. Two publications have provided an integrated consideration of research from the manual therapy professions (Lederman 2004, Seffinger & Hruby 2007) and also suggest that there is substantial support for the application of manual therapy in the treatment of musculoskeletal pain and musculoskeletal disorders. Since the publication of those books, more research has been published, some of

which is included in this book. Based on the review of the evidence from the perspective of the authors of this chapter, as stated above, the conclusion is that there is substantial evidence for the benefit of manual therapy. Furthermore, from the perspective of the individual manual therapy professions this conclusion is justified; however, the argument is even stronger when the evidence from all the manual therapy professions is considered.

Manual therapy in musculoskeletal disorders – the rest of the body and mind

A number of clinical trials reported in the clinical chapters of this book reported benefit of manual therapy for appendicular (upper and lower extremities) musculoskeletal and perispinal conditions. In Chapter 12, research was reported for the benefit of manual therapy for restricted and painful shoulder function in the elderly (Knebl et al. 2002), reduction of carpal tunnel syndrome pain, and improved wrist range of motion (Sucher 1993, Sucher & Hinrichs 1998, Sucher et al. 2005), and relief of pain in patients with fibromyalgia syndrome (Gamber et al. 2002).

Also from the osteopathic literature, Eisenhart et al. (2003) reported statistically significant reductions in pain and ankle swelling from the application of manual therapy. Osteopathic manipulation has shown benefits in the treatment of Achilles tendonitis (Howell et al. 2006) and plantar fasciitis (Wynne et al. 2006). The therapeutic massage literature reports benefit for patients with osteoarthritis of the knee (Perlman et al. 2006), as does the physical therapy literature (van den Dolder & Roberts 2006).

Albeit not an exhaustive review, the studies cited above constitute a significant body of research on the application of manual therapy for pain in appendicular skeletal structures. Manual therapy is applied to the whole body, and the tendency in reviews is to cite only those studies pertaining to axial skeleton (spinal) structures. Indeed, when the research demonstrating the benefit of manual therapy for musculoskeletal extremity disorders is added to that for axial skeleton disorders, the evidence base for the benefit on manual therapy is both broadened and strengthened.

Pregnant women also experience musculoskeletal disorders and pain. As discussed in Chapter 12, osteopathic manipulative treatment (OMT) has been shown to reduce back pain and disability during the third trimester of pregnancy (Guthrie & Martin 1982, Licciardone et al. 2010) as well as improve vagal control of heart rate after just one OMT visit (Hensel 2009). One investigation (King et al. 2003) found that pregnant women who received OMT had significantly fewer preterm deliveries and instances of meconium-stained amniotic fluid, and suggested large cost savings if the morbidity and mortality from these disorders could be reduced. The nature of these results is also suggestive of viscerosomatic interaction effects, in addition to any postural improvements alleviating pain.

As Kahn reports in Chapter 15, the application of therapeutic massage has been shown to result in reductions in state anxiety, blood pressure, and heart rate, but not in cortisol levels, and that multiple massage treatments produced reductions in pain and depression comparable to those following psychotherapy (Moyer et al. 2004). Kahn also describes the research of Hodge et al. (2002) in which therapeutic massage was applied in the workplace, and states, 'Findings indicate that compared with those in the control group, the massage group had significant improvement in cognition scores ($p < 0.001$), as assessed by the Symbol Digit Modalities Test, a 90-second timed instrument providing indices of normal capacities in adults as well as improvement resulting from specific therapeutic interventions. The massage subjects also showed lower anxiety (state $p < 0.009$, trait $p < 0.04$), improved emotional control ($p < 0.05$), and a reduction in sleep disturbance for massage subjects on 12-hour shifts ($p < 0.02$).' These results show the effects of manual therapy on cortical functions and add to the discussion by Goehler in Chapter 10.

Manual therapy effects on physiologic function and systemic disorders

Those conditions that have been systematically reviewed – asthma, vertigo, dysmenorrhea/PMS (premenstrual syndrome), infantile colic, and nocturnal enuresis – are summarized by Hawk in Chapter 13, and she quotes from her 2007 review (Hawk et al. 2007, p. 506):

'1) *The adverse effects reported for spinal manipulative therapy (SMT) for all age groups and conditions were rare and, when they did occur, were transient and not severe.*

2) *Evidence from both controlled studies and usual practice is adequate to support the 'total package' of chiropractic care, including SMT, other procedures, and unmeasured qualities such as belief and attention, as providing benefit to patients with asthma, cervicogenic vertigo, and infantile colic.*

3) *Evidence was promising for the potential benefit of manual procedures for children with otitis media and for hospitalized elderly patients with pneumonia.*

4) *Evidence did not appear to support chiropractic care for the broad population of patients with hypertension, although it did not rule out the possibility that there may be subpopulations of hypertensives which might benefit.*

5) Evidence was equivocal regarding chiropractic care for dysmenorrhea and PMS; it is not clear as to the level of biomechanical force most appropriate for patients with these related conditions. It does appear that an extended duration of care, over at least 3 menstrual cycles, is more likely to be beneficial.

6) There is insufficient evidence to make conclusions about chiropractic care for patients with other conditions.'

We suggest that the strongest evidence for the impact of manual therapy on physiologic function and systemic disorders may be in the conditions of pneumonia, asthma, and otitis media. Although Hawk mentions them in her 2007 review article quoted above, she did not specifically review the studies on manual therapy applied to the treatment of hospitalized elderly patients with pneumonia and children with otitis media. These studies, including research in press and available only from abstracts and posters, are reviewed by King in Chapter 12 and constitute some of the strongest evidence for the impact of manual therapy on systemic disorders. As detailed in Chapter 12 the studies on manual therapy for pneumonia in the hospitalized elderly by Noll et al. (Noll et al. 1999, 2000, Noll 2009) constitute a promising line of research, with the possibility to affect standards of care for these patients if subsequently substantiated in a larger clinical trial. For the treatment of otitis media in children, the studies by Mills et al. (2003) and Degenhardt and Kuchera (2006) show strong treatment effects, and have led to a subsequent clinical trial currently in analysis.

When the pneumonia studies are taken together with the asthma studies (Chapter 13), there is a broadening of the concept of manual therapy for pulmonary function and disorders. As suggested by King in Chapter 12, immune system function mediated by improved lymphatic flow due to manual therapy may account for much of the benefit seen in asthma and pneumonia patients. Specifically, we refer to the work of Knott et al. (2005) and Hodge et al. (2007) showing increased lymphatic flow in dogs during various manual therapy pump techniques. Several other studies confirm the finding of increased immune system cell counts as a consequence of lymphatic and visceral pump techniques of manual therapy (Measel 1982, Mesina et al. 1998, Jackson et al. 1998).

Another area of research common to both the osteopathic and therapeutic massage research is that as applied to pediatrics. Besides the aforementioned osteopathic research showing the benefit of OMT for pediatric otitis media, OMT has also been shown to reduce the symptoms of infantile colic (Hayden & Mullinger 2006) and sleep apnea (Vandenplas et al. 2008). Therapeutic massage research has shown the benefit of massage for premature infants in that neonates receiving massage gained weight faster (Field 2001), were able to leave hospital sooner (Field 1995), and while still in hospital were calmer and showed fewer stress behaviors (Hernandez-Reif et al. 2007).

This section would not be complete without mention of the osteopathic literature, described in more detail in Chapter 12. OMT significantly reduced the hospital stay for patients with postoperative ileus (Crow & Gorodinsky 2009) and pancreatitis (Radjieski et al. 1998). OMT also reduced the amount of analgesia in patients who received hysterectomies (Goldstein et al. 2005), improved pulmonary funtion in hospitalized patients (Sleszynski & Kelso 1993), and improved cardiac function and oxygen saturation in patients who had just undergone coronary artery bypass surgery (Yurvati et al. 2005).

Although there have been relatively few clinical trials on the impact of manual therapy on systemic disorders and physiological functions, the results thus far are intriguing and hold the prospect of great benefit, meriting top priority for further clinical investigation. There are enough manual therapy professionals to provide a meaningful service for these and related systemic disorders. In current times, when healthcare reform is being considered in the US and elsewhere, the cost savings of manual therapy applications, both in preventive healthcare and in the reduction of hospital stays, merits serious consideration at all levels of clinical research.

The authors of this chapter contend that the manual therapy research described above more than meets the requirements of evidence-based medicine for acceptance as a valid mode of treatment for musculoskeletal disorders, and is an impressive start in the process of establishing an evidence base. However, the fact remains that more research needs to be done to provide enough evidence for systematic review statements that have the potential to affect standards of practice in the treatment of musculoskeletal disorders. Research related to the question of which specific manual therapy techniques are more effective than others for certain musculoskeletal conditions is also needed. It is recognized that different manual therapy techniques have not always been effective for certain individual patients and conditions.

Interwoven with research on the effects of manual therapy on systemic disorders and physiological functions is the question of mechanism of action for the effects. This topic is considered next.

Evidence for concepts underlying the mechanism of actions for manual therapy

Chapters 12–15 provide a broad review of clinical research done in the medical professions that use manual therapy in some form or other. As suggested by King (Langevin et al. 2009), leading researchers from all professions utilizing manual therapy acknowledge the tenets of osteopathic medicine as being consistent with those promulgated in their training. Included in these is the concept of somatovisceral and viscerosomatic interactions, which is now generally accepted and supported with evidence-based research (see Chapters 2–5 and 7–10).

However, it is now becoming clear that the concept of simple spinal somatovisceral and viscerosomatic interactions must be abandoned, and the effects of higher centers on these interactions taken into account in any explanation of manual therapy effects on systemic and even pain syndromes. Goehler, in Chapter 10, delineates the 'multiple pathways viscerosensory information takes in the brain, how it interfaces with other systems, and possible mechanisms by which viscerosensory systems influence mood and behavior.' Uvnäs-Moberg and Petersson in Chapter 9 'suggest that all types of therapy involving gentle skin contact will lead to activation of a basic psychophysiological reaction in response to activation of cutaneous sensory nerves.' It may be necessary to refine or reformulate some concepts along the way, but evidence supporting the underlying principles of manual therapy appears to be increasing. In Chapter 16, Jänig has made it clear that any attempt to explain the effects of manual therapy on systemic and pain syndromes will necessarily have to involve not only spinal but also supraspinal interactions, and cortical influences in particular.

In the studies and formulations by Denslow and Korr (e.g., Korr 1947) that resulted in the concept of the facilitated segment and to the extensions of the somatic dysfunction concepts, Korr made several simplifying assumptions, the basic one of which was that the facilitated state of the spinal center was maintained by continued input from some peripheral source. Denslow (1944) initially referred to this facilitated state as a 'central excitatory state.' There was no other activating source that he knew that could explain such a continued hyperexcitability. As Jänig rightly points out in Chapter 16, it is most likely that such a mechanism to maintain spinal hyperexcitability is not such a simple feedback loop. It is much more likely that alterations in actual cellular function now known as 'central excitation' (see Latremoliere & Woolf 2009 for a recent review) may be the actual basis for alterations seen by Denslow and Korr in their studies of somatic dysfunction, possibly compounded by influences from higher centers of the brain stem and cortex. In addition, the evidence for simple effects of autonomic outflows and of somatic afferent influences on autonomic system function put forward by Korr as a main determinant of systemic disease and dysfunction are most likely not nearly as simple as Korr postulated (again, see Chapter 16). As seen in Chapters 7–10, the interactions between spinal and supraspinal centers is both vast and very complex. As pointed out by Jänig in Chapter 16, the descending tracts from the brain stem to the spinal cord are far greater than those going from the cord to the brain, suggesting the tremendous influence of encephalization in the human over simpler spinal function.

In addition to direct influences on spinal function, the influences of the frontal cortex on lower function are becoming more evident. The so-called 'placebo' and 'nocebo' effects usually thought of as influences apart from physiologically meaningful effects are being shown to have powerful effects on physiological function (see Chapter 11, Patterson; Enck et al. 2008), with ideational and emotional effects on the belief systems of the patient actually directly influencing nociceptive processing at the spinal level, possibly through the endogenous opioid system (Eippert et al. 2009). In addition, evidence is accumulating that what happens to infants shortly after birth can influence how they react to nociceptive stimuli as adults, and that being male or female can make a difference in response to pain. Ruda et al. (2000) reported that neonatal chronic inflammation produced adults with a lower

threshold to nociceptive stimulation, and with greater numbers of spinal interneurons and synapses processing nociceptive information. In contrast, LaPrairie and Murphy (2007) reported that acute injury in neonatal rats produced adults that were less responsive to nociceptive inputs, and that females were more influenced than males. These studies may begin to explain some of the differences seen in response to such syndromes as low back pain between individuals, and even between males and females.

Taken together, these lines of evidence show that the formulations made by Korr need to be rethought, as stated by Jänig (Chapter 16). The influences of higher centers need to be somehow brought into the mix of thinking in manual medicine. They will have to be taken into account in attempting to deduce the mechanisms of action of the various manual techniques used by practitioners of manual therapies.

Thus, the search for mechanisms underlying manual therapies, and especially their effects on systemic disease, seem to necessitate a broader scope than traditionally spinal and/or mechanistic interpretations. It seems likely from the evidence that the efficacy of manual therapies on processes that involve more than simple mechanical musculoskeletal problems must be envisaged in terms of interactions between afferent input disturbances and the effects of subsequent local (e.g. integument), segmental, and supraspinal influences on the mechanics of complex networks of spinal pathways. Thus, the efficacy of manual therapies on systemic disease would involve both the direct effects of the manual procedure on local tissues and joints and the far-reaching effects of altered afferent neural inputs from involved tissues of supraspinal and cortical centers that mediate conscious and non-conscious processes, which in turn provide powerful descending effects on the spinal networks influencing both somatic and autonomic function.

Albeit quite complex, the reformulation of Korr's theories undertaken by Jänig in

Chapter 16, when considered in the context of what is now known about the alterations of spinal neural networks, can assist in reformulating a global hypothesis of dysfunction that involves both local and global neural function and dysfunction that can lead to testable hypotheses about actual mechanisms of action of manual therapies in systemic disease. The rapid advances in imaging technologies such as fMRI that allow visualization of CNS function may provide vital information about system changes following manual therapy, and as such constitutes a potential major source of state-of-the-art empirical data. Such non-invasive technologies can be used in human patients and healthy subjects to detect normal and abnormal neural function and responses to manual techniques. Thus, it is necessary that we move from strictly mechanically oriented formulations as the underpinnings for the effects of manual therapies to a more system-wide and dynamic hypothesis for such effects.

Obviously, our understanding of the efficacy of manual therapies must continue to be a high priority in research. As shown in the reviews here, there are few areas in which efficacy has been rigorously shown, and evidence is accumulating for several other areas. However, new formulations of the basis for the clinical findings that drive manual therapies are necessary to drive further tests of hypotheses as to mechanism, especially in the area of efficacy in systemic syndromes. Building on and adding to what Korr and Denslow provided, as well as redoing some of their studies to confirm or not confirm their empirical findings, is essential to provide new directions for thinking about mechanisms of all forms of manual therapy.

Discussion groups at the 2008 symposium

At the end of the 2008 Symposium, attendees were assigned to one of three discussion groups and asked four identical questions.

The *first question* was to identify key clinical observations that need to be studied. There were three distinct categories of answer common to the three groups:

A. Observations of effects on clinical entities such as GI syndromes, cardiac syndromes, pulmonary disease, etc. This group of answers showed the need for continued efficacy studies on all types of syndrome.

B. Observations on the effects of manual therapies on the natural history of diseases and disease prevention. These answers were clearly aimed at the need to understand the effects of manual therapies on the course of function, rather than on disease itself.

C. Observations about the process of manual therapy itself, such as defining the therapy or intervention, how it is done, and what forces are used.

Taken together, these responses suggested that there could be a productive dialog between the various practitioners represented about what they think they are treating and how their therapies are understood to work. This dialog should include the basic scientists.

The *second question* asked about assumed mechanisms of therapies. Again, the answers were varied across the three groups, but essentially, most dealt with the belief that manual therapies do something to affect function, either directly by effects on a specific dysfunctional element, or by helping to restore some aspect of function that presumably helped the body restore normality and health. These answers reflected the belief common to manual therapy practitioners that this type of therapy is mainly aimed not at a disease itself, but at normalizing function and hence allowing the system to restore health.

The *third question* asked participants to name approaches and tools available to address the assumed mechanisms. This question was answered by two general categories of tool: one, emerging technologies such as fMRI and other imaging techniques, ultrasound, laser Doppler, quality of life measures, etc.; and two, databases, such as insurance databases, electronic medical records, and so forth. These answers indicated that the participants saw the need to use emerging technologies and data to address the questions facing the manual therapy community, but seemed to indicate a lack of knowledge of how to do so, as little was said about what such instruments would contribute.

The *fourth question* asked about research priorities for the manual therapy community for the next 10 years. Interestingly, the answers fell into two interdependent categories, one being that more efficacy studies are needed (of various types, including establishing better outcome measures, retrospective studies of data, and hospital and outpatient outcome studies); and studies to look at such factors as reliability of palpatory data, treatment mechanics (force, etc.), and characteristics and intraprofessional application characteristics. *Only once was there mention of a need for more studies of mechanisms underlying manual therapies. This question highlighted the continuing preoccupation of the professions with showing the efficacy of manual therapies and that the need for better theories about mechanisms of action, leading to testable hypotheses, has yet to gain widespread support.*

Perhaps the answers to this last question do highlight the grip the prevailing theories have held on thinking in the manual therapy world, and the need for renewed thinking about what is really happening in the common syndromes treated with manual therapies. The recognition was obviously there that new tools need to be used to begin to understand mechanisms, but the real need for new approaches to thinking about what underlies those conditions has yet to be realized.

It is our hope that this book will help to emphasize the need for new ways of thinking about manual therapies and their mechanisms, and will interest more of the scientific community in the search for the underpinnings of the obvious clinical successes of the various forms of manual therapy.

Synopsis and outlook

Chapters 16 and 17 summarize the basic and clinical science and theory underlying manual therapy. Clinical research has shown the effects of manual therapy on musculoskeletal disorders as well as physiologic processes and systemic disorders. Each of the manual therapy professions contributing to this book has generated research sufficient to justify continuance of their unique standards and styles of manual therapy in their respective clinical settings. Taken together, the research effort in manual therapy has achieved an evidence base sufficient for such services to be considered as primary or adjuvant modalities in a number of musculoskeletal conditions. Indeed, manual therapy services are included in many medical centers and clinics throughout the world. This book may serve as a resource for those looking for direction in research efforts and a summary of the relevant research that justifies the proposed research. Besides summarizing clinical research data, this chapter has followed on suggestions from Chapter 16 about the reformulation of certain mechanism of action concepts such as the 'facilitated segment.' Clearly, phenomena such as viscerosomatic interactions, as described in Chapters 16 and 17, involve the total nervous system, not just segmental interactions. As suggested in Chapter 16, the measured changes in physiologic function as a result of manual therapy need further exploration before definitive mechanisms of action can be asserted. However, the potential of a fuller understanding of total psychoneuroendocrine–immune system interactions mediated by spinal, supraspinal, and cortical structures, as affected by manual therapy, appears to be taking on some semblance of organization and enough research findings to refine and direct future research.

References

Assendelft, W.J., Morton, S.C., Yu, E.I., et al., 2004. Spinal manipulative therapy for low-back pain. Cochrane Database Syst. Rev. (1) CD000447. DOI: 10.1002/14651858.CD000447.pu.

Bigos, S.J., Bowyer, O.R., Braen, G.R., et al., 1994. Acute low back problems in adults: assessment and treatment. US Department of Health and Human Services, Public Health Services, Agency for Health Care Policy and Research, Rockville, MD Clinical practice guideline number 14. Publication no. 95-0643, December, 1994.

Bronfort, G., Haas, M., Evans, R., Kawchuk, G., Dagenais, S., 2008. Evidence-informed management of chronic low back pain with spinal manipulation and mobilization. Spine J. 8, 213–225.

Cherkin, D.C., Eisenberg, D., Sherman, K.J., et al., 2001. A randomized trial comparing traditional Chinese medical acupuncture, therapeutic massage and self-care education for chronic low back pain. Arch. Intern. Med. 161, 858–1856.

Cherkin, D.C., Sherman, K.I., Deyo, R.A., et al., 2003. A review of the evidence for the effectiveness, safety, and the cost of acupuncture, massage therapy, and spinal manipulation for low back pain. Ann. Intern. Med. 138, 898–906.

Cherkin, D.C., Sherman, K., Cook, A., et al., 2009. A randomized trial comparing relaxation massage, focused structural massage, and usual care for chronic low back pain. Altern. Ther. Health Med. 15, S99–S100.

Crow, W.T., Gorodinsky, L., 2009. Does osteopathic manipulative treatment (OMT) improve outcomes in patients who develop postoperative ileus: a retrospective chart review. International Journal of Osteopathic Medicine 12, 32–36.

Degenhardt, B.F., Kuchera, M.L., 2006. Osteopathic evaluation and manipulative treatment in reducing the morbidity of otitis media: a pilot study. J. Am. Osteopath. Assoc. 106, 327–334.

Denslow, J.S., 1944. An analysis of the variability of spinal reflex thresholds. J. Neurophysiol. 7, 207–216.

Denslow, J.S., Hassett, C.C., 1942. The central excitatory state associated with abnormalities. J. Neurolphysiol. 5, 393–402.

Eippert, F., Finsterbusch, J., Bingel, U., Buchel, C., 2009. Direct evidence for spinal cord involvement in placebo analgesia. Science 326, 404.

Eisenhart, A.W., Gaeta, T.J., Yens, D.P., 2003. Osteopathic manipulative treatment in the emergency department for patients with acute ankle injuries. J. Am. Osteopath. Assoc. 103, 417–421.

Enck, P., Benedetti, F., Schedlowski, M., 2008. New insights into placebo and nocebo responses. Neuron 59, 195–206.

Field, T., 1995. Massage therapy for infants and children. J. Dev. Behav. Pediatr. 16, 105–111.

Field, T., 2001. Massage therapy facilitates weight gain in preterm infants. Current Directions in Psychological Science 10, 51–54.

Furlan, A.D., Imamura, M., Dryden, T., et al., 2009. Massage for low back pain: An updated systematic review within the framework of the Cochrane back review group. Spine Jun 25 Epub ahead of print.

Gamber, R.G., Shores, J.H., Russo, D.P., et al., 2002. Osteopathic manipulative treatment in conjunction with medication relieves pain associated with fibromyalgia syndrome: results of a randomized clinical pilot project. J. Am. Osteopath. Assoc. 102, 321–326.

George, S.Z., Bishop, M.D., Bialosky, J.E., Zeppieri Jr., G., Robinson, M.E., 2006. Immediate effects of spinal manipulation on thermal pain sensitivity: an experimental study. BMC Musculoskelet. Disord. 7, 68.

Goldstein, F.J., Jeck, S., Nicholas, A.S., et al., 2005. Preoperative intravenous morphine sulfate with postoperative osteopathic manipulative treatment reduces patient analgesic use after total abdominal hysterectomy. J. Am. Osteopath. Assoc. 105, 273–279.

Guthrie, R.A., Martin, R.H., 1982. Effect of pressure applied to the upper thoracic (placebo) versus lumbar areas (osteopathic manipulative treatment) for inhibition of lumbar myalgia during labor. J. Am. Osteopath. Assoc. 82, 247–251.

Hawk, C., Khorsan, R., Lisi, A.J., Ferrance, R.J., Evans, M.W., 2007. Chiropractic care for nonmusculoskeletal conditions: a systematic review with implications for whole systems research. J. Altern. Complement. Med. 13, 491–512.

Hayden, C., Mullinger, B., 2006. A preliminary assessment of the impact of cranial osteopathy for the relief of infantile colic. Complement. Ther. Clin. Pract. 12, 83–90.

Hensel, K.L., 2009. Osteopathic manipulative medicine in pregnancy: acute physiological and biomechanical effects. Unpublished doctoral dissertation. University of North Texas Health Science Center, Fort Worth, TX.

Hernandez-Reif, M., Field, T., Krasnegor, J., et al., 2001. Lower back pain is reduced and range of motion increased after massage therapy. Int. J. Neurosci 106, 3–4 131–145.

Hernandez-Reif, M., Diego, M., Field, T., 2007. Preterm infants show reduced stress behaviors and activity after 5 days of massage therapy. Infant. Behav. Dev. 30, 557–561.

Hodge, M., Robinson, C., Boehmer, J., et al., 2002. Employee outcomes following work-site acupressure and massage. In: Rich, G.J. (Ed.), Massage therapy: the evidence for practice. Mosby, St. Louis.

Howell, J.N., Cabell, K.S., Chila, A.G., Eland, D.C., 2006. Stretch reflex and Hoffman reflex responses to osteopathic manipulative treatment in subjects with Achilles tendinitis. J. Am. Osteopath. Assoc. 106, 537–545.

Hurwitz, E., Morgenstern, H., Harber, P., Kominski, G.F., Belin, T.R., Yu, F., Adams, A.H., 2002. A randomized trial of chiropractic manipulation and mobilization for patients with neck pain: clinical outcomes from the UCLA neck-pain study. Am. J. Public Health 10, 1634–1641.

Hurwitz, E.L., Carragee, E.J., van der Velde, G., et al., 2008. Treatment of neck pain: noninvasive interventions. Spine 33, S123–S152.

International Bone and Joint Decade, 2006. Press release Department of Orthopaedics. University Hospital, Lund, Sweden. http://www.boneandjointdecade.org/HTML/musconline/images/2006_BJD_Conference/BJDPressRealeaseSpine16.10.06.pdf Accessed October 31, 2009.

Jackson, K.M., Steele, T.F., Dugan, E.P., et al., 1998. Effect of lymphatic and splenic pump techniques on the antibody response to hepatitis B vaccine: a pilot study. J. Am. Osteopath. Assoc. 98, 155–160.

King, H.H., Tettambel, M.A., Lockwood, M.D., et al., 2003. Osteopathic manipulative treatment in prenatal care: A retrospective case control design study. J. Am. Osteopath. Assoc. 103, 577–582.

Knebl, J.A., Shores, J.H., Gamber, R.G., et al., 2002. Improving functional ability in the elderly via the Spencer technique, an osteopathic manipulative treatment: a randomized, controlled trial. J. Am. Osteopath. Assoc. 102, 387–396.

Knott, E.M., Tune, J.D., Stoll, S.T., et al., 2005. Increased lymphatic flow in the thoracic duct during manipulative intervention. J. Am. Osteopath. Assoc. 105, 447–556.

Korr, I.M., 1947. The neural basis of the osteopathic lesion. J. Am. Osteopath. Assoc. 47, 191–198.

Langevin, H., Goertz, C., King, H.H., Khalsa, P., Dryden, T., Woodhouse, L.J., 2009. Synergistic research goals for manual treatments of musculoskeletal and soft tissue disorders. Symposium presented at North American Research Conference on Complementary and Integrative Medicine, Minneapolis, MN. May 12–15, 2009 [CD of Symposium available from Conference Recording Service, Inc., 1308 Gilman St., Berkeley, CA 94706. www.conferencerecording.com Ask for CD #318].

LaPrairie, J.L., Murphy, A.Z., 2007. Female rats are more vulnerable to the long-term consequences of neonatal inflammatory injury. Pain 132 (Suppl. 1), 124–133.

Latremoliere, A., Woolf, C.J., 2009. Central sensitization: a generator of pain hypersensitivity by central neural plasticity. J. Pain 10, 895–926.

Lederman, E., 2004. The Science and Clinical Practice of Manual Therapy. Elsevier, Edinburgh.

Licciardone, J.C., Brimhall, A., King, L.N., 2005. Osteopathic manipulative treatment for low back pain: a systematic review and meta-analysis of randomized controlled trials. BMC Musculoskelet. Disord. 6, 43–54.

Licciardone, J.C., Buchanan, S., Hensel, K., et al., 2010. Osteopathic manipulative treatment of back pain and related symptoms during pregnancy: a randomized controlled trial. Am. J. Obstet. Gynecol. 202 (43), e1–e8.

McReynolds, T.M., Sheridan, B.J., 2005. Intramuscular ketorolac versus osteopathic manipulative treatment in the management of acute neck pain in the emergency department: a randomized clinical trial. J. Am. Osteopath. Assoc. 105, 57–68.

Measel, J., 1982. The effect of the lymphatic pump on the immune system response: I. Preliminary studies on the antibody response to pneumococcal polysaccharide assayed by bacterial agglutination and passive hemagglutination. J. Am. Osteopath. Assoc. 82, 28–31.

Mesina, J., Hampton, D., Evans, R., et al., 1998. Transient basophilia following the application of lymphatic pump techniques: A pilot study. J. Am. Osteopath. Assoc. 98, 91–94.

Mills, M.V., Henley, C.E., Barnes, L.L., et al., 2003. The use of osteopathic manipulative treatment as adjuvant therapy in children with recurrent acute otitis media. Arch. Pediatr. Adolesc. Med. 157, 861–866.

Moyer, C.A., Rounds, J., Hannum, J.W., 2004. A meta-analysis of massage therapy research. Psychol. Bull. 130, 3–18.

Noll, D.R., 2009. Pneumonia study presented in Washington, DC. Aging Well Newsletter 1, 1–4.

Noll, D.R., Shores, J.H., Bryman, P.N., et al., 1999. Adjunctive osteopathic manipulative treatment in the elderly hospitalized with pneumonia: a pilot study. J. Am. Osteopath. Assoc. 99, 143–144.

Noll, D.R., Shores, J.H., Gamber, R.G., et al., 2000. Benefits of osteopathic manipulative treatment for hospitalized elderly patients with pneumonia. J. Am. Osteopath. Assoc. 100, 776–782.

Osteopathic Research Center, 2008. International Research Symposium on Somatovisceral Interactions and Autonomic Mechanisms of Manual Therapy http://www.hsc.unt.edu/orc/svressymp.htm Accessed October 31, 2009.

Perlman, A.L., Sabina, A., Williams, A., Njike, V., Katz, D., 2006. Massage therapy for osteoarthritis of the knee: a randomized controlled trial. Arch. Intern. Med. 166, 2533–2538.

Preyde, M., 2000. Effectiveness of massage therapy for subacute low-back pain: a randomized controlled trial. Can. Med. Assoc. J. 162, 1815–1820.

Radjieski, J.M., Lumley, M.A., Cantieri, M.S., 1998. Effect of osteopathic manipulative treatment on length of stay for pancreatitis: a randomized pilot study. J. Am. Osteopath. Assoc. 98, 264–272.

Ruda, M.A., Ling, Q.D., Hohmann, A.G., Peng, Y.B., Tachibana, T., 2000. Altered nociceptive neuronal circuits after neonatal peripheral inflammation. Science 289, 628–631.

Seffinger, M.A., Hruby, R.J., 2007. Evidence-Based Manual Medicine. Saunders Elsevier, Philadelphia.

Sherman, K.J., Cherkin, D.C., Hawkes, R.J., et al., 2009. Randomized trial of therapeutic massage for chronic neck pain. Clin. J. Pain 25, 233–238.

Sleszynski, S.L., Kelso, A.F., 1993. Comparison of thoracic manipulation with incentive spirometry in preventing postoperative atelectasis. J. Am. Osteopath. Assoc. 93, 834–836.

Sucher, B.M., 1993. Myofascial manipulative release of carpal tunnel syndrome: documentation with magnetic resonance imaging. J. Am. Osteopath. Assoc. 93, 1273–1278.

Sucher, B.M., Hinrichs, R.N., 1998. Manipulative treatment of carpal tunnel syndrome: biomechanical and osteopathic intervention to increase the length of the transverse carpal ligament. J. Am. Osteopath. Assoc. 98, 679–686.

Sucher, B.M., Hinrichs, R.N., Welcher, R.L., et al., 2005. Manipulative treatment of carpal tunnel syndrome: biomechanical and osteopathic intervention to increase the length of the transverse carpal ligament: part 2. Effect of sex differences and manipulative 'priming'. J. Am. Osteopath. Assoc. 105, 135–143.

United States Bone and Joint Decade, 2009. Burden of musculoskeletal diseases in the United States. http://www.boneandjointburden.org/ 30 Aug 2009.

Van den Dolder, P.A., Roberts, D.L., 2006. Six sessions of manual therapy increase knee flexion and improve activity in people with anterior knee pain: a randomized controlled trial. Aust. J. Physiother. 52, 261–264.

Vandenplas, Y., Denayer, E., Vandenbossche, T., et al., 2008. Osteopathy may decrease obstructive apnea in infants: a pilot study. Osteopathic Medicine and Primary Care 2, 8.

Wynne, M.M., Burns, J.M., Eland, D.C., Conaster, R.R., Howell, J.N., 2006. Effect of counterstrain on stretch reflexes, Hoffman reflexes, and clinical outcomes in subjects with plantar fasciitis. J. Am. Osteopath. Assoc. 106, 547–556.

Yurvati, A.H., Carnes, M.S., Clearfield, M.B., et al., 2005. Hemodynamic effects of osteopathic manipulative treatment immediately after coronary artery bypass graft surgery. J. Am. Osteopath. Assoc. 105, 475–481.

Index

T

Printed in the United States
By Bookmasters

Printed in the United States
By Bookmasters